Clinical Cases for General Practice Exams

4e

T0357950

Acknowledgments

I am delighted that Dr Andrew Moreton, Dr Leela Arthur, Dr Rebekah Ledingham and Dr Lucas Wheatley were willing to join me in writing this fourth edition. They are experienced and compassionate clinicians with a great desire and ability to help doctors learn through the process of passing exams. Their cases challenged and taught me when I tried them out, and they are a very welcome addition.

I would also like to express my appreciation to all those who helped with the previous editions of this book. Dr Linda Samera, Professor John Wakerman, Dr Ethel Gilbert, Dr Patrick Mutandwa, Dr Nina Kilfoyle, Dr Chris Lesnikowski, Dr Rob Roseby, Dr Peter Tait and Dr Rupa Vedantam were a great help with the first edition. The second edition benefited from input from Dr Pat Giddings, Dr Louise Baker, Dr Trudi Cullinan, Dr Tyler Schofield, Dr Daniel Cloughton, Dr Danielle Butler, Dr Katrina Page, Dr Louise Butler, Dr Sarah Koh, Dr Charles Mutandwa, Dr Ann Dunbar, Angela Beilby and Dr Tim Henderson. For the third edition I was helped by Dr Andrew Moreton, Dr Genevieve Yates, Dr Bambi Ward, Dr Robert Menz, Dr Sarah Kloeden and Dr Sally Banfield.

The photographs in Figures 1 and 3 were supplied by iStockphoto; the Eczema Association of Australasia Inc. provided the photograph for Figure 2; Dr Andrew Moreton supplied the photographs in Figures 4, 6 and 7; and Dr Brendan Bell supplied the ECG in Figure 5.

CLINICAL CASES SERIES

Clinical Cases for General Practice Exams

4e

ASSOCIATE PROFESSOR SUSAN WEARNE

NOTICE

Medicine is an ever-changing science. As new research and clinical experience broaden our knowledge, changes in treatment and drug therapy are required. The editors and the publisher of this work have checked with sources believed to be reliable in their efforts to provide information that is complete and generally in accord with the standards accepted at the time of publication. However, in view of the possibility of human error or changes in medical sciences, neither the editors, nor the publisher, nor any other party who has been involved in the preparation or publication of this work warrants that the information contained herein is in every respect accurate or complete. Readers are encouraged to confirm the information contained herein with other sources. For example, and in particular, readers are advised to check the product information sheet included in the package of each drug they plan to administer to be certain that the information contained in this book is accurate and that changes have not been made in the recommended dose or in the contraindications for administration. This recommendation is of particular importance in connection with new or infrequently used drugs.

This fourth edition published 2019

First published 2005, second edition 2010, third edition 2015

Reprinted 2011, 2012, 2013 (twice), 2016

Text © 2019 Susan Wearne

Illustrations and design © 2019 McGraw-Hill Australia Pty Ltd

Every effort has been made to trace and acknowledge copyrighted material. The authors and publishers tender their apologies should any infringement have occurred.

Reproduction and communication for educational purposes

The Australian *Copyright Act 1968* (the Act) allows a maximum of one chapter or 10% of the pages of this work, whichever is the greater, to be reproduced and/or communicated by any educational institution for its educational purposes provided that the institution (or the body that administers it) has sent a Statutory Educational notice to Copyright Agency (CA) and been granted a licence. For details of statutory educational and other copyright licences contact: Copyright Agency, 66 Goulburn Street, Sydney NSW 2000. Telephone: (02) 9394 7600. Website: www.copyright.com.au

Reproduction and communication for other purposes

Apart from any fair dealing for the purposes of study, research, criticism or review, as permitted under the Act, no part of this publication may be reproduced, distributed or transmitted in any form or by any means, or stored in a database or retrieval system, without the written permission of McGraw-Hill Australia including, but not limited to, any network or other electronic storage.

Enquiries should be made to the publisher via www.mcgraw-hill.com.au or marked for the attention of the Rights and Permissions Manager at the address below.

National Library of Australia Cataloguing-in-Publication Entry

A catalogue record for this book is available from the National Library of Australia

Author: Wearne, Susan
Title: Clinical cases for general practice exams
Edition: 4th edition
ISBN: 9781743767450 (paperback)

Published in Australia by
McGraw-Hill Australia Pty Ltd
Level 33, 680 George Street, Sydney NSW 2000

Publisher: Diane Gee-Clough
Production Editor: Lara McMurray
Editor: Yani Silvana
Cover design: ChristaBella Designs
Internal design: SPi, India
Proofreader: Meredith Lewin
Typeset in 10/12 pt Nimbus by SPi , India
Printed in China by 1010 Printing International Limited on 80gsm matt art

Contents

Acknowledgments ii
Preface viii
About the author and contributing authors ix
List of abbreviations xi
Introduction xv
How to use this book xxi

Section 1	Aboriginal health	1
Case 1	Kasey Kox	2
Case 2	Sharon Price	8

Section 2	Adolescent health	13
Case 3	Erin Campbell	14
Case 4	Amanda Porter	18

Section 3	Aged care	23
Case 5	Elsie Humphries	24
Case 6	Flora McMillan	32
Case 7	Nell Worthington	36
Case 8	Margaret Wilson	40

Section 4	Cardiovascular system	45
Case 9	Helen Berkovic	46
Case 10	Dilip Patel	50
Case 11	Jackie Maloney	55
Case 12	Eric Schmidt	60

Section 5	Challenging consultations	65
Case 13	Doug Sullivan	66
Case 14	Jeanette Wilkinson	73
Case 15	Craig Kelly	79
Case 16	Wazza Wainright	84
Case 17	Hope Briganza	88

Section 6	Child health	95
Case 18	Kylie Chong	96
Case 19	Brandon Harkness	99
Case 20	Natalie Jones	103
Case 21	Latu O'Donnell	107

Section 7	Dermatology	113
Case 22	Sammy Burnside	114

CONTENTS

Case 23	Robert Kerslake	119
Case 24	Ken Anderson	123

Section 8	**Ear, nose and throat**	127
Case 25	Ruby Chan	128
Case 26	Jane Matthews	132
Case 27	Pamela Taylor	136
Case 28	Trevor Watts	140
Case 29	Clayton Dixon	144

Section 9	**Emergency medicine**	151
Case 30	Catriona Chryssides	152
Case 31	Carrie Patterson	157

Section 10	**Endocrinology**	161
Case 32	Veronica Richards	162

Section 11	**Eyes**	167
Case 33	Edward Galloway	168
Case 34	Henrik Schneider	172
Case 35	Roger Chin	176

Section 12	**Gastroenterology**	183
Case 36	Jenna Banks	184
Case 37	Enrico Castallani	189
Case 38	Kirrilee DeMarco	193
Case 39	Mohammed Noor	199
Case 40	Annie Nguyen	205
Case 41	Kathy Jones	209
Case 42	Jack Kingsley	215
Case 43	Neil Dawson	220

Section 13	**Men's health**	227
Case 44	Kim Hosking	228
Case 45	Jock Palmer	233
Case 46	Costa Rinaldi	238

Section 14	**Mental health**	243
Case 47	Phyllis Brown	244
Case 48	Shirley Hill	248
Case 49	Monica Middlethorpe	253
Case 50	Tom Newton	257

Section 15	**Musculoskeletal medicine**	261
Case 51	Anthony Campbell	262
Case 52	Martin Chatterjee	266
Case 53	Sarah Cosgrove	271
Case 54	Jeremy King	275
Case 55	Geoff Sharp	279
Case 56	Anna Wong	283

Section 16	Neurology	289
Case 57	Wilma Burns	290
Case 58	Sybil Clarke	294
Case 59	Rosie Inkamala	299
Case 60	Joe Summers	305
Section 17	Palliative care	309
Case 61	Liz Ross	310
Case 62	Frank Stanley	314
Case 63	Katrina Carroll	318
Section 18	Preventive health	323
Case 64	Bill Ferguson	324
Case 65	Taylor Jordan	328
Case 66	Ali Turnbull	332
Section 19	Professional practice	337
Case 67	Vincent Butler	338
Case 68	Stephanie Clark	344
Case 69	Debra and Declan Poole	347
Section 20	Respiratory medicine	351
Case 70	Andrew Bond	352
Case 71	Kerrie Griffiths	357
Case 72	Paul Jackson	361
Case 73	Nicholas Morris	366
Case 74	Jonty McLeod	372
Section 21	Sexual health	377
Case 75	Ben Ramsay	378
Case 76	Vinay Singh	383
Case 77	Samantha Heyward	390
Section 22	Travel health	397
Case 78	Tanya Hardy	398
Case 79	Betty Ward	404
Section 23	Women's health	409
Case 80	Jenny Butterfield	410
Case 81	Vikki Nicolaides	414
Case 82	Shantelle Kickett	418
Case 83	Zahra Mohammed Ibrahim	424
Section 24	Vivas	431
Case 84	Lori Dalton	432
Case 85	Kaitlin Johansen	436
Section 25	Vulnerable populations	441
Case 86	Jill Krecher	442
Case 87	Marcus Petrovic	448

Preface

This is the book that I looked for when I first moved to Australia. A group of GP registrars wanted help preparing for their Fellowship exam and examples of clinical cases did not exist, so I began writing questions. This book is the teaching material that I have developed and refined since then.

It has been rewarding to hear many stories of doctors who found the book useful. Doctors have persuaded non-medical friends, partners and spouses to role-play patients and the instructions have proved adequate to provide realistic exam practice.

One GP registrar expressed concern that the book was too 'cook book' or formulaic. Forgive me if I have unintentionally promoted uniformity. Each time I see a GP at work or in a role-play, I see new ways of being a GP. Each of us brings our personality and experience to our role, but some core principles apply to each consultation. I hope that my practice will forever include the formula of an introduction, building rapport to understand something of the person's life and situation, hearing their concerns, assessing the problem in bio–psycho–social terms and working with them to create a plan that they understand and want to implement.

We have to judge each situation, without being judgemental, listen intently and be supportive without being patronising. How I achieve this varies for different patients and makes the job both challenging and satisfying. This 'how' of calibrating words and actions to individuals is crucial in exams and in practice; the 'what' of creating therapeutic relationships, and explaining medical terms is different for fractious children, over-stretched middle-aged professionals or an elderly person facing losing health and their independence.

Most of the cases are adapted from my clinical practice and identifying details have been changed to protect the patient's identity. If you think you can spot yourself or a friend it is only because these cases cover common clinical conditions. I appear in them and, with their permission, so do many of my family.

I hope that this book assists medical students, GP registrars and GPs to learn more about the art and science of being an effective GP.

About the author and contributing authors

Associate Professor Susan Wearne
BM PhD MMedSci FRACGP FACRRM MRCGP DRCOG DCH DFFP GCTEd
Susan Wearne is a GP in Canberra and a Clinical Associate Professor at the Australian National University (ANU). She is Senior Medical Adviser for the Commonwealth Department of Health, in the Division which manages general practice training.

Susan is from England; she grew up in Alderley Edge, Cheshire and qualified in medicine from Southampton University. After GP training in Kettering, Northamptonshire and Wilmslow, Cheshire, she was a partner in training practices in Manchester and York. She started her academic career teaching communication skills at Leeds University, and then moved to the Centre for Remote Health in Alice Springs. Susan was a medical educator for the Royal Australian College of General Practitioners, Northern Territory General Practice Education and the Remote Vocational Training Scheme. She is an examiner for ANU, the Royal Australian College of General Practitioners and the Australian College of Rural and Remote Medicine. She has published over 40 articles on general practice and medical education.

Susan is married to Tim Henderson, an ophthalmologist at Alice Springs Hospital. Their married daughter Charlotte lives in England and their son Michael works in Adelaide. Susan is a member of the Alice Aussi Swimming Club and enjoys needlework. Since her job moved to Canberra she has taken up rowing and knitting—but not simultaneously!

Contributing authors

Dr Andrew Moreton
Andrew Moreton graduated from the University of Queensland in 1987 and became a Family Medicine trainee with the Royal Australian College of General Practitioners (RACGP) in Bourke, New South Wales, where he went on to practise for 15 years. Having completed his FRACGP he became involved in case-writing, examining and quality assurance for the FRACGP exams. He is passionate about teaching and learning in medicine and has enjoyed roles teaching GP registrars, GP supervisors and medical students for almost 20 years. He has special interests in communication skills, Indigenous and rural health, exam preparation and doctor's self-care. His cases are drawn from the rich tapestry of life that is general practice.

Dr Leela Arthur
Leela Arthur BSc (Hons 1), MBBS, FRACGP, DCH graduated from the University of Queensland in 2008, then completed her FRACGP in Hervey Bay in 2015. She

has since moved back to her home town of Brisbane where she is now working both in general practice, and as a 'GP with Special Interest' in an irritable bowel syndrome clinic within the hospital system. She has a keen interest in teaching medical students and registrars and has been a medical educator for Queensland Rural Medical Education for several years. More recently, she has become an examiner for the RACGP. She has a particular interest in chronic disease management and refugee health.

In her spare time, Leela enjoys going on adventures with her husband and children, and singing women's barbershop with her quartet Kit'n'Kaboodle, and chorus Brisbane City Sounds.

Dr Rebekah Ledingham

Rebekah Ledingham Bsc (Nursing); BMBS; DRANZCOG; DCH; FRACGP is a GP and medical educator in Broome, Western Australia. She is passionate about Aboriginal health and committed to Closing the Gap and supporting an increasing number of Aboriginal and Torres Strait Islander people in the health workforce. She is also a keen advocate for the well-being of medical students and doctors in training, and would like to see a more nurturing, flexible system in which to grow our future workforce. She founded the online group Medical Mums and Mums to be, now a support network for more than 7000 doctors, after struggling with the prospect of being a junior doctor and a mum simultaneously, but remains eternally thankful that she ignored the (ridiculous) advice not to have babies, as they are growing into fabulous humans who help it all make sense.

Dr Lucas Wheatley

Lucas Wheatley BBiomedSc, MBBS, FRACGP, GDipClinEd, GDipSurgAnat, MPH qualified in Medicine in 2009 and entered service with the Royal Australian Air Force. After completing his FRACGP and MPH, with several tours overseas working in Primary Care and Aeromedical Retrievals, Lucas returned to Brisbane, Queensland. Furthering his scope of practice with additional training in surgery and critical care, Lucas splits his time between working for Queensland Health and the Australian Defence Force. Focusing on clinical and procedural training, Lucas has an interest in medicine in austere and rural environments, with a passion for registrar and medical student education, examining for the University of Queensland and Bond University.

Dr Genevieve Yates

Genevieve Yates is Associate Director of Training for North Coast GP Training, a general practitioner and medical writer. She also delivers medico-legal education sessions and develops resource materials for MDA National and is an examiner for the RACGP and a member of the RACGP Fellowship Support Panel. In 2014, she was named GPET Medical Educator of the Year. She has particular interests in doctors' health and wellbeing, ethics and professionalism, and the medical humanities.

List of abbreviations

Abbreviation	Meaning
24hrECG	24 hour electrocardiogram
ABPI	ankle blood pressure index
ACE	angiotensin converting enzyme
ACR	albumin-creatinine ratio
ACRRM	Australian College of Rural and Remote Medicine
ACS	acute coronary syndrome
ADHD	attention deficit hyperactivity disorder
ADLs	activities of daily living
ADT	adult diphtheria-tetanus vaccine
AFB	acid fast bacilli (tuberculosis)
AF	atrial fibrillation
alb	albumin
Anti CCP	anti-cyclic citrullinated peptide antibody
ARB	angiotensin receptor blocker
b.d.	twice a day (*bis die*)
bHCG	beta human chorionic gonadotropin
bili	bilirubin
BMI	body mass index
BP	blood pressure
bpm	beats per minute
BSL	blood sugar level
CABG	coronary artery bypass grafting
CHA_2DS_2VASc	calculates risk of ischaemic stroke
Chol	cholesterol
CI	confidence interval
CK	creatine kinase
Cl	chloride
Coags	coagulation tests
COPD	chronic obstructive pulmonary disease
COX2 inhibitors	cyclo-oxygenase 2 inhibitors
CPD	continuing professional development
Creat	creatinine
CRP	C-reactive protein
CST	cervical screening test
CT	computerised tomography
CXR	chest X-ray
dTp_a	diphtheria, tetanus and pertussis vaccine adult formulation

DNA	did not attend
DMARDs	disease-modifying anti-rheumatic drugs
DVT	deep venous thrombosis
ECG	electrocardiogram
ED	emergency department
EDNOS	eating disorder not otherwise specified
ELISA	enzyme linked immunosorbent assay
EPDS	Edinburgh Postnatal Depression Score
ERCP	endoscopic retrograde cholangiopancreatography
ESR	erythrocyte sedimentation rate
FAI	free androgen index
FBC/E	full blood count/examination
FEV1	forced expiratory volume in 1 second
FODMAPs	fermentable oligosaccharides, disaccharides, monosaccharides and polyols
FSH	follicle stimulating hormone
FVC	forced vital capacity
GA	general anaesthetic
GCS	Glasgow coma scale
GGT	gamma-glutamyl transferase
GP	general practitioner
GPM	gravida, parity, miscarriages
GTN	glyceryl trinitrate
GTT	glucose tolerance test
HAS-BLED	calculates the risk of bleeding from anticoagulation in patients with atrial fibrillation
Hb	haemoglobin
HbA1c	haemoglobin A1c
HCO_3	bicarbonate
HDLChol	high density lipoprotein cholesterol
Hep B	hepatitis B
Hep C	hepatitis C
Hib	haemophilus influenzae type B vaccination
HIV	human immunodeficiency virus
HPV	human papillomavirus
HRT	hormone replacement therapy
HZV	herpes zoster vaccine
IBS	irritable bowel syndrome
IM	intramuscular injection
INR	international normalised ratio
IUCD	intrauterine contraceptive device
IV	intravenous
JVP	jugular venous pulse
K	potassium
kg	kilogram

LBP	lower back pain
LDH/LH	lactate dehydrogenase
LDLChol	low density lipoprotein cholesterol
LFTs	liver function tests
LH	luteinising hormone
LMP	first day of last menstrual period
LSCS	lower segment Caesarean section
LUTS	lower urinary tract symptoms
m	metre
mane	in the morning
MCS	microscopy, culture and sensitivity
MCP	metacarpophalangeal joints
MCV	mean cell volume
mg	milligram
MRI	magnetic resonance imaging
MSU	midstream urine
MTHFR	methylenetetrahydrofolate reductase
MTP	metatarsophalangeal joints
MVA	motor vehicle accident
Na	sodium
NAAT	nucleic acid amplification test
NAD	no abnormality detected
NH&MRC	National Health and Medical Research Council
NIDDM	non-insulin dependent diabetes mellitus
NIPT	non-invasive pre-natal testing
nocte	at night
NPS	National Prescribing Service
NRT	nicotine replacement therapy
NSAIDs	non-steroidal anti-inflammatory drugs
OA	osteoarthritis
OCP	oral contraceptive pill
ocp	ova, cysts and parasites
od	once a day
OGTT	oral glucose tolerance test
OTC	over the counter—medication bought from a pharmacy without a prescription
Pap	Papanicolaou
PBS	Pharmaceutical Benefit Scheme
PCOS	polycystic ovarian syndrome
PCR	polymerase chain reaction
PEFR	peak expiratory flow rate
PMH	past medical history
PND	paroxysmal nocturnal dyspnoea
PR	per rectum
PrEP	pre-exposure prophylaxis

prn	as and when needed (*pro re nata*)
Prot	protein
PSA	prostate specific antigen
qds	four times a day (*quarter die sumendus*)
RACGP	Royal Australian College of General Practitioners
RDW	red cell distribution width
RFDS	Royal Flying Doctor Service
RPR	rapid plasma reagin test for syphilis
RR	relative risk
sc	subcutaneous
SHBC	steroid hormone binding globulin
SLR	straight leg raising
SOB	shortness of breath
SSRI	selective serotonin reuptake inhibitor
STI	sexually transmitted infection
SVD	spontaneous vaginal delivery
TB	tuberculosis
TCA	tricyclic antidepressant
tds	three times a day (*ter die sumendus*)
temp	temperature
TFTs	thyroid function tests
TIA	transient ischaemic attack
TMJ	temporomandibular joint
TSH	thyroid stimulating hormone
TURP	transurethral resection of prostate
UEC	urea, electrolytes and creatinine
Vit D	Vitamin D
WHO	World Health Organization
WONCA	World Organization of National Colleges, Academies and Academic Associations of General Practitioners/Family Physicians aka World Organization of Family Doctors

Introduction

The aim of this book is to help you prepare for Australian general practice exams using clinical case role-plays.

General practice activity data[1] indicate that general practitioners' work has become increasingly complicated: patients have multiple comorbidities and are prescribed more drugs. My impression is that more research information can counter-intuitively create less certainty. GPs spend more time assessing patients' personal risk-benefit of any particular intervention. Screening for prostate cancer and prescribing hormone replacement therapy are prime examples of where there is a high risk of iatrogenic disease. The GP needs to be an expert in reading patients' personalities and fears, as well as scientific data. The cases in this book test the skill of taking a holistic approach to managing uncertainty in a complex context.

Most doctors find the time restrictions of the exam difficult. Three minutes is not long to read a patient's notes but may be longer than many doctors take to do this in clinical practice. Likewise, dealing with a problem in eight minutes, challenges some candidates, while others expertly breeze through with time to spare to include opportunistic health promotion, confirming that the examiners do not ask the impossible. Cases should be quicker than in real life as the 'patient' knows in advance the answers to the important questions and candidates are not required to make clear, contemporaneous written notes.

Definitions of general practice

Before you take a general practice exam you need to have a clear understanding of general practice. Let's look at some definitions of general practice (also called family practice in some countries).

The Royal Australian College of General Practitioners (RACGP) says:[2]

General practice is part of the Australian health care system and operates predominantly through private medical practices, which provide universal unreferred access to whole person medical care for individuals, families and communities. General practice care means comprehensive, coordinated and continuing medical care drawing on biomedical, psychological, social and environmental understandings of health.

The World Organization of Family Doctors (WONCA Europe) defines the competencies and characteristics of general practitioners as:[3]

- normally the point of first medical contact within the health care system, providing open and unlimited access to its users, dealing with all health problems regardless of the age, sex or any other characteristic of the person concerned
- making efficient use of health care resources through coordinating care, working with other professionals in the primary care setting and by managing the interface with other specialties, taking an advocacy role for the patient when needed

- developing a person-centred approach, orientated to the individual, his/her family and their community
- having a unique consultation process, which establishes a relationship over time through effective communication between doctor and patient
- being responsible for the provision of longitudinal continuity of care as determined by the needs of the patient
- having a specific decision-making process determined by the prevalence and incidence of illness in the community
- managing simultaneously both acute and chronic health problems of individual patients
- managing illness that presents in an undifferentiated way at an early stage in its development, which may require urgent intervention
- promoting health and wellbeing both by appropriate and effective intervention
- having a specific responsibility for the health of the community
- dealing with health problems in their physical, psychological, social, cultural and existential dimensions.

Doctors working in rural and remote Australia can face clinical situations that require skills in a wider scope of practice. Doctors can now choose to qualify as a general practitioner via the Australian College of Rural and Remote Medicine (ACRRM) Fellowship examination. ACRRM expects Fellows to be performing all the functions of a GP listed by RACGP and WONCA plus:

- responding to emergencies including stabilisation and definitive management as appropriate; providing hospital-based secondary care where required; delivering obstetric care; and undertaking a range of population health interventions at the practice and community level.[4]

Those planning to sit the ACRRM exam may still find the cases useful by thinking through what they would do in each case if the nearest hospital or referral centre was more than an hour's flight away, or they were the only doctor in town running both a general practice and a small hospital.

The above definitions demonstrate the breadth of the general practice specialty and remind me why it is such an interesting profession. The illnesses we see are common but we are also alert for potentially serious conditions. For this we need a system of diagnosis that differentiates the headache caused by a brain tumour from a tension headache or a hangover and, if it is a tension headache, we need ways of exploring possible causes of the tension and discussing with the patient how to manage them.

Consultation frameworks

The traditional consultation framework comprises history, examination, investigation, diagnosis, treatment and follow-up. While suitable for emergency care, this model is inadequate for the complexity of general practice.

I recommend the following texts that suggest some task-based and some process-based consultation frameworks:

- Pendleton, D, Schofield, T, Tate, P, et al. 2003, *The new consultation: developing doctor-patient communication*, Oxford.

- Neighbour, R 2004, *The inner consultation: how to develop an effective and intuitive consulting style,* 2nd ed, Oxford.
- Stewart, M, Brown, J. B., Weston, W. W., et al. 2003, *Patient-centred medicine: transforming the clinical method,* 2nd ed, Oxford.

In 2001 a meeting of medical educators and communication skills experts reached a consensus on the essential elements of communication in medical encounters (Kalamazoo Consensus Statement).[5] In this book I have adopted the elements of their suggested approach to cases, summarised as:

- build the doctor–patient relationship
- open the discussion
- gather information
- understand the patient's perspective
- share information
- reach agreement on problems and plans
- provide closure.

General practice exams

General practice exams need to ensure that, to be effective, GPs have the appropriate attitude and a broad range of knowledge and skills. So prepare to be tested on any of the characteristics outlined in the above definitions. Reading a textbook on clinical medicine is not enough, you have to apply the textbook knowledge to a particular person in their particular context, making the best use of the resources available.

One way to do this is to consider the domains of general practice. The RACGP domains are:[6]

1. Communication skills and the doctor–patient relationship
2. Applied professional knowledge and skills
3. Population health and the context of care
4. Professional and ethical roles
5. Organisational and legal dimensions.

The ACRRM domains are:[7]

1. Core clinical knowledge and skills
2. Extended clinical practice
3. Emergency care
4. Population health
5. Aboriginal and Torres Strait Islander health
6. Professional, legal and ethical practice
7. Rural and remote contexts.

Applying the domains to a particular situation

Imagine that you have just completed your reading on diabetes. You are now up-to-date with the latest research and the signs of early diabetic retinopathy. How will you apply this as a GP?

RACGP domain 1. Communication skills and the doctor-patient relationship

Domain 1 reminds you that diabetes affects a person. In consultations you will focus on the patient and their experience of life with diabetes. You will communicate clearly in terms they understand and that are free of medical jargon.

A trap for doctors, particularly those from non-English speaking backgrounds, is to assume that patients whose first language is English understand all English. This is a myth: it is said that first-year medical students learn more new words than first-year language students. We need to constantly distinguish between medical English and colloquial Australian English, and use each when appropriate.

Another aspect of practice that varies between countries is how much patients direct consultations. In Australia, GPs do not automatically have patients' agreement to give advice or recommendations. This right has to be earned by first listening carefully to patients' ideas, concerns, and expectations. Only then can doctors outline their ideas and plans, and negotiate with patients a management plan. There are exceptions, such as emergencies, but in general shared decision-making is expected(1). Learning this skill is essential and requires a considerable shift in approach if you trained in a system where doctors were expected to give advice and patients passively acquiesced.

Domain 1 also includes health promotion, so discuss immunisations, smoking, alcohol and maintaining health, as well as the illness of diabetes, with your patient.

RACGP domain 2. Applied professional knowledge and skills

This is the most familiar domain, in which you ensure your patient has good diabetic control and you work to prevent complications.

RACGP domain 3. Population health and the context of general practice

'Population health' requires you as a GP to broaden your thinking beyond your patient to encompass the wider community. What is your role in preventing or screening for diabetes? Is there a group of patients with an increased risk of diabetes—Torres Strait Islander people, for instance—who need culturally appropriate screening?

'The context of general practice' includes consideration of your patient's life circumstances. Can they get fresh fruit and vegetables easily? What exercise can they safely do? Does their family or religious background influence their health? For example, how would you advise a Muslim patient with diabetes on hypoglycaemics to cope during Ramadan?

RACGP domain 4. Professional and ethical role

Your role as a GP requires you to look at the standard of care that you provide for patients with diabetes. Use clinical audit to check that you are following the national guidelines. Consider how your care integrates with the rest of the health care system: what are your links with the local optometrist who could screen your patients for diabetic retinopathy? Are you making the best use of resources? Could a practice nurse do routine diabetic care so that you can focus on complex cases?

Your ethical role might include such dilemmas as a case where a diabetic patient whose livelihood depends on holding a commercial driving licence also requires insulin.

RACGP domain 5. Organisational and legal dimensions

Are you using information technology to improve the quality of care for your patients with diabetes? What are the recall systems? How do you ensure patient confidentiality when they attend for repeat prescriptions? When did you last calibrate your glucometer and sphygmomanometer? Do you make comprehensive and comprehensible notes? Is yours an accredited practice eligible for Service Incentive Payments?

ACRRM domains. Emergency care, rural and remote context and Aboriginal and Torres Strait Islander health

For diabetes this may mean managing diabetic ketoacidosis in a small rural hospital, starting newly diagnosed diabetic children on insulin or running a screening program at a football carnival in a remote Aboriginal community.

Long and short cases

In this book, long cases usually test a whole consultation. Short cases usually test part of a consultation, perhaps focusing on taking a history, performing a physical examination, giving a diagnosis or negotiating management. This challenges doctors who are used to conducting full consultations.

In cases that require management only, both students and doctors often still begin with a history and examination. This is a normal (and good) clinical response but it wastes precious time because it isn't required. Several cases in this book give you practice at picking up the consultation halfway through.

GPs would never finish our day's work if we took a full history and performed a complete examination on every patient. We take appropriate short cuts and focused histories, examining the patient for specific information to rule a diagnosis in or out. Our expertise 'is the ability to access knowledge and make connections across seemingly disparate fields and life experiences'.[8] The art of exams is to demonstrate this expertise.

Medical students can eventually reach the answer but only experienced clinicians can connect the disparate elements of a scenario into a diagnostic approach in the time available. This 'elaborated knowledge' is essential for an independent general practitioner.[9]

For example, what diagnosis comes to mind when you read 'headache', 'fever', 'rash'? The safe, experienced GP asks, 'Is this meningitis?' The clinical encounter will focus on excluding meningitis by a short, focused history and an immediate look at the rash. If it is purpuric they would exclude an allergy, give parenteral antibiotics and arrange immediate hospital admission. By contrast, a student might approach this case using a systematic, hypothetico-deductive method,[10] first taking a detailed history of the presenting symptoms, then a review of current medication and allergies, followed by a social history, family history, systems review and finally conducting a top-to-toe clinical examination. Once all the data is gathered the student will begin to piece together a possible hypothesis or diagnosis and deduce the most likely diagnosis from the evidence available, or perhaps decide that further information is needed. By this time the experienced GP will have given the patient antibiotics. In this extreme example, the speed of the GP's diagnosis may be life-saving. This is rare in clinical practice but it illustrates the efficiency of pattern recognition as a diagnostic process. There is no short cut to this. It requires considerable study and experience and underlines the need for GPs to undergo supervised clinical practice.

Summary

Clinical practice is still the best preparation for general practice and general practice exams. My hope is that this book will supplement your clinical work so that during exams you can demonstrate that you have the knowledge, skills and attitudes necessary for general practice in Australia.

References

1. Britt, H, Miller, G. C., Henderson, J, Bayram, C, Valenti, L, Harrison, C, et al. 2014, *A Decade of Australian General Practice Activity 2004-05 to 2013-14,* General Practice Series no. 37.
2. Royal Australian College of General Practitioners, 'Definition of general practice and general practitioner'. Available at: www.racgp.org.au/ whatisgeneralpractice, accessed 1 June 2010.
3. WONCA Europe, 'The European definition of general practice/family medicine'. Available at: www.euract.org/index.php?folder_id=24, accessed 1 June 2010.
4. Australian College of Rural and Remote Medicine, 'The ACRRM position on the specialty of general practice'. Available at: www.acrrm.org.au, accessed 22 April 2015.
5. Participants in the Bayer-Fetzer conference on physician–patient communication in medical education 2001, 'Essential elements of communication in medical encounters: the Kalamazoo consensus statement'. Academic Medicine vol. 76, pp. 390-3.
6. Royal Australian College of General Practitioners 2011, 'The RACGP Curriculum for Australian General Practice'. Available at: http://curriculum. racgp.org.au/, accessed 27 February 2015.
7. Australian College of Rural and Remote Medicine 2013, *Primary Curriculum,* Fourth ed.
8. Fraser S. W. and Greenhalgh, T 2001, 'Coping with complexity: education for capability', *British Medical Journal,* vol. 323, pp. 799-803.
9. Bordage G 1994, 'Elaborated knowledge: a key to successful diagnostic thinking', *Academic Medicine,* vol. 69, issue 11, pp. 883-5.
10. Hays, R 1999, *Practice-based Teaching: a Guide for General Practitioners,* pp.19-21.

How to use this book

This book is designed to help medical students and doctors practise clinical cases likely to be seen by general practitioners in Australia. Each case consists of instructions for the doctor and role-playing patient, a suggested approach, case commentary and references, or recommended further reading. The cases are written in note form as is usual practice in clinical records.

It is based on my experience of facilitating case-based learning groups for medical students and general practice registrars. Trial and error helped establish what worked and what did not, but everyone is different, so if you find a new way of practising please let me know.

Don't read this book!

You will learn more by using this book rather than reading it from cover to cover. Come to each case fresh, so that you can test your knowledge and skills in general practice and identify your learning needs. If you read through the book when you practise cases you will distract yourself with trying to remember the suggested approach. This would test your recall rather than the application of your knowledge and clinical skills to a particular context.

Do read the instructions

The easiest way to fail a clinical exam is to ignore the instructions as marks are pre-allocated according to the instructions. Time management is crucial to ensure you cover the requirements. For example, you need to take a 'good enough', safe history before moving on to the clinical examination and planning management, if all three elements are requested in the scenario. Taking eight minutes to do a complete history will lead to a fail if the examination and management are omitted.

Find a group

Most people find it is easier to study with a group rather than in isolation. A group motivates you to persevere and learning from your mistakes in a safe environment is far better than learning from making mistakes with patients.

If you are in isolated practice you can still join a group. I have run practice consultation groups over the phone, via Skype or video-conference. It presents some challenges but can be done. I do not know of any technology for remote physical examination, but all other aspects of the consultation can be practised. If you have not been observed conducting physical examinations you could videorecord consultations with patients (with their written consent), friends or relatives. Send password-protected copies to your group and ask them for constructive feedback. Your physical examination of each system and body part must be so automatic that you can focus and interpret what you find.

Groups work better if group rules have been agreed to. The group needs to develop trust so that ignorance leads to learning rather than embarrassment. Confidentiality is an important issue. Participants will learn more if learning is derived from and related to their own clinical practice, so everyone needs to know that they can safely share their experiences.

Allocate roles

Allocate the roles to the role-players ahead of the session if possible. This lets the role-players familiarise themselves with the scenario and search out more information about the clinical problem, which adds to their learning. Props can help role-players give a more authentic look and mimic the sorts of clues that prompt GPs in clinical practice.

These scenarios are about common problems; at some stage one of the scenarios could be about a condition that the role-player, or a friend or relative, suffers from. This may enhance their performance but equally it could create a tense situation. By allocating roles in advance, the role-player can decline the case before major issues develop.

Observers

Observers of the role-play will learn more if they see only the 'Instructions for the doctor'. Encourage observers to make notes on how they would approach the case, which helps them to be active learners rather than passive observers. They can also give constructive feedback to the role-playing doctor and patient.

Facilitator

One person can facilitate the case and have access to all the information. The checklists are designed for the facilitator to tick off as the doctor deals with a particular aspect of the case.

Please give the doctor the examination findings only on specific request. Doctors should demonstrate their reasoning by asking for the findings that will confirm or refute the diagnosis. For example 'what are the neurological findings' is too broad a question to ask about a patient with a suspected stroke. Instead questions should be asked about the expected changes in tone, power, sensation, coordination and reflexes in the affected limbs.

Timing

Allocate a timekeeper for each scenario. Students and junior general practice registrars may decide to use the material without a time limit but more experienced doctors should complete the short cases in eight minutes and the long cases in nineteen minutes, following three minutes to read through the case scenario.

Allow time for discussion after each scenario: usually twenty minutes for short cases and thirty minutes for long cases is adequate.

Room setup

Set up the room like a consulting room, with chairs for the patient and doctor, a desk, examination couch and standard consultation equipment. The patient should be sitting on the chair at the beginning of the consultation even if they will need to be examined. It gives too big a clue if the doctor walks in and finds the patient dressed ready for a physical examination! Role-playing patients may prefer to wear bathers or shorts under their clothes to ease their potential embarrassment at being examined BUT remember that this is about learning, not humiliation. If the patient role-player does not wish to be examined, please accommodate this.

In physical examination cases you should demonstrate in a deliberate way that you are performing the examination correctly. Talking yourself through the examination, making a running commentary of your actions and findings, can increase your awareness of what you are doing and why, and demonstrate your clinical reasoning to observers.

Doctors training in the Australian College of Rural and Remote Medicine pathway

One component of the Australian College of Rural and Remote Medicine (ACRRM) assessment is 'StAMPS': structured assessment using multiple patient scenarios. This is an examination via video-conference where each scenario lasts for ten minutes. Doctors are asked questions in a viva or role-play format. Physical examination and practical skills are assessed separately from StAMPS.

The cases in this book were primarily designed for doctors preparing for the Royal Australian College of General Practitioners (RACGP) Clinical Examination but doctors preparing for the ACRRM Fellowship may find them a useful resource to practise via video-conference or webcam (see Introduction on page xv).

Suggested approach

The suggested approach to each case includes the essential elements of medical consultations as outlined in the Kalamazoo Consensus Statement[1] but does not exhaust all the possibilities. When you are reading this section you will probably think of your own additions, but for each addition you need to remove an item to avoid the cases becoming impossibly long for the time available. You will find that additions are easy but taking something out is not; discuss these issues with your group—the process of considering what to do in each case greatly improves your clinical reasoning. If your group does agree on a significant addition, please let me know.

Mnemonics pose a particular risk. They help us to remember what to ask but are best used as a framework for a conversation. Too often a doctor is working hard to remember the mnemonic rather than focusing on the patient's response to the questions. While this is understandable we must be more than questionnaires on legs! There is no point asking the right questions if you don't listen and respond to the answers.

Case commentary

There is a commentary on the relevant issues in each case as well as references and suggestions for further reading.

Let the show go on

Doctors will usually learn more from the scenario if it runs for the allotted eight or nineteen minutes. However, maintaining someone's self-esteem may be more important. The response to a doctor getting stuck or suffering from stage fright mid-consultation will depend on their level of experience. For doctors early in training, you can ask for volunteers to take over the consultation. For more experienced doctors, the facilitator can make suggestions such as, 'Try reading through the scenario again; it might prompt you on how to proceed,' or 'If this happened in your surgery, what would you do?'

This gives the doctor a framework for what to do if they get stuck in either an exam situation or in clinical practice.

If the role-playing patient is disturbed or upset, the scenario may need to be stopped.

Guidelines for giving constructive feedback

Giving feedback constructively is a skill that will be useful for all general practitioners. Confidence can quickly evaporate in someone who has done badly in a scenario and it helps to have guidelines to avoid feedback being perceived as judgemental and destructive. It may feel contrived but it is safe. Once the group has grown and is learning well together you can focus more quickly on the aspects for improvement.

Pendleton's guide to giving feedback

- Briefly clarify matters of fact
- The doctor says what was done well, and how
- The rest of the group says what was done well, and how
- The doctor says what could be done differently, and how
- The rest of the group says what could be done differently, and how.

I follow Pendleton's guide and ask the doctor to start the discussion by outlining what they did well.[2] Doctors invariably focus on their mistakes and fail to notice what worked well. I have waited on occasion for several minutes for some doctors to say just one good thing about their consultations. This is important, so that learning builds on what is already good and gives practitioners a realistic framework for self-reflection throughout their career.

Once the positives have been recognised I ask the doctor to outline what they might do differently if they had another chance. This gives me insight into their perceptions of their performance, and allows them to self-correct before group members comment. I know that I am facing a major teaching challenge when someone is unaware that they have performed poorly.

If there is time and the doctor has noticed an error, you can re-run the role-play and allow them to practise their new learning. Once they have shared their ideas on how to improve their consultations, the observers can join in. Again, it is a good principle to ensure that feedback is balanced. *Descriptive* feedback should reduce defensiveness and promote learning. It is:[3]

- non-judgemental
- specific
- directed towards behaviour rather than personality
- checked with the recipient
- outcome-based
- problem-solving
- in the form of suggestions rather than prescriptive comments.

Let me give you an example. You have just watched a colleague's consultation. During the consultation the doctor wrote a script for an anti-hypertensive, asking the patient about her exercise regime at the same time. You observed the patient go red in the face and mumble an answer. The doctor did not raise the issue of exercise again and did not notice the patient blush.

Judgemental feedback might be something like this:

Facilitator: 'You missed your chance to hear about her exercise. It is bad practice to ask questions while you are writing scripts. You'll never make a decent doctor. Don't they teach you anything at medical school?'

The alternative *descriptive* feedback might be:

Facilitator: 'Well done for asking about exercise. She did not say very much. Why do you think that might be?'

Doctor: 'Maybe she was embarrassed because she does so little. Why do you ask?'

Facilitator: 'I noticed that you asked about exercise while you were writing the script. When you asked the question she blushed, looked embarrassed and mumbled an answer. What do you think that was about?'

Doctor: 'I guess asking about exercise is a delicate issue. Maybe I gave the impression that I wasn't interested in the answer when I asked her at the same time as writing the script. No wonder she didn't say much. In future I'll try to give patients my full attention when I ask important questions.'

Facilitator: 'Would you like to re-run the scenario?'

Reluctant participants

Role-play has an established place in facilitating learning in general practice and in assessing the competency of practitioners in Australia.[4] However, many students and doctors are reluctant to participate. This is understandable. Consulting is central to our effectiveness as practitioners but it is also very personal.

International medical schools may have different approaches to teaching consultation skills. Several doctors that I have taught had not been observed consulting during their training. When they moved to Australia they found this method of learning new and frightening—an added challenge was consulting in English. My tip for this situation is to suggest that international medical graduates come to groups and just watch at first. When they are more familiar with the process they may be prepared to role-play as patients. Once confident in this, they can be invited to play the doctor.

Have fun

Lastly, do enjoy your practice sessions. This is NOT about ritual humiliation. I learn something new each session about clinical practice, which improves the quality of care I give as a GP and increases my interest in the profession.

References

1. Elwyn, G, Frosch, D, Thomson, R, Joseph-Williams, N, Lloyd, A, Kinnersley, P, et al. 2012, 'Shared decision making: a model for clinical practice', *Journal of general internal medicine,* vol. 27, issue 10, pp. 1361–7.
2. Participants in the Bayer-Fetzer conference on physician–patient communication in medical education 2001, 'Essential elements of communication in medical encounters: the Kalamazoo consensus statement', *Academic Medicine,* vol. 76, pp. 390–3.
3. Pendleton, D, Schofield, T, Tate P & Havelock, P 2003, '*The new consultation: developing doctor-patient communication,* Oxford.
4. Silverman, J, Draper, J & Kurtz, S. M. 1997, 'The Calgary–Cambridge approach to communication skills teaching II: the SET-GO method of descriptive feedback', *Education for General Practice,* vol. 8, pp. 16–23.

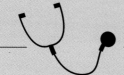

Section 1
Aboriginal health

Case 1
Kasey Kox

Instructions for the doctor

This is a long case.

Please take a history from Kasey. When you are ready, request examination findings and the results of surgery tests from the examiner and outline your differential diagnosis. Outline your immediate investigations and negotiate a management plan with Kasey. Please answer the examiner's questions.

Scenario

Kasey is a 17-year-old Aboriginal girl who has not been seen at your Melbourne practice before.

The following is on her summary sheet:

Past medical history
Grommets as a child

Medications
Etonorgestrel contraceptive implant (Implanon)

Allergies
Nil known

Immunisations
As per schedule

Family history
Nil recorded

Social history
From Balgo in WA
Moved to Melbourne last year for boarding school.

Instructions for the patient, Kasey Kox

You are a 17-year-old Aboriginal girl from Balgo in WA who has a scholarship to complete year 12 in Melbourne. Over the past few days you have been unwell with aches and pains. Five days ago, your left wrist was sore and warm. Then both wrists were affected, but they have improved. Now your right knee has become really painful. It is difficult to walk or bend your knee so you couldn't go to school today. You have a headache and feel thirsty.

You feel cold even though it's warm outside. You have had no skin sores, no diarrhoea or vomiting, no abdominal pain, and no urinary symptoms.

You like boarding school but you do get homesick. You spend a lot of time on social media connecting with your family back home.

You've recently been at home for the holidays and, if asked, you did have a sore throat a few weeks ago. As usual your three-bedroom house was packed; there are often 12 people living there, depending on who is in the community.

Sexual health

You were sexually active with a boyfriend last year (aged 16) and would accept an STI check if offered.

You had the cervical cancer vaccines at school and haven't had any screening tests yet.

Your periods are regular and very light since the contraceptive implant went in.

Social (home and education)

You are one of five children. Your older sister is studying medicine in Melbourne and you hope to be a teacher. You are fit and a keen Aussie rules footballer.

Drugs and alcohol

You don't smoke.
You've tried marijuana and alcohol at parties but take nothing regularly.

Family history

Your dad has diabetes and kidney problems.

Your mum had a heart operation in her 30s for her valves. If asked for more detail say, 'rheumatic heart' and that she takes blood thinners.

Your sister also has heart problems; if asked specifically, say she gets a monthly injection to prevent it getting worse.

The following is on your summary sheet:
Past medical history
Grommets as a child
Medications
Etonorgestrel contraceptive implant (Implanon)
Allergies
Nil known
Immunisations
As per schedule
Family history
Nil recorded
Social history
From Balgo in WA
Moved to Melbourne last year for boarding school.

Questions for the doctor

Will I need to go to hospital?

Information for the facilitator

Vital signs
Temperature 38.3°C
Pulse 80 bpm
BP 100/60
SpO2 99% room air
RR 20/min
BMI 22
ENT throat NAD
No cervical lymphadenopathy
Ears—bilateral scarred tympanic membranes
Chest clear
Heart sounds—systolic murmur
JVP normal
Abdomen soft and non-tender
Right knee warm to touch, obvious effusion, mild limitation in range of
    motion in all directions
Antalgic gait, significant limp but can weight bear
Left wrist—warm, mild tenderness to palpation
Skin NAD
U/A normal

BSL 4.5 mmol
ECG—see page 6.

With three minutes to go, or when the candidate finishes speaking, ask
the following:
1. What are your differential diagnoses? Tell me your favoured diagnosis.
2. What blood tests are you going to do?
3. What immediate management will you provide?
4. What are the criteria for diagnosing acute rheumatic fever?

Suggested approach to the case

History

History of presenting complaint and risk factors for acute rheumatic fever
need to be solicited.

A HEADDSSS (Home situation; Employment, Education, Economic situation; Activities, Affect, Ambition, Anxieties; Drugs, Depression; Sexuality;
Suicide, Self-esteem, Stress) approach is also valuable for this young woman
who finds herself far from home and is unknown to the practice. Offering
a chaperone or an Aboriginal health worker if available would be helpful.

Examination

Vital signs
Joint examination—including other joints
Skin examination looking for skin sores (alternative source of Group A
    Strep) and erythema marginatum or subcutaneous nodules (both rare)
Cardiovascular, particularly auscultation of the heart and looking for signs
    of heart failure.

Investigations

FBC, UEC, CRP/ESR
Blood culture
Throat swab and swab any infected skin sores
Anti-DNase B
Anti-streptolysin O titre
Echocardiogram
STI screen
Surgery tests
    ECG
    Urinalysis.

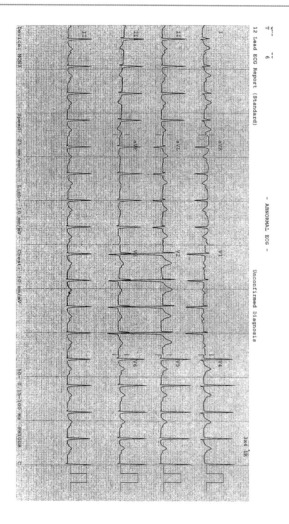

Major criteria (need two major or one major and two minor for diagnosis plus evidence of preceding Group A streptococcal infection)
—Carditis, including subclinical evidence of rheumatic vasculitis on echocardiogram
—Polyarthritis or aseptic monoarthitis or polyarthralgia
—Erythema marginatum
—Subcutaneous nodules
—Chorea (Sydenham's chorea does not need evidence of preceding Group A streptococcal infection, providing other causes of chorea are excluded).

Minor criteria
—Monoarthralgia
—Fever (>38°C)
—ESR > 30 or CRP >30
—Prolonged PR interval on ECG.

Management

Given the differentials in this case, hospital referral for further workup is appropriate. If septic arthritis can be excluded, benzathine penicillin would be given for acute rheumatic fever and aspirin or NSAIDs would be first-line treatment for pain.

Ongoing management would include four-weekly benzathine penicillin as secondary prophylaxis of recurrent episodes of acute rheumatic fever with the aim of preventing rheumatic heart disease.

COMMON PITFALLS

Doctors working outside areas with a high prevalence of acute rheumatic fever may not have this diagnosis at the forefront of their minds. Untreated acute rheumatic fever leads to rheumatic heart disease, which causes significant morbidity and mortality, so it is an important disease not to miss.

Online resources

ARF/RHD Guideline app
www.rhdaustralia.org.au
http://kamsc.org.au/wp-content/uploads/2016/11/Acute-Rheumatic-Fever-October-2016.pdf.

References

Bossingham, D 2015, 'Case study: Atypical arthritis: a young woman presents with fever and joint pains.' *How to Treat—Australian Doctor*, Available at: https://www.howtotreat.com.au/case-report/case-study-atypical-arthritis, accessed 18 March 2019.
Karthikeyan, G & Guilherme, L 2018, 'Acute rheumatic fever', *Lancet*, vol. 392 (10142), pp. 161–74.

Case 2
Sharon Price

Instructions for the doctor

This is a short viva.

Please answer the questions of a GP supervisor about your consultation with Sharon.

Scenario

Sharon, a 39-year-old Aboriginal woman who works in retail, has just moved to your area. She was seen by a colleague last week for some scripts and your colleague suggested Sharon book in for an Aboriginal adult health check.

The limited summary in her file is as follows:

Past medical history

Diabetes

Medications

Metformin XR 2 g daily

Sitagliptin 100 mg daily.

Instructions for the facilitator

The doctor is expected to talk with you as a professional colleague. During the viva please ensure you ask the following questions:

1. Why is it important to identify Aboriginal and Torres Strait Islander patients in your practice?
2. What would you do to check Sharon's diabetes?
3. Sharon has just moved interstate as a newly single parent. The cost of her diabetes medications is overwhelming. What could you do to assist?

4. What other screening would be important for Sharon at this point?
5. You realise the practice does not see many Aboriginal patients. How could you ensure your practice is culturally safe and welcoming to Aboriginal and Torres Strait Islander patients?
6. What resources or guidelines might help you deliver the most appropriate care for Sharon?

 CASE COMMENTARY

1. Identifying Aboriginal and Torres Strait Islander patients is important for many reasons, including:
   - providing culturally safe medical care, e.g. male or female doctors to provide care for men's and women's business respectively
   - offering interpreters or cultural mentors to attend appointments
   - different disease prevalence leading to
     - Aboriginal and Torres Strait Islander specific immunisation and chronic disease screening schedules
     - Medicare incentives for practices and patients to improve access to care and treatment.
2. Sharon has diabetes and needs:
   - assessment of her current wellbeing and how she is handling her diabetes
   - consideration of the suitability of her medication regime, her coherence and any barriers to taking medications
   - exploration of her modifiable risk factors: smoking, nutrition, alcohol, physical activity (SNAP) and check of BMI, waist circumference, lipid profile
   - screening for end-organ damage of her eyes (retinal screening), heart (BP, ECG), kidneys (UEC, urine ACR) and feet (skin, peripheral pulses, monofilament testing of sensation).
3. Sharon could register for the Medicare 'Closing the Gap' initiative. This reduces the cost of her medications if she has no Health Care Card or eliminates costs if she has one. A combined preparation of her medications would reduce the cost and the number of pills she takes.

   She is eligible for a Medicare rebate on an Aboriginal and Torres Strait Islander adult health check (715) and GP Management Plan and Team Care Arrangement (721/723). The latter would give her subsidised access to a diabetes educator and/or podiatrist.

4. Documentation of past medical history, immunisation status, family and social history, allergies and physical examination if this was not done when seen last week. Plus cervical and STI screening if appropriate.

5. To create a culturally safe practice, all staff should undertake cultural training, ideally offered by local Aboriginal or Torres Strait Islander providers. Aboriginal and Torres Strait Islander flags or acknowledgement of the traditional owners can make the practice more welcoming as can local Aboriginal artworks and culturally appropriate pamphlets and resources. Increasing the numbers of Aboriginal and Torres Strait Islander health professionals and staff members is also important for ongoing improvements in providing culturally safe and appropriate care.

6. There are resources designed to assist GPs to provide appropriate care for Aboriginal and Torres Strait Islander people. These include:
   - *National resources*, for example the National guide to a preventative health assessment for Aboriginal and Torres Strait Islander people.[1]
   - *Local guidelines* developed in collaboration with local Aboriginal people and community controlled health organisations, for example the CARPA manual (NT)[2] and *Kimberley Aboriginal Medical Services guidelines.*[3]

References

1. National Aboriginal Community Controlled Health Organisation and The Royal Australian College of General Practitioners 2018, *National guide to a preventive health assessment for Aboriginal and Torres Strait Islander people,* 3rd ed, RACGP, East Melbourne, Vic.

2. Centre for Remote Health, *CARPA standard treatment manual,* 7th ed., Alice Springs, NT.

3. Kimberley Aboriginal Health Planning Forum 2018, *Kimberley Aboriginal Medical Services guidelines.* Available at: https://kahpf.org.au/clinical-protocols, accessed 18 March 2018.

Further reading

Australian Indigenous Health InfoNet at healthinfonet.ecu.edu.au, accessed 10 February 2019.

Liaw, ST, Hasan, I, Wade, V, Canalese, R, Kelaher, M, Lau, P & Harris, M 2015, 'Improving cultural respect to improve Aboriginal health in general practice: a multi-methods and multi-perspective pragmatic study', *Australian Family Physician,* vol. 44, no. 6, pp. 387–92.

RACGP Aboriginal and Torres Strait Islander Health, *Five steps toward excellent Aboriginal and Torres Strait Islander healthcare.* Retrieved from: www.racgp. org.au/FSDEDEV/media/documents/Faculties/ATSI/Five-steps-guide.pdf, accessed 26 February 2019.

The Royal Australian College of General Practitioners 2016, 'General practice management of type 2 diabetes: 2016–18', RACGP, East Melbourne, Vic.

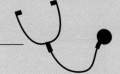

Section 2
Adolescent health

Case 3
Erin Campbell

Instructions for the doctor

This is a short case.

Please take a history from Erin. A clinical photograph of Erin's face will be available to you on request (refer to Figure 1, centre insert page A).[1] Please then outline the most likely diagnosis and negotiate a management plan with her.

Scenario

Erin Campbell is a 14-year-old girl who presents to you with moderate facial acne. Her mum has come with her to the surgery but lets Erin see you on her own.

The following information is on her summary sheet:

Past medical history
Nil significant
Medication
Nil
Allergies
Nil
Immunisations
Up-to-date
Social history
Lives with parents.

Instructions for the patient, Erin Campbell

You are 14 years old and attend the local high school. Your pimples dominate your life. Each morning your mum shouts at you to get dressed and ready for school, while you stare at your pimples in the mirror. You are convinced that you will never have a boyfriend like all your other friends. You used to take comfort in eating chocolate and cheese but have stopped since a friend said that was causing your pimples.

You are embarrassed to be going to see the GP and hope the doctor will be kind.

The following information is on your summary sheet:

Past medical history
Nil significant
Medication
Nil
Allergies
Nil
Immunisations
Up-to-date
Social history
Lives with parents.

Suggested approach to the case

Establish rapport with Erin
Open-ended questions to explore Erin's concerns and expectations about her acne.

Specific questions

Duration of acne
Location of acne
Impact of acne on social life and relationships
What has she tried so far as treatment?
What does she think causes the acne?
General health, e.g. are her periods regular?
Request permission to examine.

Examination

Examine the face
    —Confirm acne
    —Describe signs: comedones, pustules, erythema or scarring.

Management

Explain medical understanding of cause of acne without using jargon
Reassure that acne can be controlled, should not stop her socialising
Advise against picking or squeezing
Offer treatment depending on what Erin has already tried
Advise regular washing with soap
Avoid oily or greasy skin preparations
Recommend healthy diet
Treatment takes four to eight weeks to be effective, can combine topical and oral treatments

Reduce excess cells (hyperkeratinisation)[2]
Topical retinoids, azelaic acid

Reduce bacteria (propionibacterium acnes)
Benzoyl peroxide, strength according to skin type
Course of topical antibiotics (combine with Benzoyl peroxide or topical retinoids).[3] Courses of oral antibiotics are indicated for severe cystic acne—tetracyclines not recommended until bone and teeth development complete

Rebalance hormones (reduce androgen excess)
Oral contraceptives

Reduce sebum hypersecretion
Oral isotretinoin—high risk of teratogenicity

Arrange follow-up.

 CASE COMMENTARY

Adolescent acne is a common problem and can lead to physical and psychological scarring.[4] Acne is a problem of pilosebaceous ducts caused by, duct obstruction from keratinocytes, androgen-induced increase in sebum, *Propionibacterium acnes* proliferation and inflammation. The mainstay of treatment is topical retinoids as there is concern that the prolonged use of topical and oral antibiotics is contributing to the problem of antimicrobial resistance.[2] Antibiotics can be used for courses of three to four months to control cystic acne; once under control topical retinoids are used to maintain control.[3]

Typically many treatments will have been tried at home prior to consulting a GP. It is important to find out what Erin has tried so you are offering something new rather than a treatment that has already been tried and failed. Diets with a high glycaemic index may exacerbate acne so it is worth encouraging a healthy diet.[2]

For some teenagers, the hidden agenda of an acne presentation is a request for contraception. This requires sensitive exploration. A phrase that I find useful is: 'Some people who come to see me know that the contraceptive pill helps with their skin; is this the case with you?' The question about Erin's periods is to assess the likelihood of polycystic ovarian syndrome.

COMMON PITFALLS

Teenagers determine the severity and impact of their acne, not doctors. This case tests the doctor's ability to practise in a patient-centred framework. Low marks will be given to doctors who dismiss Erin as having a few pimples which are insignificant and which she should learn to live with.

References

1. Usatine, RP, Smith, MA & Mayeaux Jr, EJ 2009, *The Color Atlas of Family Medicine,* McGraw-Hill, New York, NY, p. 439.
2. Dawson, AL & Dellavalle, RP 2013, 'Acne vulgaris', *British Medical Journal,* vol. 346, p. f2634.
3. Zaenglein, AL 2018, 'Acne vulgaris', *New England Journal of Medicine,* vol. 379, no. 14, pp. 1343–52.
4. Goodman, G 2006, 'Acne and acne scarring: the case for active and early intervention', *Australian Family Physician,* vol. 35, no. 7, pp. 503–4.

Case 4
Amanda Porter

Instructions for the doctor

This is a short case.

Please take a history from Amanda and then negotiate an initial management plan with her. Your management plan will include explaining the need for a physical examination.

Scenario

Amanda Porter is a 16-year-old girl who has been coming to the practice for a long time. Last week during a school trip her class teacher caught Amanda making herself sick after the evening meal. With Amanda's consent the teacher phoned to make this appointment.

The following information is on her summary sheet:

Past medical history
Greenstick fracture left radius aged eight
Medication
Nil
Allergies
Nil
Immunisations
Fully immunised
Social history
Lives with parents.

Instructions for the patient, Amanda Porter

Your family have always had 'big bones'. As a child you accepted the fact that your mum and dad were on the sidelines at sports day rather than entering in the parents' races. You are used to being part of a big family and shopping at the plus size stores. Whenever friends visit they can't finish the amount of food they are given. About three months ago you had a really bad attack of gastroenteritis. You were amazed to find that you lost weight. Losing weight made you feel great.

You found that if you made yourself vomit just after the evening meal at home you could lose weight without having to diet. Although the vomiting is not pleasant it makes you feel good because your figure is better and you are getting attention from the boys at the youth club.

Last week during a school trip your class teacher caught you making yourself sick after the evening meal. Your teacher phoned to make this appointment with your consent. You are 1.67 m tall and weighed 95 kg three months ago, giving you a BMI of 34 kg/m^2. You now weigh 89 kg (BMI 29 kg/m^2).

You are very scared about seeing the GP.

The following information is on your summary sheet:

Past medical history
Greenstick fracture left radius aged eight
Medication
Nil
Allergies
Nil
Immunisations
Fully immunised
Social history
Lives with parents.

Suggested approach to the case

Establish rapport
Confirm confidentiality assured—unless disclosure required by law
Sensitively explore Amanda's ideas, concerns and expectations regarding the consultation.

Specific questions

Establish facts about the vomiting and weight loss
Exclude significant physical pathology
    —Energy and general health
    —Diet, appetite

–Fever, cough, sputum

–Nausea, vomiting, diarrhoea, bowel disturbance, abdominal pain, amenorrhoea

–Thirst, polyuria

Explore symptoms of an eating disorder using the **SCOFF** questionnaire:[1]

1. Do you make yourself **S**ick because you feel uncomfortably full?
2. Do you worry you have lost **C**ontrol over how much you eat?
3. Have you recently lost more than **O**ne stone (approx 6.4 kg) in a three-month period?
4. Do you believe yourself to be **F**at when others say you are too thin?
5. Would you say **F**ood dominates your life?

Exercise regime

Drugs such as laxatives

Or **HEADSS**[1] screen:

- **–H** Home situation
- **–E** Employment, Education, Economic situation
- **–A** Activities, Affect, Ambition, Anxieties
- **–D** Drugs, Depression
- **–S** Sexuality
- **–S** Suicide, Self-esteem, Stress

Explain that a physical examination is needed.

Most likely diagnosis

Explain most likely diagnosis–purging disorder.

Management

Explain reasons for concern about vomiting

Raise possibility of an eating disorder

Perform physical examination and urinalysis

Recommend blood tests to exclude electrolyte disturbance

Assure of ongoing support and follow-up

Reassure that assistance is available.

 CASE COMMENTARY

The aim of this case is for the doctor to develop a trusting relationship with Amanda and establish that she has an eating disorder. Sensitive questioning and active listening is needed to get Amanda to admit that she is making herself vomit. She does not meet the criteria for either anorexia or bulimia; however, the self-induced vomiting, or purging disorder, is classified as Other specified feeding or eating disorder (OFSED).[2] Eating disorders affect 2–3% of people in Australia and are presenting earlier and in more boys than previously.[3]

The SCOFF questionnaire provides a framework for asking about food and its place in people's lives.[1] Appropriate management is a combination of the medical aspects, such as a physical examination and investigations, and the psychosocial aspects.[2] HEADSS[4] is another useful framework for conversation with adolescents.

A poor or inexperienced doctor will focus solely on the medical implications of her purging and not consider the person and their situation and the emotion surrounding the problem. Feedback to the teacher can only be given with Amanda's permission.

The doctor is not expected to give details of the proposed management in the time available, but should reassure Amanda that there are options for assistance which usually involve her family and a psychologist, and maybe a psychiatrist, paediatrician, dietitian, social worker or psychiatric nurse.[2]

References

1. Morgan, JF, Reid, F & Lacey, JH 1999, 'The SCOFF questionnaire: assessment of a new screening tool for eating disorders', *British Medical Journal,* vol. 319, pp. 1467–8.
2. Rowe, E 2017, 'Early detection of eating disorders in general practice', *Australian Family Physician,* vol. 46, no. 11, pp. 833–8.
3. Madden, S, Morris, A, Zurynski, YA, Kohn, M & Elliot, E. 2009, 'Burden of eating disorders in 5–13-year-old children in Australia', *Medical Journal of Australia,* vol. 190, no. 8, pp. 410–4.
4. Goldenring, J & Cohen, E 1988, 'Getting into adolescents' heads', *Contemporary Paediatrics,* July pp. 75–80.

Further reading

Hay, P, Chinn, D, Forbes, D, Madden, S, Newton, R, Sugenor, L et al. 2014, 'Royal Australian and New Zealand College of Psychiatrists clinical practice guidelines for the treatment of eating disorders', *Australian & New Zealand Journal of Psychiatry,* vol. 48, no. 11, pp. 977–1008.

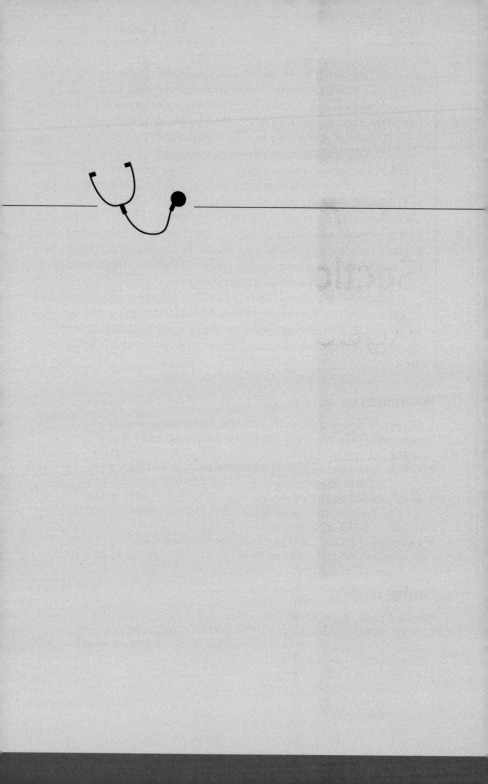

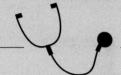

Section 3
Aged care

Case 5
Elsie Humphries

Instructions for the doctor

This is a long case.

Please take a history from Mrs Humphries. Then ask the facilitator for the results of the physical examination. Discuss your management plan with Mrs Humphries.

Alternative instructions

Medical students and junior doctors might learn more from this scenario if they are asked to conduct the physical examination and negotiate a management plan with Mrs Humphries without a time restriction.

Scenario

You are called to see Mrs Elsie Humphries, an 85-year-old woman, at home. Her family phoned for the visit because she has told them that she has had several falls recently. They run a business interstate and visit her twice a year. The family want reassurance that Mrs Humphries is safe.

The following information is on her summary sheet:

Current medical problems
Diverticular disease
Congestive heart failure
Atrial fibrillation (AF)
Past medical history
Burnt-out rheumatoid arthritis
First child 1959
Second child 1961

Medication
Warfarin as directed
Digoxin   0.625 mg od
Frusemide   20 mg od
Perindopril   5 mg od
Allergies
Nil
Immunisations
Up-to-date
Social history
Widowed 2007
Husband was an Australian Football League coach
Non-smoker
Alcohol intake—two standard drinks per week.

Instructions for the patient, Elsie Humphries

You are a rural battler. You have survived several droughts and floods and had rheumatoid arthritis during middle life. You are determined not to let old age beat you. You have coped since you were widowed and, while you do not enjoy getting old, you are proud of managing despite having only your cat for company.

You gave up expecting your children to be of any help to you long ago. They visit for just long enough to ease their guilt and run back to the city. If the children had their way they would parcel you up and put you in a home. It has worried them that you have mentioned a couple of recent falls. The children have asked your doctor to make a home visit to check that you are still safe.

You have fallen three times in your home in the past two months. The most recent fall was last week when you tripped over a door mat going to hang your washing out. You hit the side of your head on the door frame, but did not sustain any other injuries or lose consciousness. Your other falls have been similar. You have had no dizziness and are currently otherwise well.

You have noticed it is harder to see details on the TV, and you stopped buying the newspaper a couple of years ago when you couldn't read the small print. You haven't noticed any changes in your hearing.

You have given up driving and catch a taxi once per week to the local shops to buy your groceries, have your blood test for warfarin and pay your bills at the post office. You manage to cook simple meals at home, although you are buying microwave meals more and more often. You struggle with your housework, particularly heavy work such as vacuuming, and you haven't changed the sheets on your bed since you fell changing them a few months ago. You are mostly continent of urine with the very occasional accident when you struggle to get out of your chair easily, and you shower daily although this tires you out. Your doctor has mentioned getting some home help in the past, but you have brushed off these suggestions, feeling that it would just be a step towards losing your independence and ending up in a nursing home.

You have had limited local supports since your close friend passed away shortly after your husband.

You don't smoke but you do still enjoy your 50-year habit of a sherry on a Friday and Saturday night before bed.

Your house is full of a lifetime of collected trinkets and memorabilia, which makes moving without tripping difficult. You have an alarm, which you carry round your neck.

Clinical examination findings

You have cataracts and your toenails are so long you cannot wear shoes. You are wearing slippers, and a headscarf to cover up the bruise on your left temple from a recent fall.

Your blood pressure is 140/90 mmHg with no postural drop and your pulse is 72 and irregularly irregular. There is no evidence of congestive cardiac failure. You have some ulnar deviation of the fingers following your rheumatoid arthritis.

All other physical examination findings are within normal limits.

The following information is on your summary sheet:

Current medical problems
Diverticular disease
Congestive heart failure
Atrial fibrillation (AF)

Past medical history
Burnt-out rheumatoid arthritis
First child 1959
Second child 1961

Medication
Warfarin as directed
Digoxin   0.625 mg od
Frusemide   20 mg od
Perindopril   5 mg od

Allergies
Nil

Immunisations
Up-to-date
Social history
Widowed 2007
Husband was an Australian Football League coach
Non-smoker
Alcohol intake—two standard drinks per week.

Information for the facilitator

Clinical examination findings

Mrs Humphries has cataracts, her visual acuity is 6/18 left eye 6/12 right eye not correctable by glasses, and her toenails are so long she cannot wear shoes. She is wearing slippers, and a headscarf to cover up the bruise on her left temple from a recent fall.

Her blood pressure is 140/90 mmHg with no postural drop and her pulse is 72 and irregularly irregular. There is no evidence of congestive cardiac failure. She has some ulnar deviation of the fingers following her rheumatoid arthritis.

All other physical examination findings are within normal limits.

Mrs Humphries' house is full of trinkets and memorabilia, which makes moving without tripping difficult. She has an alarm, which she carries round her neck.

Suggested approach to the case

Establish rapport
Open-ended questions to explore Mrs Humphries' ideas, concerns and
    expectations.

Specific questions

Ask about the falls
    —Frequency of the falls
    —Timing of the falls
    —Mrs Humphries' ideas on the cause of the falls
    —Have any of the falls been witnessed?
    —Have any injuries been sustained?
    —Any history of fits, incontinence or loss of consciousness?
Obtain further history exploring possible causes of falls
    —Environment related/accommodation
    —Impaired sensory input

−Drugs and alcohol
−Locomotor disorders
−Lower cerebral perfusion−postural hypotension, syncope, uncontrolled atrial fibrillation
−Epilepsy
−Systemic illness, e.g. infection
Explore her response to the falls, how she sees her future
Social history−current support mechanisms, how is she managing activities of daily living, driving, continence
Request permission to examine.

Examination

Ask the facilitator for specific examination findings or seek permission to examine
Assess the home
- Causes of falls−loose rugs, obstacles, poor lighting, footwear
- Safety items−personal alarm

Assess Mrs Humphries
- Temperature
- Inspect for evidence of injury such as multiple bruises of different ages
- Cardiovascular system
  −Pulse, rate and rhythm
  −BP standing and sitting
  −Jugular venous pulse
  −Heart sounds
  −Carotid bruits
  −Ankle oedema
- Respiratory system
  −Respiratory rate
  −Chest auscultation
- Neurological system
  −Cognitive function
  −Hearing and visual acuity, including type of glasses worn
  −Tremor
  −Weakness
  −Proprioception and balance: Romberg's test
  −Coordination
- Movements
  −Walking

—Neck movements
—Falls risk-assessment tests, e.g. sit-to-stand test, 6-metre walk
• Mental health
—Depression
—Anxiety
• Miscellaneous
—Thyroid
—Toenails
—Metabolic.

Investigations

FBC   ECG
UEC   24 hr ECG
BSL   TFTs
Vitamin D
LFTs   Exclude underlying urine infection—MSU for MCS
CT head To exclude cerebral haemorrhage.

Management

Outline to Mrs Humphries that her cataracts and her toenails may be
    causing the falls
Explain treatment is available for both
Seek Mrs Humphries' consent for referral and treatment:
• ophthalmologist for cataracts
• podiatrist for toenails.
Drug therapy:
• monitor current therapy
• consider risk–benefits of warfarin with CHA_2DS_2-VASc and HAS-
    BLED calculators.[1]
Maintain activity and mobility
With Mrs Humphries' permission, she should be referred to My Aged
    Care (www.myagedcare.gov.au) for assessment. Some reassurance that
    services can help her maintain her independence may encourage this.
Other options to consider will depend on the services available locally
    but could include occupational therapy, physiotherapy, group exercise/
    balance programs, continence services, social services, volunteer services
    such as Meals on Wheels, trial of hip protectors, referral to a falls clinic.
The issues to include regarding home safety are:
• current likelihood of fall—is she safe staying at home?
• ability to feed, dress and bathe safely

- clear passageways of trinkets and memorabilia
- remove loose rugs
- get frame/walking aid
- telephone near bed
- regular visitors.

Bone density scan should be considered

Arrange follow-up

Ask Mrs Humphries if she wishes you to discuss the outcome of the visit with her family.

 ## CASE COMMENTARY

This is a common general practice scenario: an elderly, independent lady who is at risk of losing her independence. Assessing Mrs Humphries at home is key to determining her level of risk and seeing life from her perspective. This richer understanding of the person and their life, compared to the impression gleaned in a clinic room, provides a good foundation for discussing her ability to continue living independently.

Doctors are expected to demonstrate a systematic approach to the problem of falls in the elderly, addressing the physical, psychological and social issues. Interventions can help elderly people to live safely and independently and can delay admission to hospital or nursing home care. The history should focus on the details of the falls and on identifying a potential cause together with a risk assessment of the likelihood of further falls and significant injury for Mrs Humphries. Mrs Humphries' perspective on the falls must be explored. Is she frightened and seeking residential care? Or would she prefer to stay at home despite the risks? Mrs Humphries' past history of rheumatoid arthritis is a risk factor for osteoporosis.

In this case the examination reveals cataracts and long toenails. The facilitator will only mention this pathology if asked. These are treatable and the doctor can be optimistic that Mrs Humphries can maintain her independence once these issues are dealt with appropriately. I have seen one doctor offer to cut the toenails that day. Before the cataracts are treated, the doctor may need to offer short-term residential care. If Mrs Humphries goes outside, it is worthwhile for her to have a single-lens pair of spectacles to avoid falls that can be caused by multifocal lenses.

Referral to allied health services through the Enhanced Primary Care items can follow completion of a care plan. Mrs Humphries might benefit from a Home Medicines Review; it is imperative that her warfarin is reviewed—does the risk of warfarin therapy now outweigh its potential benefits?

COMMON PITFALLS

This case requires the doctor to focus their questions and examination on the common causes of falls in the elderly. Doctors who take an overly-detailed history or examination will run out of time and not progress to discussing management with Mrs Humphries.

Mrs Humphries is the doctor's patient but the family have asked for the visit. It is important to involve her family in her care, however, her consent is needed before discussing the outcome of the visit with them.

There is a risk of either bowing to the relatives' pressure and arranging admission for Mrs Humphries or colluding with Mrs Humphries' denial of the issues and not taking action where it is needed.

Reference

1. National Prescribing Service 2017, *Predicting risk with oral anticoagulants.* Available at: www.nps.org.au/medical-info/clinical-topics/news/predicting-risk-with-oral-anticoagulants, accessed 24 June 2018.

Further reading

Gillespie, LD, Robertson, MC, Gillespie, WJ, Sherrington, C, Gates, S, Clemson, LM, et al. 2012, 'Interventions for preventing falls in older people living in the community', *Cochrane Database of Systematic Reviews,* doi: 10.1002/14651858.CD007146.pub3.

Mackenzie, L & Clemson, L 2014, 'Can chronic disease management plans including occupational therapy and physiotherapy services contribute to reducing falls risk in older people?', *Australian Family Physician,* vol. 43, pp. 211-5.

The Royal Australian College of General Practitioners 2018, *Guidelines for preventive activities in general practice,* 9th ed, updated, RACG, East Melbourne, Vic.

Waldron, N, Hill, AM & Barker, A 2012, 'Falls prevention in older adults—assessment and management', *Australian Family Physician,* vol. 41, pp. 930-5.

Case 6
Flora McMillan

Instructions for the doctor

This is a short case.

Please explain the test results to Flora and develop a management plan with her for the prevention of further osteoporotic fractures.

Scenario

In January of this year Flora McMillan, aged 73, fell on her left arm and sustained a Colles fracture. She recently had a bone densitometry scan done and the results are:

Scan	BMD g/ cm²	T-score	Fracture risk	Z-score	Peer relationship
Lumbar spine	0.854	−2.6	Marked	−1.2	Lowest quartile
Total femur (L)	0.686	−2.6	Marked	−1.5	Lowest quartile

T-score—comparison with young normal adult
Z-score—comparison with aged matched controls

The following information is on her medical record:

Past medical history
Hyperlipidaemia

Medication
Simvastatin 40 mg od

Allergies
Nil known

Immunisations
Up-to-date

Family history
Father died of a myocardial infarction, aged 45
Social history
Teacher, semi-retired
Non-smoker
Height 1.6 m
Weight 53 kg
BMI 20.7 kg/m².

Instructions for the patient, Flora McMillan

You are a 73-year-old teacher. You work part-time in the school library. In January of this year, you tripped over while on a walking holiday and broke your left wrist. (You did not quite hear the name of the fracture—it sounded like a Collie fracture but you though Collies were dogs.)

You are now back at work. Your wrist is apparently healed but it feels stiff in the morning and aches after a long day of carrying books.

Your GP arranged a bone density scan. You are here to find out the results and want to hear about anything you can do to prevent further fractures.

The following information is on your medical records:
Past medical history
Hyperlipidaemia
Medication
Simvastatin 40 mg od
Allergies
Nil known
Immunisations
Up-to-date
Family history
Father died of a myocardial infarction, aged 45
Social history
Teacher, semi-retired
Non-smoker
Height 1.6 m
Weight 53 kg
BMI 20.7 kg/m².

Suggested approach to the case

Establish rapport
Check reason for attendance—to obtain results of bone density scan

Give results

—Explain results in terms that Flora understands—scan demonstrates osteoporosis ('thinning of the bones')

—Link osteoporosis with recent fracture

—Explain risk of further fractures and need to prevent

Maintain/improve bone density

—Calcium intake—recommended 1000–1500 mg calcium per day, ideally through low-fat dietary sources; may need supplement if unable to meet requirements in diet

—Vitamin D—assess sun exposure, check and replace Vitamin D if at risk

—Weight-bearing exercise 30–60 minutes, three to four days per week

—Initiate treatment with anti-osteoporosis medication, e.g. bisphosphonate or denosumab

—Avoid excess alcohol and caffeine. Don't start smoking

Fracture prevention

—Preventing falls—regular exercises to maintain sense of balance and proprioception, appropriate footwear, safety at home, caution at night. (For higher risk patients, consider occupational therapy assessment, walking aids and hip protectors)

—Review of medications that predispose to bone loss/falls, e.g. steroids, sleeping tablets, anti-hypertensives can cause postural drop

Consider referrals to allied health professionals, e.g. exercise physiologist, dietician, occupational therapist to provide further assistance with addressing the above issues

Plan follow-up to review medication and reinforce lifestyle advice

—A repeat BMD is generally not required unless considering a change to or cessation of anti-osteoporosis medication.

 CASE COMMENTARY

This case requires the GP to interpret Flora's bone density scan results and give her understandable, practical information about osteoporosis and preventing falls and further fractures. The Z-score compares Flora's bone mineral density to that of other women of her age whereas the T-score compares Flora's bone mineral density to that of normal young women. The T-score relates more closely to fracture risk. A T-score less than –2.5 is consistent with the diagnosis of osteoporosis and each standard deviation reduction in bone density is associated with an approximate doubling of the risk of hip fracture.

Osteoporosis prevention and treatment characterises much of modern general practice: the evidence regarding best practice is changing rapidly and can be contradictory for different conditions. Flora's osteoporosis needs good calcium and vitamin D levels, but in the low-fat diet needed for her hyperlipidaemia many of the foods that contain these are reduced. An association between calcium supplements and heart disease adds further complications. Prevention of skin cancer requires patients to avoid sun exposure–just the very thing needed to produce vitamin D! Balancing these competing guidelines is difficult.

Pharmacological treatment options include an oral or intravenous bisphosphonate or denosumab, and second-line options are raloxifene, strontium or teriparatide. Careful consideration should be given to prescribing strontium for people at increased risk of cardiovascular disease. The recommended daily intake of calcium for women over 50 is 1300 mg/day. This requires at least three serves of dairy foods per day, with one of these being calcium fortified.

COMMON PITFALLS

There is a risk of seeing osteoporosis and fracture prevention purely in terms of medication. Drugs play an important role but are only one aspect of management. Simple advice about maintaining fitness and balance, safety at home, a healthy diet and adequate but not excessive sun exposure is also needed. The challenge is to say this in a way that Flora does not feel patronised. She sees herself as a working teacher, not an old lady!

Further reading

Ewald, D 2012, 'Osteoporosis–prevention and detection in general practice', *Australian Family Physician,* vol. 41, pp. 104–8.

The Royal Australian College of General Practitioners and Osteoporosis Australia 2017, *Osteoporosis prevention, diagnosis and management in postmenopausal women and men over 50 years of age,* 2nd ed, RACGP, East Melbourne. Available at: www.osteoporosis.org.au/sites/default/files/files/20439%20Osteoporosis%20guidelines.pdf, accessed 23 November 2018.

Therapeutic Drugs Administration 2014, 'Strontium ranelate (Protos) and risk of adverse events'. Available at: www.tga.gov.au/alert/strontium-ranelate-protos-and-risk-adverse-events-0, accessed 23 November 2018.

Therapeutic Guidelines 2014, 'Treating osteoporosis: calcium and vitamin D supplements and osteoporosis therapy', in *eTG complete* [Internet], TG, Melbourne.

Winzenberg, T, van der Mei, I, Mason, RS, Nowson, C & Jones, G 2012, 'Vitamin D and the musculoskeletal health of older adults', *Australian Family Physician,* vol. 41, pp. 92–9.

Case 7
Nell Worthington

Instructions for the doctor

This is a short case.

Please take a history as if you were in clinical practice and then outline your plans to Mrs Worthington.

Scenario

Mrs Nell Worthington is an 80-year-old retired legal secretary. She has hypertension. She has just moved to your area to be nearer to her daughter. She has brought her summary sheet from her previous practice.

The following information is on her summary sheet from her previous practice:

Past medical history
Hypertension diagnosed 2013
Osteoarthritis of neck and hips
Vaginal hysterectomy for prolapse 1995
Four children

Medication
Spironolactone 25 mg od
Ramipril 10 mg od
Potassium chloride 600 mg slow release 1 tab od

Allergies
Nil known

Immunisations
Up-to-date

Social history
Widowed 2008.

Instructions for the patient, Nell Worthington

You are an 80-year-old retired legal secretary. You have just moved to be nearer your daughter. Life has been hard since Vince, your husband, died in 2008. You are feeling lost as you try to establish your new life in this town. You had attended the same doctor back home for years and are nervous about coming here today.

You have been feeling lethargic recently but have put this down to the move. Your opening line will be, 'Doctor I'm feeling tired, but maybe this is because I have just moved here.'

The following information is on your summary sheet:

Past medical history
Hypertension diagnosed 2013
Osteoarthritis of neck and hips
Vaginal hysterectomy for prolapse 1995
Four children
Medication
Spironolactone 25 mg od
Ramipril 10 mg od
Potassium chloride 600 mg slow release 1 tab od
Allergies
Nil known
Immunisations
Up-to-date
Social history
Widowed 2008.

Suggested approach to the case

Establish rapport
Welcome Mrs Worthington to the practice
—Ask about the move, is she settling in?
Explore patient's ideas, concerns and expectations regarding this consultation.

Specific questions

Enquire about current symptoms
Brief systems review—any problems with your breathing, your appetite, your bowels, your 'waterworks', sleep, energy level, weight changes?
Sensitively explore any mood symptoms

Review information on summary sheet with Mrs Worthington
Confirm current medication
Explore other cardiac risk factors
  —Exercise
  —Smoking
Other preventive health measures
  —Immunisation status
  —Alcohol consumption
Full physical examination—needed, but not part of this consultation.

Investigations

Explain need for investigations
Surgery tests: BSL or urine dipstick, ECG
Lab tests
  —Arrange urgent UEC—drug regimen risks hyperkalaemia, can cause
    tiredness
  —Non-urgent BSL, FBC, LFTs, TFTs.

Management

Cease potassium supplement and explain why
Arrange follow-up—how Mrs Worthington will get the results.

CASE COMMENTARY

The first consultation for a new patient at a practice provides a good opportunity for a thorough medical review. Mrs Worthington's drug regimen puts her at risk of hyperkalaemia and she needs urgent assessment of her electrolytes.

Mrs Worthington's lethargy could be due to the recent relocation but, given her age, it is important to exclude other pathology. Doctors are expected to deal with the immediate issue of potential hyperkalaemia and then make arrangements for further review. This prioritisation of 'what do I need to do today, what do I need to do in the next week, what do I need to do in the next month' is an important skill for GPs to learn and demonstrate. The cost of admission creates a tendency to do everything at once for hospitalised patients, but in general practice the best use of resources and the best way to help patients to change is to establish priorities and work through them systematically over time.

This case is based on a true story. The patient was admitted to hospital because of the hyperkalaemia—a preventable admission. The rates of morbidity and mortality associated with hyperkalaemia have risen with the increased use of angiotensin-converting enzyme inhibitors, angiotensin receptor blockers and aldosterone receptor antagonists. Adverse drug reactions were reported in 10% of patients seen in Australian general practice over a six-month period, in 16% of patients presenting to emergency departments, and in up to 20% of hospital admissions.

COMMON PITFALLS

Doctors should avoid unfair criticism of the doctor who instigated Mrs Worthington's drug regimen. The ideal would be to discreetly contact the prescriber and find out why this regimen was chosen, enabling the person to learn from the experience.

Further reading

Kalisch, LM, Caughey, GE, Barratt, JD, Ramsay, EN, Killer, G, Gilbert, AL et al. 2012, 'Prevalence of preventable medication-related hospitalizations in Australia: an opportunity to reduce harm', *International Journal for Quality in Health Care,* vol. 24, pp. 239–49.

Miller, GC, Britt, HC & Valenti, L 2006, 'Adverse drug events in general practice patients in Australia', *Medical Journal of Australia,* vol. 184, pp. 321–4.

Nyirenda, MJ, Tang, JI, Padfield, PL & Seckl, JR 2009, 'Hyperkalaemia', *British Medical Journal,* vol. 339, p. b4114.

Phillips, AL, Nigro, O, Macolino, KA, Scarborough, KC, Doecke, CJ, Angley, MT et al. 2014, 'Hospital admissions caused by adverse drug events: an Australian prospective study', *Australian Health Review,* vol. 38, pp. 51–7.

Case 8
Margaret Wilson

Instructions for the doctor

This is a short case.

Please take a history from Margaret Wilson and discuss your management plan with her.

Scenario

Margaret and Don Wilson have been your patients for many years. Don has developed Alzheimer's disease. You made the diagnosis on the basis of a typical history and an unremarkable organic screen. Don has been seeing a geriatrician who has started him on donepezil (Aricept) with little response to date. Margaret is generally healthy but is carrying Don's care almost single-handedly and you are concerned about how she is coping.

The following information is on her summary sheet:

Age
74
Past medical history
Osteoarthritis
Medication
Paracetamol 665 mg 2 tds
Allergies
Nil known
Immunisations
Up-to-date
Social history
Married
Non-smoker
Alcohol intake—two standard drinks per week.

Instructions for the patient, Margaret Wilson

You and your husband, Don, have been coming to see this doctor for many years. Don is 76 and has recently been diagnosed with Alzheimer's disease. He sees a visiting geriatrician (Dr Sue Davies), who has prescribed a medication—Aricept—but so far there doesn't seem to be any improvement. You are finding his care very draining and are worried about how you are going to manage. Don is anxious when you are not nearby, so he follows you around the house or garden and seems to need your reassurance all the time. He asks the same things over and over again and needs assistance with all but the most basic activities. You have found yourself getting increasingly frustrated with him and have lost your temper with him lately. You have never been physically violent, but you worry about what might happen if things continue the way they are. Dr Davies suggested Don go to home group once or twice a week, but he doesn't want to go and usually refuses. You have stopped going out to most of your usual activities (walking, croquet and bridge) because you don't feel you can leave Don alone. You have lost contact with most of your friends and can feel yourself being worn down emotionally.

Your appetite is normal and you are sleeping reasonably well, but you often worry about what is going to happen to Don. Your mood is dominated by worry about Don but is otherwise OK and your energy levels seem normal. Your children live interstate and are busy with their own lives. You don't have anyone you feel you can share your worries with, and you are grieving the relationship you previously had with Don where you could talk about things. If the doctor raises possible placement in care, you respond by saying, 'Oh, I could never do that'. Don needs almost constant help, and you have heard stories about people being neglected in nursing homes. You can't bear to imagine Don wasting away by himself in one of those places—besides you took a vow to stay with him in sickness and in health. You have not had any suicidal thoughts but you feel lonely and trapped in an impossible situation with no way out. You are hopeful the doctor will have some answers for you.

The following information is on your summary sheet:

Age
74
Past medical history
Osteoarthritis
Medication
Paracetamol 665 mg 2 tds
Allergies
Nil known

Immunisations
Up-to-date
Social history
Married
Non-smoker
Alcohol intake—two standard drinks per week.

Suggested approach to the case

Establish rapport
Open questions to explore Margaret's concerns.

Specific questions

Explore Margaret's ability to cope
Establish whether Don and Margaret are safe
How is she currently managing her stress
Explore Margaret's supports
Sensitive questioning regarding option of applying for carer's pension.

Management

Reflect on your concerns about Margaret's current stress
Demonstrate empathy and acknowledge the difficulties her role entails
Education about carer stress and its management principles:
* need for regular respite, offer referral to arrange
* involvement in a carer support group
* making time for herself for social and physical activities and connecting with others.
Ensure regular and close follow-up.

CASE COMMENTARY

About 1.2 million Australians care for someone with dementia. GPs play a crucial role in managing the needs of people with dementia and caregivers, by providing ongoing support and by facilitating access to evidence-based care. Scheduled, regular reviews of people with dementia and their caregivers should be standard practice, and this case allows those skills to be demonstrated. It is common for caregivers to feel trapped as their partner's demands increase and their own coping ability diminishes. Margaret's situation has many of the recognisable risk factors for elder abuse, and the safety of both patients needs to be sensitively explored. Margaret needs education, resources and practical assistance in order to become a healthy caregiver.

Many carers find that the experience of a carer support group is invaluable, mainly because it connects them with others who have faced similar circumstances and challenges and who can share their struggles and solutions. This can help combat a carer's feelings of isolation, guilt, uncertainty and helplessness. Margaret needs assistance in developing a strong support network of her own, as well as regular, quarantined time-out for herself. She should be encouraged to resume her activities—both social and physical—that have been set aside as the demands of caring for Don have increased.

 COMMON PITFALLS

If we approach the situation with the single focus of convincing Margaret to place Don in residential care, we miss the opportunity to explore other fruitful areas like carer stress and its management. Elder abuse is a serious and all-too-common problem and needs to be explored in a situation like this. Utilising the various community supports for Margaret without losing the central, caring role of the GP can also be a challenge.

Further reading

Alzheimer's Association 2014, 'Caregiver stress'. Available at: www.alz.org/care/alzheimers-dementia-caregiver-stress-burnout.asp, accessed 25 September 2014.

Brooks, D, Ross, C & Beattie, E 2015, *Caring for someone with dementia: the economic, social and health impacts of caring and evidence based supports for carers,* Alzheimers Australia. Available at: www.dementia.org.au/files/NATIONAL/documents/Alzheimers-Australia-Numbered-Publication-42.pdf, accessed 16 August 2018.

Burke, D 2012 'Carer stress', *Australian Doctor,* 15 May 2012. Available at: www.ausdoc.com.au/therapy-update/carer-stress, accessed 23 May 2019.

Commonwealth of Australia 2006, *Dementia: the caring experience. A guide for families and carers of people with dementia,* Canberra, ACT.

Strivens, E & Craig, D 2014, 'Managing dementia-related cognitive decline in patients and their caregivers', *Australian Family Physician,* vol. 43, no. 4, pp. 170–4.

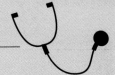

Section 4
Cardiovascular system

Case 9
Helen Berkovic

Instructions for the doctor

This is a short case.

Please negotiate a management plan with Helen.

Scenario

Helen Berkovic is a 53-year-old prison officer. You have just returned from leave and in your absence Helen has been seeing your locum. The locum has diagnosed essential hypertension as blood pressure readings have been over 180/110 on three different occasions.

The following information is on her summary sheet:

Past medical history

Nil

Medication

Nil

Allergies

Nil

Immunisations

Up-to-date

Family history

Father—on blood pressure medication

Social history

Smokes 10 cigarettes per day.

Instructions for the patient, Helen Berkovic

You are a 53-year-old prison officer. Your own GP has been on leave and you have been seeing the locum. The locum has diagnosed high blood pressure but you don't know what this means or what can be done about it. Your dad has been taking medication for his blood pressure for years.

You have now come to see your own doctor to plan what to do.

The following information is on your summary sheet:
Past medical history
Nil
Medication
Nil
Allergies
Nil
Immunisations
Up-to-date
Family history
Father—on blood pressure medication
Social history
Smokes 10 cigarettes per day.

The locum conducted a physical examination that was normal. Your BMI is 27 kg/m^2 and urine dipstick was normal, with no evidence of micro/macro-albuminuria. The CXR, ECG, echocardiogram, FBC, UEC, LFTs, fasting blood glucose and fasting lipids were normal.

Suggested approach to the case

Management

Re-establish rapport
Confirm diagnosis of essential hypertension
Confirm with Helen that investigations and examination were normal
Explore Helen's understanding of hypertension and treatment.

Treatment options

Non-pharmacological
   —Exercise
   —Weight loss
   —Salt reduction
   —Reduce alcohol intake
   —Address potential life stressors—work
   —Treatment of obstructive sleep apnoea
Discuss smoking and assess readiness to quit
Pharmacological
   —Start medication.

Follow-up

Document BP and suggest mechanism for patient to record readings, for example, manually on a card or using an app on a smartphone or tablet
Add to recall system to recheck UEC and BP on treatment
Provide sources for further information for the patient.

CASE COMMENTARY

This is a common general practice situation. The first aim of this case is to ensure that the doctor has the skill to take over management of a patient from a colleague.

Traditional medical training is for doctors to plan patient management after taking a history and conducting an examination themselves. The increase in team practice requires doctors to pick up a consultation at different stages of the process. Reading the patient's notes was considered 'cheating' prior to seeing patients as a medical student: now it is a prerequisite of every consultation. Scanning notes with an attitude of critical trust is needed.

The second aim is to ensure the doctor can think holistically about hypertension and cardiovascular risk. Helen needs tailored, practical assistance to lower her risk of cardiovascular disease both through medication and via non-pharmacological interventions such as quitting smoking and increasing physical activity.

Helen meets the criteria for starting medication for her blood pressure. ACEI, ARB, calcium-channel blockers, thiazide-like diuretics are drugs of first choice for uncomplicated hypertension in non-pregnant adults. The actual choice is influenced by individual patient factors such as associated medical conditions and the risks of adverse effects of the drug.

Lastly, arrangements for ongoing monitoring and follow-up are needed.

COMMON PITFALLS

While lifestyle advice is recommended for all patients, in patients at low absolute CVD risk ($<$10% five-year risk) with persistent blood pressure $>$ 160/100 mmHg, antihypertensive therapy should be started once the diagnosis is confirmed.

Further reading

Banks, E, Crouch, SR, Korda, RJ, Stavreski, B, Page, K, Thurber, KA & Grenfell, R 2016 'Absolute risk of cardiovascular disease events, and blood pressure- and lipid-lowering therapy in Australia', *Medical Journal of Australia,* vol. 204, no. 8, p. 320.

Blood Pressure Lowering Treatment Trialists Collaboration, Sundstrom, J, Arima, H, Woodward, M, Jackson, R, Karmali, K et al. 2014, 'Blood pressure-lowering treatment based on cardiovascular risk: a meta-analysis of individual patient data', *Lancet,* vol. 384, pp. 591–8.

National Heart Foundation of Australia 2016, *Guidelines for the diagnosis and management of hypertension in adults,* National Heart Foundation of Australia. Available at: www.heartfoundation.org.au/images/uploads/publications/PRO-167_Hypertension-guideline-2016_WEB.pdf, accessed 18 February 2019.

O'Callaghan, CJ, Goh, MY & Rong, P 2013, 'Hypertension—the difficult decisions', *Australian Family Physician,* vol. 42, pp. 376–9.

Therapeutic Guidelines Ltd 2018, 'Elevated blood pressure: pharmacological management'. In *eTG Complete* [Internet], Therapeutic Guidelines Ltd, Melbourne, Vic.

The Royal Australian College of General Practitioners 2015, *Smoking, nutrition, alcohol, physical activity (SNAP): A population health guide to behavioural risk factors in general practice,* 2nd ed, RACGP, East Melbourne, Vic.

The Royal Australian College of General Practitioners 2018, *Guidelines for preventive activities in general practice,* 9th ed, updated, RACGP, East Melbourne, Vic, pp. 85–91.

Case 10
Dilip Patel

Instructions for the doctor

This is a short case.

Please respond appropriately to Dilip's questions.

Scenario

Dilip Patel is a 44-year-old plumber who lives in your rural town. Four weeks ago he had severe chest pain while working and was admitted to hospital with acute coronary syndrome. Tests confirmed myocardial infarction and triple vessel disease for which he had coronary artery bypass graft (CABG) surgery in a metropolitan tertiary hospital. Dilip is now on the following medications:

- Atorvastatin 80 mg od
- Glyceryl trinitrate spray prn
- Aspirin 100 mg od
- Clopidogrel 75 mg od
- Perindopril 5 mg od
- Metoprolol 50 mg od.

The following information is on his summary sheet:

Past medical history
Nil
Allergies
Nil
Immunisations
Nil recorded
Family history
Nil recorded
Social history
Plumber
Ex-smoker.

Instructions for the patient, Dilip Patel

You are a 44-year-old plumber in a rural town. Four weeks ago you had severe chest pain while working and you were admitted as an emergency to the local hospital. You were told that you had had a heart attack. After lots of tests you had urgent bypass surgery in a big city hospital.

You are now back home. On discharge from the hospital you were given a long list of medications to take. You have never needed tablets before and keep forgetting to take them.

You are unsure what the tablets are for as you assumed the bypass surgery cured the problems. You have all the tablets with you in a shopping bag in case the GP asks you what you are taking. You have the following questions for the GP:

- why do I need to take tablets when the operation fixed the problem?
- what does each tablet do?
- how long will I be on these tablets?
- do they have any side effects?

You take:

- Atorvastatin 80 mg once per day
- Glyceryl trinitrate spray as required for chest pain
- Aspirin 100 mg once per day
- Clopidogrel 75 mg once per day
- Perindopril 5 mg once per day
- Metoprolol 50 mg once per day.

You quit smoking 10 years ago and do not drink alcohol. You do no regular exercise.

Once the GP has discussed your worries about the medication you will be interested to hear any other advice the GP offers. If the GP starts to give other advice before answering your concerns about the medication you will get quite cranky and irritable.

The following information is on your summary sheet:
Past medical history
Nil
Allergies
Nil
Immunisations
Nil recorded
Family history
Nil recorded

Social history
Plumber
Ex-smoker
Alcohol—nil.

Suggested approach to the case

Establish rapport
Explore Dilip's understanding and concerns about his medication
Ask if there are any other queries today:

Why do I need to take tablets when the operation fixed the problem?
The operation has bypassed the blocked blood vessels or 'pipes'. You need to keep the new vessels or 'pipes' open and prevent blockages in any other of your blood vessels. This is best done with a healthy lifestyle and medication.

What does each tablet do?
- Atorvastatin 80 mg tablets help to stop fat build-up in the blood vessels along with a healthy diet that includes five serves of vegetables and two serves of fruits per day.[1]
- Glyceryl trinitrate spray prn helps to open up the blood vessels to get more oxygen to the heart if you have any chest pain.[2]
- Aspirin 100 mg od and Clopidogrel 75 mg od both 'thin' the blood. They reduce the risk of blood clots and another heart attack.[1]
- Perindopril 5 mg od is an ACE inhibitor. It works on a chemical in the kidney that makes your blood pressure go up. An ACE inhibitor protects the kidneys and keeps your blood pressure down, which reduces the risk of another heart attack.[1]
- Metoprolol is a beta-blocker. This blocks any excess adrenaline from damaging your heart and blood vessels by slowing your heart rate and lowering your blood pressure.[1]

How long will I be on these tablets?
You will be able to stop the Clopidogrel a year after your surgery provided there are no further risks. Normally it is best for people to stay on the other medication. This will be reviewed at regular intervals.

Do they have any side effects?
All medications have potential side effects. If you are concerned if something might be a side effect either phone or come in for advice. The common ones are:[2]
- Atorvastatin—muscle pains
- Glyceryl trinitrate spray prn—headaches, dizziness
- Aspirin—stomach pains (gastritis)

- Clopidogrel—bleeding, diarrhoea
- Perindopril—cough, reduced kidney function
- Metoprolol—tiredness, cold hands and feet, impotence.

If you have time, raise other common concerns—understanding of procedure done, return to driving (minimum four weeks post-CABG for private car), return to work, advice about sexual activity, mood disturbance post-heart attack.

Summarise information

Surgery was needed to bypass the blocked blood vessels
Aim now to get fit and stay healthy by:
- taking medication as prescribed
- regular check-ups—blood pressure, lipids
- not smoking
- graded increase in exercise
- healthy diet—offer dietician referral
- establish cardiac rehabilitation program.[2]

Offer to provide printed patient handout on any of these topics.

 CASE COMMENTARY

Despite overwhelming evidence of the effectiveness of secondary prevention therapies, surveys indicate poor adherence to medical treatments and lifestyle recommendations after an acute coronary syndrome.[3, 4]

Dilip is a plumber who spends his life fixing blocked pipes. He understands the principles of coronary artery bypass grafting well but needs to also understand the risk of re-blockage and what can be done to prevent it.

The GP should be able to explain the role of each medication and its potential side effects in straightforward lay terms, avoiding jargon, as this will increase Dilip's chances of following the advice being given.[5] The GP will also need to discuss other cardiovascular risk factors such as levels of activity and smoking.[6] Patients recovering from surgery have many concerns. Dilip firstly wants his questions answered about the drugs but will also be grateful to a GP who raises more sensitive issues, such as mood disorders[5] and when it is safe to resume sexual intercourse, work and driving.

 COMMON PITFALLS

Dilip wants to be treated with respect. He needs more than just being told to take the tablets because 'the hospital said so'.

The GP may be tempted to criticise the hospital for not giving Dilip enough information about his medication. Experience suggests that patients remember less than half of what they are told. Factors that make this worse are fear, pain, recent anaesthesia and anxiety, all of which may apply to Dilip. It's important to give him information politely and not to assume that the hospital made no effort. But if this is a consistent gap with a particular hospital unit it is worth phoning the consultant to let them know your observation and ask what systems are in place. If Dilip continues to be perplexed or uncertain about his medication, the GP can ask if he would like a Home Medicines Review with a pharmacist.

References

1. National Heart Foundation of Australia 2012, *Reducing risk in heart disease; an expert guide to clinical practice for secondary prevention of coronary heart disease.* Available at: www.heartfoundation.org.au/images/uploads/publications/Reducing-risk-in-heart-disease.pdf, accessed 18 February 2019.
2. Therapeutic Guidelines Ltd 2018, 'Secondary prevention of cardiovascular events'. In: *eTG complete* [Internet], Melbourne, Vic.
3. Thakkar, JB & Chow, CK 2014, 'Adherence to secondary prevention therapies in acute coronary syndrome', *Medical Journal of Australia,* vol. 201, pp. S106-9.
4. Stroke Foundation 2012, *Guidelines for the management of absolute cardiovascular disease risk;* National Vascular Disease Prevention Alliance. Available at: www.heartfoundation.org.au/images/uploads/publications/Absolute-CVD-Risk-Full-Guidelines.pdf, accessed 24 June 2018.
5. Stafford, L, Jackson, HJ & Berk M 2008, 'Illness beliefs about heart disease and adherence to secondary prevention regimens', *Psychosomatic Medicine,* vol. 70, pp. 942-8.
6. The Royal Australian College of General Practitioners 2018, *Guidelines for preventive activities in general practice,* 9th ed, updated, RACGP, East Melbourne, Vic.

Case 11
Jackie Maloney

Instructions for the doctor

This is a short case.

Please take a history from Jackie. Ask for the results of a focused examination from the facilitator. Tell Jackie the most likely diagnosis and your management plan.

Scenario

Jackie Maloney is a 50-year-old taxi driver. She smokes 30 cigarettes a day. She has asked for an appointment to see you today because she has noticed some pain in her chest when she lifts heavy suitcases or has to go up stairs.

The following information is on her summary sheet:

Past medical history
Mechanical low back pain—recurrent
Hiatus hernia—gastro-oesophageal reflux disease
Medication
Omeprazole 40 mg od
Allergies
Nil
Immunisations
Nil known
Family history
Irish family
Mother died of myocardial infarction aged 60
Social history
Taxi driver.

Instructions for the patient, Jackie Maloney

You are a 50-year-old taxi driver. You feel heaviness in your chest on exercise. The heaviness lasts for less than a minute if you stop what you are doing.

You are worried that this heaviness comes from your heart. It has been getting worse and you have finally admitted that you need help. At the back of your mind is the fact that your mother died of a heart attack. You have not had any palpitations but when pressed admit that you have some shortness of breath at the same time as you get the chest pain. You last had pain two days ago.

The most likely diagnosis is angina.

The following information is on your summary sheet:

Past medical history
Mechanical low back pain—recurrent
Hiatus hernia—gastro-oesophageal reflux disease
Medication
Omeprazole 40 mg od
Allergies
Nil
Immunisations
Nil known
Family history
Irish family
Mother died of myocardial infarction aged 60
Social history
Taxi driver.

Instructions for the facilitator

Clinical examination findings

Looks well
No cyanosis
Height 1.65 m
Weight 87 kg
BMI 32 kg/m^2
Waist circumference 94 cm
Blood pressure 130/80 mmHg
Pulse 72
Apex beat not displaced
Heart sounds normal, no added sounds
Chest clear
Peripheral pulses present, no oedema.

Please have a copy of *Assessing Fitness to Drive* available and pass to the candidate on request. Please keep the copy out of sight until requested.

Suggested approach to the case

Establish rapport
Open questions to explore patient's ideas, concerns and expectations.

Specific questions

Detail about the heaviness/pain
Shortness of breath
Palpitations
Cough
    —Relieving factors
Assess cardiac risk factors
    —Smoking
    —Diabetes
    —Hypertension
    —Hyperlipidaemia
    —Family history
Explore lifestyle contributing factors, diet and exercise
Request permission to examine.

Examination

Looks well
No cyanosis
Height 1.65 m
Weight 87 kg
BMI 32 kg/m^2
Waist circumference 94 cm
Blood pressure 130/80 mmHg
Pulse 72
Apex beat not displaced
Heart sounds normal, no added sounds
Chest clear
Peripheral pulses present, no abnormalities found, no oedema.

Most likely diagnosis

Angina—sensitive explanation without using medical jargon.

Planned management

Investigations
FBC, UEC, LFTs, fasting blood glucose, lipids—fasting, resting ECG, consider troponin (see Case Commentary).

Treatment

–GTN spray
–Aspirin low dose
–Beta-blocker or nitrate or long-acting calcium-channel blocker
Check emotional impact of possible diagnosis
Arrange cardiology referral and further testing according to local protocols and facilities (see below)
Recommend urgent attendance at hospital/call ambulance if pain not settling at 10 minutes[1]
Check and discuss implication for driving[2]
Ensure follow-up and offer health promotion (smoking cessation, immunisations, check alcohol intake, advice regarding exercise).

 CASE COMMENTARY

This is a case of angina. In the time available the doctor should be able to state angina as the most likely diagnosis. When this probable diagnosis is mentioned for the first time, a good doctor will watch carefully for Jackie's reaction and allow her to vent her feelings.

Aspirin is recommended in angina but caution is needed because of the past history of gastro-oesophageal reflux and Jackie will need to be asked about recurrences of pain in follow-up. Beta-blockers, nitrates and calcium-channel blockers appear to be equally effective for relieving angina.

Knowing when to test troponin is difficult. It is indicated in suspected acute coronary syndrome (ACS)[3] but not in chronic stable angina. Urgent hospital admission and assessment are appropriate for the management of ACS, not troponin testing in the surgery. Jackie's symptoms do not meet the criteria for ACS and her angina is not yet classified as stable, so it may be reasonable to do a troponin test to rule out ACS, provided follow-up is in place to ensure the result arrives and is actioned urgently if indicated.[4] The role of imaging in ischaemic heart disease is evolving,[5] and decision rules have limited validation in primary care.[5, 6]

Jackie needs an early referral to a specialist cardiologist for probable exercise stress test, stress echocardiography, coronary angiography or computerised tomography (CT) coronary angiography to assess her potential for coronary revascularisation.[7] A telehealth consultation is an option in rural or remote areas without ready access to cardiology services.

A safety point is to consider the impact of angina on Jackie's work as a taxi driver. Doctors are not expected to remember the rules regarding angina and commercial vehicle drivers, but must be aware that this is an issue and tell the facilitator that they would check the regulations and advise Jackie accordingly. Jackie meets the standards for private driving but not the commercial standard. Jackie would need to be off work until a cardiologist assesses the severity of the angina.[2]

COMMON PITFALLS

Jackie's livelihood is her ability to drive a taxi; the candidate should approach the medical and licensing considerations for cardiovascular disease delicately. The seriousness of Jackie's symptoms should be emphasised, not trivialised; an excellent candidate will be able to alert but not alarm the patient. Critically, the candidate should provide a safety net for the patient and outline circumstances where ACS is a risk and they should seek immediate medical attention.

References

1. Heart Foundation. *Heart attack symptoms. Will you recognise your heart attack?* (serial online). Available at: www.heartfoundation.org.au/your-heart/ heart-attack-symptoms/, accessed 1 November 2018.
2. Austroads and National Transport Commission 2017, *Assessing Fitness to Drive,* 5th ed, Sydney.
3. Parsonage, WA, Cullen, L & Younger, JF 2013, 'The approach to patients with possible cardiac chest pain', *Medical Journal of Australia,* vol. 199, pp. 30-4.
4. Mauro, M, Nelson, A & Stokes, M 2017, 'Troponin testing in the primary care setting', *Australian Family Physician,* vol. 46, pp. 823-6.
5. Storey, P 2014, 'Imaging for cardiac disease: a practical guide for general practitioners', *Australian Family Physician,* vol. 43, pp. 260-3.
6. Stokes, M, Nerlekar, N, Moir, S & Teo, K 2016, 'The evolving role of cardiac magnetic resonance imaging in the assessment of cardiovascular disease', *Australian Family Physician,* vol. 45, pp. 761-4.
7. Therapeutic Guidelines Ltd 2018, 'Secondary prevention of cardiovascular events'. In: *eTG complete* (Internet), Melbourne, Vic.

Further reading

Australian cardiovascular risk charts, *Australian absolute cardiovascular disease risk calculator.* Available at: www.cvdcheck.org.au, accessed 18 February 2019.
Stroke Foundation 2012, *Guidelines for the management of absolute cardiovascular disease risk,* National Vascular Disease Prevention Alliance. Available at: www. heartfoundation.org.au/images/uploads/publications/Absolute-CVD-Risk-Full-Guidelines.pdf, accessed 18 February 2019.

Case 12
Eric Schmidt

Instructions for the doctor

This is a long case.

Please take a history and conduct an appropriate examination. Outline the most likely diagnosis and negotiate a management plan with Mr Schmidt.

Scenario

Mr Eric Schmidt is a retired farmer aged 76. He is used to hard physical work and is worried that he can no longer walk very far. He did not want to bother the doctor about it but finally let his daughter make an appointment when she saw him struggling at the weekend.

The following information is on his summary sheet:

Past medical history
Deep laceration to right arm from farm machinery 1984
Declined to attend recent men's health screening held at surgery
Medication
Nil recorded
Allergies
Nil recorded
Immunisations
Nil recorded
Family history
Father died of myocardial infarction aged 50
Mother died of 'old age'
Social history
Farmer
Married with two children.

Instructions for the patient, Eric Schmidt

You are a retired farmer aged 76. You are used to hard physical work and are worried because you can no longer walk very far. You did not want to bother the doctor about it but finally let your daughter make an appointment when she saw you struggling at the weekend.

You get a cramp-like pain in your right leg after walking a certain distance. Once you stop and rest for five minutes you can continue on further. Currently you can get to the first paddock, about 500 m, but then have to lean on the gate for a while until the pain in your leg goes away.

You do not have any nocturnal pain or any other symptoms of cardio-vascular disease.

You roll your own cigarettes and get through about 20 a day. You drink two or three cans of beer at the weekend. You have considered giving up smoking and would like advice from the doctor on how to do this, particularly if the doctor thinks that this will improve your leg pain.

Instructions for the facilitator

The candidate should perform a cardiovascular examination.

Clinical examination findings

On examination, there are absent popliteal, posterior tibial and dorsalis pedis pulses on the right leg. There are no bruits. All other findings are within the normal range.

The following information is on your summary sheet:

Past medical history
Deep laceration to right arm from farm machinery 1984
Declined to attend recent men's health screening held at surgery
Medication
Nil recorded
Allergies
Nil recorded
Immunisations
Nil recorded
Family history
Father died of myocardial infarction aged 50
Mother died of 'old age'
Social history
Farmer
Married with two children.

Suggested approach to the case

Establish rapport
Open-ended questions to explore Mr Schmidt's ideas, concerns and expectations.

Specific questions

Establish claudication distance and how quickly pain eases with rest
Absence of pain at night or at rest
Check for other symptoms of cardiovascular disease—angina, TIAs, shortness of breath, fatigue
Effect of low temperature on symptoms
Impact of symptoms on function
Recent worsening of symptoms
Cardiovascular risk factors—smoking history and readiness to change
Past medical history
Family history
Medication—ask about over-the-counter medication, complementary or alternative medicines
Request permission to examine.

Examination

Height 1.80 m
Weight 80 kg
BMI 24.7 kg/m^2
Waist circumference 82 cm
Blood pressure 135/80 mmHg right arm, 132/78 mmHg left arm
Pulse 65 Apex beat not displaced
Heart sounds normal
No signs of heart failure
No carotid bruits
Peripheral pulses
Skin
  —Note colour, distribution of hair
  —Postural colour change
  —Capillary filling
Urinalysis
  —Glycosuria, proteinuria.

Most likely diagnosis

Intermittent claudication.

Investigations

FBC
UEC
Lipids—fasting with ratio
ECG
Fasting BSL
Exclude arteritis/thrombophlebitis—ESR or CRP
Doppler study of peripheral arteries—ankle-brachial pressure index.

Management

'Keep walking, stop smoking'
Explain the pathophysiology of intermittent claudication and the rationale
   for exercise and giving up smoking
Offer practical advice on quitting smoking; schedule follow-up
Treat any dyslipidaemia, diabetes, hypertension
Start aspirin[1]
Advise on urgent symptoms that would need early review: critical ischaemia
   (gangrene, rest pain, ulcers) and features of acute coronary syndrome
Plan follow-up including review of need for immunisations, particularly
   tetanus
Referral for intervention such as angioplasty, stenting or surgery if femoral
   pulses absent, critical ischaemia (urgent) or persistent symptoms despite
   medical treatment.

 CASE COMMENTARY

Mr Schmidt gives a clear history and typical examination findings of a
person with intermittent claudication. Doctors need to demonstrate that
the leg is not critically ischaemic and measure/discuss the ankle-brachial
pressure index (ABPI) to confirm peripheral arterial disease—an ABPI
less than 0.9 is diagnostic.[1, 2] The 'risk to the limb is low but the risk
to life is high'[3] as intermittent claudication is an independent marker
for other cardiovascular problems, such as myocardial infarction or
cerebrovascular disease.[4] The focus of management should be on the

reduction of cardiovascular risk[1] by treating any dyslipidaemia, diabetes and hypertension and by quitting smoking, exercising regularly[5] and dietary modification.[2]

The doctor will need to explain the link between the current pain and cardiovascular risk factors and use motivational interviewing techniques to discuss smoking cessation. Vasoactive medication may be used if symptoms persist after initial interventions.[1, 2]

Mr Schmidt has an occupational risk of tetanus but there is no information in the summary sheet about his immunisations. Good doctors will notice this and arrange a review of Mr Schmidt's immunisations at another appointment.

References

1. Au, T, Golledge, J, Walker, P, Haigh, K & Nelson, M 2013, 'Peripheral arterial disease, diagnosis and management in general practice', *Australian Family Physician,* vol. 42, pp. 397–400.
2. Peach, G, Griffin, M, Jones, KG, Thompson, MM & Hinchliffe, RJ 2012, 'Diagnosis and management of peripheral arterial disease', *British Medical Journal,* vol. 345, p. e5208.
3. Burns, P, Gough, S & Bradbury A 2003, 'Management of peripheral arterial disease in primary care', *British Medical Journal,* vol. 326, pp. 584–8.
4. Lakshmanan, R, Hyde, Z, Jamrozik, K, Hankey, GJ & Norman, PE 2010, 'Population-based observational study of claudication in older men: the Health in Men Study', *Medical Journal of Australia,* vol. 192, pp. 641–5.
5. Handbook of Non-Drug Intervention (HANDI) Project Team 2013, 'Exercise for intermittent claudication and peripheral arterial disease', *Australian Family Physician,* vol. 42, pp. 879.

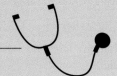

Section 5
Challenging consultations

Case 13
Doug Sullivan

Instructions for the doctor

This is a short case.

Please take a focused history from Doug. Request the findings of an appropriate physical examination and investigations. Explain your provisional diagnosis and initial management plan to Doug.

Scenario

Doug Sullivan is a 32-year-old man who has been a patient of the practice for 12 months.

He has a history of intravenous drug use (mainly opiates) and alcohol dependence. He has been off illicit drugs and alcohol for two years and is compliant with a methadone maintenance program. He is on telmisartan (Micardis) for hypertension and esomeprazole (Nexium) for gastro-oesophageal reflux.

He is divorced with three children who live with their mother on the coast. He is not working consistently but sometimes helps his father who runs a contract construction crew.

He presented last month with back pain, which he attributed to having to sleep in his car on a recent trip back from the coast. There were no neurological symptoms and physical examination was largely unremarkable apart from paraspinal muscle spasm, so you managed him with simple measures.

Last week he attended the emergency department with the same pain and the discharge letter is attached. He was asked to see you if the pain persisted.

The following information is on his summary sheet:

Age

32

Past medical history

Hypertension

Gastro-oesophageal reflux

Alcohol abuse/dependence

Opiate dependence IV drug use

Dental caries/poor dentition

Medication

Telmisartan 40 mg mane

Esomeprazole 40 mg mane

Methadone syrup 5 mg/ml 3ml po per day

Paracetamol 500mg 2 qid prn

Allergies

Nil known

Immunisations

Up-to-date

Social history

Divorced—has shared custody of his three children

Smokes 20 cigarettes per day

Non-drinker

Family history

Hypertension

Osteoarthritis.

Below is the letter from the local emergency department.

Dear Doctor

Re: Mr Douglas Sullivan

This 32-year-old man was seen at the emergency department with back pain. He described three to four weeks of pain in the lumbar region which was not responding to conservative measures. Further history and physical examination were consistent with mechanical back pain and there were no red flags.

He was given oxycodone (Endone) tabs 5 mg 2 tds prn and meloxicam (Mobic) 15 mg daily and was referred for physiotherapy. He has been instructed to return to see you if his symptoms do not resolve.

Kind regards,

Dr David Jones RMO

Instructions for the patient, Douglas Sullivan

You have now had almost five weeks of pretty constant upper lumbar pain, which you describe as deep and throbbing. If asked to score it, it is seven or eight out of ten. It started the day after you slept in your car returning from visiting your children on the coast. It's worse with movement but also hurts when lying down. You find yourself walking around or sitting instead of lying down. Night-times are very difficult and you often wander around unable to sleep, or try sleeping in a lounge chair. You've tried paracetamol and ibuprofen as well as a heat pack and some topical creams, none of which seem to help much.

The oxycodone from the doctor in emergency has not helped, nor has the meloxicam. You have had low back pain before but this feels different. It is higher, more constant and more severe. You worry that something else might be going on.

In answer to specific questioning: There has been no disturbance of bladder or bowel and no radiation of the pain. There's been no trauma. You've not had any fever and in fact have been otherwise pretty well other than having 'rotten teeth' which the dentist has started to work on. You have had two bad teeth removed and need several more extracted, but you are stretching it out partly because of finances and partly because there's so much work to be done. You think you might have lost a couple of kilos in the last month or two but you put that down to your rotten teeth and not being able to chew well.

There's no weakness or altered sensation. You have been tempted to try alcohol to see if it helps with the pain or with sleep but you feel you've worked hard to get on top of your drinking and don't want to go back again. Similarly, with respect to drugs, you have been tempted—especially when the pain has been bad but have resolved to stay clean for the sake of your children. You are down to 15 mL of methadone and are hoping to get off it by the end of this year.

Suggested approach to the case

A focused history and physical examination should explore possible serious causes of back pain. Most clinicians are familiar with the list of 'red flags' for low back pain but many patients with benign back pain have at least one red flag. The challenge is to evaluate the red flags in the context of the clinical presentation.

Doug has a number of risk factors for infection, and further investigation will yield the diagnosis. An initial discussion about Doug's condition and an overview of management should follow.

Points to address in the history include:
- nature of the pain
- trauma
- neurological symptoms
- constitutional symptoms (fever, weight loss)
- bladder or bowel dysfunction
- general health screen.

Physical examination should include:
- general appearance
- gait and posture
- range of movement
- palpation of the spine
- tendon reflexes, motor and sensory testing.

Further investigation:
- FBC, EUC, LFTs
- ESR/CRP
- imaging—CT lumbar spine.

Management:
- explanation of Doug's condition in simple language (spinal infection)
- outline of management—may require drainage; parenteral antibiotics followed by oral antibiotics based on specific organism(s) identified
- organise admission and communicate with receiving hospital.

Physical examination

General appearance: man of stated age in mild distress at rest
Gait: walks slowly bracing his back in the upper lumbar region
Vital signs:
- HR 85/min regular
- BP 134/85 mmHg sitting in both arms
- Temp 37.1°C
- BMI 24 kg/m^2
- RR 14/min

Spine examination: (each item to be asked for individually)
Appearance: normal
Range of movement: normal
Palpation: locally tender over L2/3 spinous processes with some paraspinal muscle spasm
Deep tendon reflexes: normal
Straight leg raising: normal
Neurological examination: power, tone and sensation testing all normal

Cardiovascular examination: normal
Respiratory examination: normal
Surgery tests: normal
Remainder of physical examination is normal.

Investigation results

FBC/EUC/LFTs: normal
ESR 52 CRP 68
CT lumbar spine: There is bony destruction at L2/3 level extending well into the body of L3 with a small intervertebral/interosseous abscess. There is loss of the disc space with circumferential soft tissue swelling at L2/3 level. No other abnormality is noted.
CONCLUSION: Acute discitis at L2/3 level with vertebral osteomyelitis and intervertebral abscess.
X-ray lumbar spine: There is loss of the disc space with circumferential soft tissue swelling at L2/3 level. There is bony destruction of the body of L3 consistent with osteomyelitis with a possible small intervertebral abscess. No other abnormality is noted.
Recommend further investigation with a CT or MRI.
Other investigations are normal.

Management

Explain that Doug has an uncommon but serious infection involving his lumbar vertebra and disc. He will require admission to hospital where he may undergo surgical drainage of his abscess to ascertain the organism(s) involved. He will require prolonged (at least several weeks) of antibiotic treatment, initially parenteral, then oral.

 CASE COMMENTARY

Low back pain is the most common musculoskeletal complaint seen in general practice in Australia. There is a growing understanding that inappropriate imaging can have a negative impact on patient attitudes and beliefs and can influence pain behaviours.[1] The concept of red flags alerts doctors to potentially serious causes among the more common benign conditions and therefore limiting imaging and further investigations to those cases where they are indicated.[2-4] This case is about applying the red flags in the overall context of a patient. Rather than learned as a list of unrelated items, red flags should be considered in clusters or groups relating to a specific serious pathology. Doug has several red flags associated with spinal infection including his serious ongoing oral sepsis, a worsening of his pain when supine and at night, as well as his previous intravenous drug use. In addition, opiates (including methadone) are known to impair immune function.

In spinal infection symptoms are frequently non-specific and fewer than 50% have an elevated white cell count. However, C-reactive protein and erythrocyte sedimentation rate are elevated in approximately 90% of patients with spinal infection and can be used to follow patient progress on treatment.[5]

Any imaging in this case would yield the diagnosis and a brief discussion of the condition and its management should follow.

 COMMON PITFALLS

Candidates will need to manage their time well in order to complete the case. Any inefficiencies in history-taking, physical examination or investigation will likely result in the candidate running out of time and not reaching management.

Some candidates may confuse this situation with that of a drug-seeker and lose important time explaining that opiates are not indicated. Although Doug is in significant pain, he is more concerned that there may be something serious going on.

It is not sufficient to rely on the assessment done on the patient in the emergency department the week before. Although the absence of red flags in the history and examination is listed, this is clearly not the case.

Doug's relatively normal physical examination should not prevent candidates from further investigation.

It is essential to identify the causative organism and antibiotics should not be commenced in the general practice setting. In addition, although Doug is not systemically unwell there should be no contemplation of outpatient management at this stage as it would significantly impact his chance of full recovery.

A variation of the case is to ask candidates to perform the examination of the spine themselves and conduct it as a long case. The significant findings of spinous tenderness can be effectively role-played.

References

1. Wheeler, L, Karran, E & Harvie, D 2018, 'Low back pain: can we mitigate the inadvertent psycho-behavioural harms of spinal imaging?', *Australian*

Family Physician, September, vol. 47, no. 9. Available at: www1.racgp.org.au/ ajgp/2018/september/low-back-pain, accessed 25 February 2019.

2. Bratton, R 1999, 'Assessment and management of acute low back pain', *American Family Physician,* 15 November, vol. 60, no. 8, pp. 2299–306.

3. Jensen, S 2004, 'Back pain–clinical assessment', *Australian Family Physician,* June, vol. 33, no. 6. Available at: www.racgp.org.au/afpbackissues/2004/2004 06/20040601jensen.pdf, accessed 25 February 2019.

4. Traeger, A, Buchbinder, R, Harris, I & Maher, C 2017, 'Diagnosis and management of low-back pain in primary care', *Canadian Medical Association Journal,* 13 November, vol. 189, no. 45, pp. E1386–95.

5. Nagashima, H, Tanishima, S & Tanida, A 2018, 'Diagnosis and management of spinal infections', *Journal of Orthopaedic Science,* January, vol. 23, issue 1, pp. 8–13.

Case 14
Jeanette Wilkinson

Instructions for the doctor

This is a long case.

Please take a history from Jeanette. Examination findings will be available from the facilitator. Discuss with Jeanette your differential diagnosis and identify her issues that need to be addressed. Negotiate a management plan with her. No investigations will be available but a request for these may be part of your management plan.

Scenario

Mrs Jeanette Wilkinson is a 48-year-old personal care worker at a residential aged care facility. Jeanette and her family have been attending your practice, in a small regional town, for several years, although Jeanette rarely attends for herself.

The following information is on her summary sheet:

Past medical history
G3P2M1: Two spontaneous vaginal deliveries (healthy babies), one miscarriage

Medication
Nil regular

Allergies
Nil known

Immunisations
None recorded

Family history
Father myocardial infarction age 65

Social history
Personal care worker at a residential aged care facility

Lives on a farm outside of town
Cervical screening
Up-to-date and normal.

Instructions for the patient, Jeanette Wilkinson

You are coming to talk to your GP about a test for the MTHFR gene. A friend of yours mentioned it and, from what you've read on the internet, it sounds like this could explain some of your problems. You have been feeling fatigued and run-down, getting progressively worse over the last two to three years. You are worried, as the website you read states the MTHFR gene can be associated with many of the symptoms and problems you or your family have experienced. For example: miscarriages (you've had one), heart attacks (your dad), fatigue, concentration problems and ADHD (your 12-year-old son has been diagnosed with this and you have struggled with his behaviour for many years). You are hopeful that there might be an answer to all your problems.

You have another child, a 15-year-old daughter. You have some worries about the friends she is starting to hang around with and the way she is dressing, but she is generally a good kid. You work full-time doing long, irregular shifts in the residential aged care facility.

You live 20 km out of town and run a small family farm with some cattle and sheep. Your time away from 'real work' is taken up with farm work. The farm is a major stress for you and is losing money financially. You are working outside of the farm to be able to cover the bills. Your husband has finally agreed to try to sell it, and it is on the market, but so far you have not had any interested buyers. You haven't been on a holiday longer than one night away in over ten years.

You feel you are depressed, probably worsening over the last six months, and you often cry in the mornings when you are alone getting ready for the day. You don't seem to enjoy the things you previously enjoyed, and you have no time for any interests outside your family and your work.

Your concentration is suffering, and you find it difficult to fall asleep. You tend to use food as a comfort when you're feeling down, and your weight has increased 5–10 kg over the last two years. You feel guilty sometimes that you're not there for your kids. You feel a sense of hopelessness that the farm will never be sold. You've had brief moments where you feel that you would be better-off dead but no real suicidal intent. You would never harm yourself because of your children. You are open to talking to a psychologist or trying medication if this is suggested.

Your relationship with your husband has deteriorated. You have a lot of resentment towards him for getting you into the mess with the farm. You have no libido and have not been sexually active in many months. You think your husband is depressed also and you tend to snap at each other rather than communicate. Your husband has taken to sleeping in a different room. Although your husband tells you this is because of your snoring, you think the relationship issues may also be contributing.

If asked, you wake feeling unrefreshed, you're fatigued during the day and you have had a couple of microsleeps driving the 20 km home from work after a 12-hour shift which have scared you.

You don't drink alcohol or smoke and have never used recreational drugs. Your diet consists of frozen/easy meals due to time constraints, and few fruit and vegetables. You do no formal exercise but are active in your roles as a personal carer and on the farm.

Your periods remain regular and you have not experienced hot flushes.

Support-wise, you have your parents in town who help sometimes with your kids.

Rest of systems review is normal.

Prompts if needed:
- there are so many things worrying me, it's really getting me down
- things with my husband haven't really been so great
- I'm so tired all the time, I even wake up feeling tired.

The following information is on your summary sheet:

Past medical history
G3P2M1: Two spontaneous vaginal deliveries (healthy babies), one miscarriage

Medication
Nil regular

Allergies
Nil known

Immunisations
None recorded

Family history
Father myocardial infarction age 65

Social history
Personal care worker at a residential aged care facility
Lives on a farm outside of town

Cervical screening
Up-to-date and normal.

Information for the facilitator

Clinical examination findings

General appearance: slightly agitated, overweight woman of middle-aged appearance
No pallor, jaundice or skin changes
Height 1.65 m
Weight 82 kg
BMI 30.1 kg/m^2
Blood pressure 152/89 mmHg
Pulse 68 beats per minute
Temperature 36.8°C
Cardiovascular and respiratory exams are normal
Thyroid exam is normal
No lymphadenopathy or hepatosplenomegaly
Finger-prick blood sugar level is 5.2 mmol/L
Urinalysis is normal
K10 score 32.

Suggested approach to the case

Establish rapport
Open-ended questions to explore Jeanette's ideas, concerns and expectations.

Specific questions

Explore why she feels she may have the MTHFR mutation
Depression—including mood, anhedonia, sleep, appetite, fatigue, motivation, concentration, thoughts of worthlessness/hopelessness/suicidal ideation and suicide risk assessment
Sleep history—falling asleep, sleep interruptions, snoring, daytime fatigue
Exploration of stressors—home, relationship, work, financial
Exclude menopause or perimenopause as a cause of symptoms
Other systems review, e.g. fever, weight loss, headaches, joint symptoms, thirst/polyuria, abdominal pains/bowel changes, genitourinary symptoms, chest pain and shortness of breath
Preventative health—smoking, alcohol, nutrition, physical activity, immunisations.

Examination

General appearance, height, weight and BMI
Blood pressure/pulse/temperature
Cardiovascular and respiratory examination

Thyroid examination
Lymph nodes/liver/spleen
Office tests including finger-prick glucose and urinalysis
Objective measure of psychological distress such as K10.

Differential diagnosis/issues that need addressing

Depression
Possible sleep apnoea, needs sleep studies
Overwork/stress
Poor libido and relationship dysfunction
Obesity
Hypertension.

The candidate should recognise the interplay between all these issues and focus on depression as the biggest issue for the patient. The candidate should recognise possible sleep apnoea as something that may be causing microsleeps and hence be potentially serious for the patient.

Management

Addressing the request for MTHFR screening—candidate should be able to explain why this is not appropriate in a sensitive manner, while leaving the consult open to exploring her issues and concerns
Management of depression:
- explanation of problem
- options for treatment—exercise, mindfulness, mental health apps/ online psychoeducation, psychology (consider Mental Health Care Plan), medication, support groups
- patient safety—discuss pros/cons of time off work, provide information about emergency assistance, such as Lifeline

Plan to investigate for sleep apnoea (recognising that this needs to be reasonably urgent given driving with microsleeps)

Plan to address her weight, assess her risk of cardiovascular disease, manage BP, check for diabetes, cholesterol and urine ACR in future consults

Further investigations for fatigue (such as thyroid function or iron studies) are not necessary at this stage without any red flags. They should not be requested unless fatigue persists, despite management of the above issues[1]

Address the relationship difficulties and poor libido. She and her husband may benefit from a referral for relationship counselling and/or assistance with parenting a child with ADHD

Extras for case—offer preventative health care, including immunisations (e.g. hepatitis B and Q fever, given her work).

CASE COMMENTARY

Fatigue is a common presentation in general practice and is often multi-factorial. Candidates should have a good approach at taking a systematic history and working through the differentials of fatigue. Cases where more than one issue needs identification and management are likewise common! Time management can be difficult, both in real life and in an exam situation. Candidates should be able to identify and prioritise issues and develop a plan to manage them in subsequent consults.

Often, when patients have symptoms of fatigue or non-specific symptoms, they will turn to the internet for answers. Jeanette presents asking for the MTHFR gene test after finding information on the internet. The MTHFR gene is responsible for the production of the enzyme methylenetetrahydrofolate reductase (MTHFR), which is important in the folate pathway. Polymorphisms of this gene are common, and it is purported by many that these polymorphisms are responsible for a raft of common symptoms, including depression and fatigue. There is, however, no good evidence that the MTHFR gene polymorphisms have any clinically important effects.[2] Often when patients turn to complementary or alternative approaches, they have not received help from conventional medicine in the past. Candidates should be able to explore the underlying reasons Jeanette is requesting this test and explain in a sensitive manner why this is not an appropriate test to order.[3]

COMMON PITFALLS

Failing to take a systematic history in this long case could mean that candidates focus on one problem only and fail to identify and manage potentially serious co-morbidities, including sleep apnoea and hypertension.

References

1. Wilson, J, Morgan, S, Magin, PJ & van Driel, M 2014, 'Fatigue—a rational approach to investigation', *Australian Family Physician,* vol. 43, pp. 457–61.
2. Long, S & Goldblatt, J 2016, 'MTHFR genetic testing: controversy and clinical implications', *Australian Family Physician,* vol. 45, pp. 237–40.
3. Royal Australian College of General Practitioners, 'Position statement: Responding to patient requests for tests not considered clinically appropriate'. Available at: www.racgp.org.au/your-practice/guidelines/position-statement-on-responding-to-patient-requests-for-tests-not-considered-clinically-appropriate, accessed 31 January 2018.

Case 15
Craig Kelly

Instructions for the doctor

This is a short case.

Please take a history from Craig. Examination findings will be available from the facilitator. You are expected to tell Craig the most likely diagnosis and negotiate a management plan with him.

Scenario

Craig Kelly is a 22-year-old man. He has not previously been seen at the clinic.

Craig filled out a new patient questionnaire with the following information:
Past medical history
Kidney stones
Current medication
Nil regularly
Allergies
Nil
Immunisations
No idea
Social history
Smokes 10 cigarettes per day
Unemployed.

Instructions for the patient, Craig Kelly

Over the past few years you have become dependent on oxycodone 5 mg tablets, which you take several times per day. You see multiple different doctors every week trying to obtain scripts.

Today you are seeing this new doctor with the intention of saying you had acute renal colic last night and that you need oxycodone 5 mg to relieve the pain. You say that the pain was right-sided and was severe enough to have you rolling around in agony. You had kidney stones previously about three years ago and were prescribed oxycodone for your pain. (This started your dependence on opioids, but do not volunteer this information straight away.) You state you had two pills still left in your cupboard from your original presentation. These helped you get through the night, but you now need more. When asked, you have some blood in your urine but no other urinary symptoms. If asked, you are happy for the doctor to contact a GP who saw you for your initial presentation. You state you have been well since and have not needed a regular GP. You are insistent that you need a 'strong painkiller' and that paracetamol/ibuprofen will not work.

If the doctor recognises you as a drug seeker, you may start to open up about your background. The initial prescription of oxycodone helped ease your physical pain but also blotted out other pains in your life. You had a difficult childhood and were sometimes beaten and often ignored. You did not achieve well at school and were an angry teen with few close friends.

You have been on various youth schemes but have never had a regular job. You moved to the city so that you could see lots of different doctors to get the oxycodone that you crave.

You have never tried other drugs but have sometimes wondered whether injecting would give you more of a hit than the tablets. You haven't considered giving up because you can't see any better way of easing the pain in your life. It is becoming harder and harder to obtain new scripts, and you are open to exploring help.

You have no other relevant past medical history. You have filled out the new patient questionnaire as below:

Past medical history
Kidney stones

Current medication
Nil regularly

Allergies
Nil

Immunisations
No idea

Social history
Smokes 10 cigarettes per day
Unemployed.

Information for the facilitator

Temperature 37°C
Pulse 88
BP 112/70 mmHg
Abdominal examination normal
No signs of opiate use or withdrawal
Urinalysis normal.

Suggested approach to the case

Establish rapport
Open-ended questions to explore Craig's ideas, concerns and expectations.

Specific questions

About renal colic
    —Frequency, duration, site, radiation etc., of pain
    —Severity of pain
    —What else has been tried?
    —Previous investigations
    —Urinary symptoms
Previous treating doctor.

Ask for the examination findings

Temperature, pulse, BP
Abdominal and renal angle examination
Urinalysis
Check for signs of opiate use or withdrawal: injection sites, pupil size, red
    eyes, runny nose.

Management

Establish/suspect that patient is a drug seeker
Negotiate permission to speak to previous GPs, specialists
Ask whether Craig has ever injected drugs
Phone Prescription Shopping Information Service
Advise of local resources to assist with addiction
Mention contacting the State/Territory poisons branch or drug
    dependence unit
Manage any anger or other emotion in the consultation
Advise on needle exchange scheme if injecting mentioned

Demonstrate commitment to provide ongoing care if the patient wishes
Consider opportunistic health promotion about smoking and need for
Hepatitis B and other immunisations.

 CASE COMMENTARY

Craig has a substance-use disorder and is seeking a script from the
doctor. GPs need to be cautious when prescribing opiates and should
have a high index of suspicion that patients are drug seeking. Warning
signs of patients seeking drugs are:

- reception and appointment: new patient recently moved, walk-ins,
  last-minute appointments
- history: very knowledgeable about condition and drugs requested,
  requests drug by name, previous doctor 'unavailable', multiple
  allergies or reactions to non-addictive medications, carries letter
  from other doctors about opiate or benzodiazepine prescriptions
  with dubious rationale
- examination: exaggerated appearance of pain, inconsistent
  behaviour and signs.

Patients who are prescribed opiates either for pain or as part of a rehabilitation scheme (usually methadone) will carry documentation with
them regarding their condition and should not be offended by probing
questions from a GP. A wise GP will still check that the supporting letter
is valid or check the patient's MyHealth electronic record, particularly
given the increase in deaths from prescription drugs obtained from
multiple prescribers.

This case tests the doctor's skill in refusing a patient's request. It
also tests the professional ethics involved in wishing to relieve pain yet
avoid perpetuating drug dependence or inadvertently facilitating the
diversion of drugs. A firm but polite no is needed. A practice policy
clearly displayed in the waiting room stating that drugs of dependence
are not prescribed on an initial visit can help. Other options for managing
this case would be offering alternative analgesia, or prescribing enough
morphine capsules to last for only the next 24 hours while gathering
further information from the previous GP.

 COMMON PITFALLS

Inexperienced or poor doctors may fail to see through Craig's story and
will issue a script for the oxycodone as requested; alternatively, they may

say no so aggressively that there is no opportunity to work with Craig on his addiction or other problems, such as the past history of abuse. Manipulative behaviour can be a symptom of substance-use disorder; recognising this is an important step in developing the rapport needed to offer treatment to these patients. Over half of dependent substance users will eventually achieve stable recovery, so it is worth offering him assistance.

Further reading

Best, DW & Lubman, DI 2012, 'The recovery paradigm—a model of hope and change for alcohol and drug addiction', *Australian Family Physician,* vol. 41, pp. 593-7.

Degenhardt, L, Whiteford, HA, Ferrari, AJ, Baxter, AJ, Charlson, FJ, Hall, WD et al. 2013, 'Global burden of disease attributable to illicit drug use and dependence: findings from the Global Burden of Disease Study 2010', *Lancet,* vol. 382, pp. 1564-74.

James, J 2016, 'Dealing with drug-seeking behaviour', *Australian Prescriber,* vol. 39, no. 3, pp. 96-100.

Kotalik, J 2012, 'Controlling pain and reducing misuse of opioids: ethical considerations', *Canadian Family Physician,* vol. 58, pp. 381-5, e190-5.

Monheit, B 2010, 'Prescription drug misuse', *Australian Family Physician,* vol. 39, pp. 540-6.

The Royal Australian College of General Practitioners 2015, 'Prescribing drugs of dependence in general practice'. Available at: www.racgp.org.au/your-practice/guidelines/drugs-landing/, accessed 26 January 2018.

Case 16
Wazza Wainright

Instructions for the doctor

This is a short case.

Please review the scenario below and take a focused history from Wazza. No further examination is required. Please discuss the issues raised and outline your management plan to Wazza. The Austroads *Assessing Fitness to Drive*[1] standards will be available in the consultation room in either hard or electronic copy.

Scenario

Wazza Wainright, aged 48, drives road trains for a living. He has booked in to see you for his commercial driving licence renewal. Wazza attends your practice but this is the first time that you have seen him. He has completed part of his driving assessment with your practice nurse, and relevant sections of this are available below.

The following information is on his summary sheet:

Past medical history
Nil significant
Medication
Nil
Allergies
Nil known
Immunisations
Up-to-date
Social history
Road train driver
Married
Non-smoker
Alcohol intake—two standard drinks weekly

The below assessments have been handed to you by your practice nurse.

Epworth Sleepiness Scale

How likely are you to doze off in the following situations, in contrast to just feeling tired?	Would never doze off (0)	Slight chance of dozing (1)	Moderate chance of dozing (2)	High chance of dozing (3)
a) Sitting and reading	☐	☐	☐	☒
b) Watching TV	☐	☐	☐	☒
c) Sitting inactive in a public place (e.g. a theatre or a meeting)	☐	☐	☐	☒
d) As a passenger in a car for an hour without a break	☐	☐	☐	☒
e) Lying down to rest in the afternoon when circumstances permit	☐	☐	☐	☒
f) Sitting and talking to someone	☐	☒	☐	☐
g) Sitting quietly after a lunch without alcohol	☐	☐	☐	☒
h) In a car, while stopped for a few minutes in the traffic	☐	☐	☒	☐

Observations

Blood pressure Pulse	136/82 mmHg 76, regular
Height Weight BMI	180 cm 149 kg 46 kg/m^2

The rest of Wazza's fitness to drive health assessment is unremarkable.

Instructions for the patient, Wazza Wainright

You are a 48-year-old road train driver. You enjoy the freedom of the open road but staying awake on long stretches has become more difficult. You keep yourself going with energy drinks, such as Red Bull, and strong coffee. Some of the younger drivers have tried to sell you amphetamines but you've resisted. Your diet is dependent on what you can buy at roadhouses, and you do little exercise.

You look forward to your days off at home but recently all you seem to do is fall asleep during the day when you try to relax. You get to sleep OK but your partner seems to spend half the night telling you to stop snoring or shouting at you to start breathing.

You have booked this consultation to renew your commercial driving licence. You are expecting the doctor to sign-off on the licence without too much fuss, as previous GPs have in the past. If the doctor refuses to sign-off on it today, you become worried and frustrated, as losing your commercial driver's licence means you risk your job.

Suggested approach to the case

Diagnostic phase

Establish rapport
Open-ended questions to explore Wazza's ideas, concerns and expectations
Calculate Epworth Sleepiness Scale score
Summarise findings of high score on Epworth Sleepiness Scale and very
    high body mass index and suspected obstructive sleep apnoea
Check Austroads *Assessing Fitness to Drive*, commercial standards.

Management phase

Explain that if commercial vehicle standards are not met, licence cannot
    be renewed
Observe for response and acknowledge any anger or frustration
Explain need for referral to specialist physician for sleep studies
Explain likely relationship between sleep apnoea and obesity
Encourage initiation of increased exercise and decreased calorie intake
Assure him of ongoing support, arrange follow-up and offer health check
Document advice in records.

 CASE COMMENTARY

Assessing fitness to drive can be a challenging aspect of general practice as the GP's public health role may need to take precedence over the role of caring for an individual patient. Doctors are not expected to remember the *Fitness to Drive*[1] standards but should be familiar with the document and find the information that shows Wazza does not meet the commercial licence standards. For Wazza this will mean loss of his livelihood until he can be treated, for example, with continuous positive airways pressure. There is no one preferred treatment for obstructive sleep apnoea but rather a range of options of proven effectiveness that can be applied individually or in combination, depending on patient preference, symptoms, severity, co-morbidities and other health risk factors.[2]

Severe obstructive sleep apnoea is strongly associated with an increased risk of stroke and cardiovascular disease. Despite this association, there is no clear evidence that treatment of sleep apnoea with continuous positive airways pressure reduces metabolic risk.[3] Wazza should be advised regarding weight reduction, as this will ameliorate obstructive sleep apnoea and is also important in managing his high metabolic risk. Wazza should be offered a preventative health check, although maintaining a therapeutic relationship when you have just removed someone's driving licence tests communication skills!

References

1. Austroads and National Transport Commission 2016, *Assessing Fitness to Drive,* 5th ed, Sydney.
2. Mansfield, DR, Antic, NA & McEvoy, RD 2013, 'How to assess, diagnose, refer and treat adult obstructive sleep apnoea: a commentary on the choices', *Medical Journal of Australia,* vol. 199, pp. S21–6.
3. Hamilton, GS & Joosten, SA 2017, 'Obstructive sleep apnoea and obesity', *Australian Family Physician,* vol. 46, pp. 460–3.

Further reading

Kee, K & Naughton, MT 2009, 'Sleep apnoea: a general practice approach', *Australian Family Physician,* vol. 38, no. 5, pp. 284–8.

Case 17
Hope Briganza

Instructions for the doctor

This is a short case.

Please take a focused history. Request the findings of an appropriate physical examination from the facilitator and explain your management plan to Hope. No further investigations are available.

Scenario

Hope Briganza is a 26-year-old child care worker who is a regular patient of the practice. She is generally healthy. She presented to your colleague 10 days ago and he diagnosed a lower back strain.

Your colleague's clinical notes from her previous visit reads:
- three days right LBP without red flags
- works in child care—lifts children all day
- past mild episodes only
- otherwise well; only on OCP
- physical examination unremarkable
- assessment: acute mechanical LBP/muscle strain
- plan: rest (medical certificate 1/7); simple analgesia prn; local heat prn
- r/v no better.

The following information is on her summary sheet:

Age

26

Past medical history

Oral contraception

Tonsillectomy (age 12)

Medication
Ethinyloestradiol 30 mcg/levonorgestrel 150 mcg (Levlen ED) 1 mane
Allergies
Nil known
Immunisations
Up-to-date
Cervical screening
Up-to-date
Social history
Non-smoker
Alcohol—one or two drinks a week
Family history
Hypertension
Ischaemic heart disease
Osteoarthritis.

Instructions for the patient, Hope Briganza

You have had about two weeks of right-sided lower back pain. You came to see another doctor at this practice 10 days ago. He diagnosed a back strain and suggested rest, heat packs and paracetamol. He thought it could be related to lifting children (you work in child care) so he gave you a day off work. The pain is in your right flank (loin) and is dull and deep. It is constant and is not affected by anything you do. It occurs at rest as well as with movement. You don't recall any particular incident or injury but you do bend and lift children all day. You've taken some paracetamol but it doesn't help much. You have had episodes of mild lower back pain previously, but they were brief and usually only when you had done too much in the garden or at sport. This pain feels different as it is higher up, and constant—you're worried it might be something serious.

If asked, you do have mild urinary frequency (day and night) and urinary urgency but no incontinence. If asked about fever or temperatures you do sometimes feel hot and cold but you haven't checked your temperature. You have been feeling tired and washed out over the last week or so. There has been some nausea and anorexia but no vomiting or change in your bowels.

You live with your boyfriend who has been your only sexual partner for the past four years. You are on the contraceptive pill (Levlen) and remember to take this every day. Your last period was about a week ago and was normal. There are no symptoms of pregnancy and your cervical screening is up-to-date.

You work full-time in child care and enjoy your work. You have an active social life playing sport (netball and touch football) with your friends regularly. You are generally healthy and well apart from the symptoms above.

When it comes to diagnosis and management, simply ask the doctor the sort of questions you think Hope would.

The following information is on your summary sheet:

Age
26

Past medical history
Oral contraception
Tonsillectomy (age 12)

Medication
Ethinyloestradiol 30 mcg/levonorgestrel 150 mcg (Levlen ED) 1 mane

Allergies
Nil known

Immunisations
Up-to-date

Cervical screening
Up-to-date

Social history
Non-smoker
Alcohol—one or two drinks a week

Family history
Hypertension
Ischaemic heart disease
Osteoarthritis.

Suggested approach to the case

Based on the scenario, the candidate should already be thinking about alternative diagnoses to mechanical low back pain in a young woman. The focused history is aimed at separating these, and the physical examination (along with surgery tests) should confirm that the doctor is dealing with a case of acute pyelonephritis. A decision will need to be made about inpatient versus outpatient treatment based on the severity of the condition and possible complications. A simple explanation of the condition and its management to Hope is required along with appropriate answers to her questions.

Points to address in the history include:
• details of the pain
• presence of any urinary symptoms

- presence of fever
- abdominal pain, nausea, vomiting
- possibility of pregnancy
- brief general health screen.

Physical examination should include:
- general appearance
- vital signs (esp. temperature, heart rate, BP)
- costovertebral angle tenderness
- possible abdominal or suprapubic tenderness
- urinalysis, pregnancy test.

Management should include:
- explanation of the significance of her symptoms and the likely diagnosis of acute pyelonephritis
- instruction regarding collection of a midstream urine for culture and antimicrobial susceptibility testing to guide possible adjustment of the initial regimen if there is no clinical improvement
- commencement of an appropriate oral antibiotic (such as amoxycillin/clavulanate, cephalosporin or trimethoprim/sulfamethoxazole) for 10 days
- imaging or blood cultures are generally not required in uncomplicated cases
- follow-up and safety netting should be outlined. It would be reasonable to review Hope in one to two days to ensure she is improving. A repeat urine culture is not usually necessary where there has been clinical resolution of the infection.

Physical examination

General appearance: young woman in no distress at rest
Vitals:
HR 94/min regular
BP 104/68 mmHg sitting
Temp 38.1°C
BMI 24 kg/m²
RR 12/min
Remainder of cardiovascular examination unremarkable
Abdominal exam: abdomen soft; no masses; mild suprapubic tenderness; bowel sounds active
Musculoskeletal: lumbar spine normal
Costovertebral angle tenderness on the right
Remainder of physical examination is normal.

Surgery tests
U/A: leucocytes ++; blood +
Urine Beta HCG: negative
BSL (random): 5.6 mmol/L
ECG: Sinus rhythm normal.

 CASE COMMENTARY

Acute unilateral back pain in a young woman should raise the possibility of pyelonephritis—a common bacterial infection of the renal pelvis and kidney that results from ascent of a bacterial pathogen up the ureter from the bladder. Because of the frequency and severity of the infection, GPs must be able to make the diagnosis, decide between inpatient and outpatient care, and select an appropriate antibiotic. In addition, because pyelonephritis is associated with adverse maternal and foetal outcomes in pregnancy, it is important to rule out pregnancy in women of child-bearing age.[1, 2]

Flank pain and lower urinary tract symptoms along with fever, costovertebral tenderness and positive urinalysis all confirm the diagnosis. Urine culture is recommended in all cases prior to empirical antibiotic prescribing. In the majority of cases in young women, *Escherichia coli* is the responsible pathogen and the spectrum of pathogens involved in acute pyelonephritis is similar to that of cystitis.[1, 2]

Australian antibiotic guidelines for mild, uncomplicated pyelonephritis differ from US and European guidelines in restricting fluoroquinolones to cases where the causative organism is resistant to first-line drugs.[3, 4]

Given the severity described in Hope's case and the absence of co-morbidities, hospitalisation is unnecessary.[1] Similarly, imaging and blood cultures are not required in uncomplicated cases and repeat urine cultures are not usually necessary where there has been clinical resolution of symptoms.

 COMMON PITFALLS

If candidates don't reconsider the initial diagnosis, significant time can be lost exploring the various red flags for low back pain with a series of closed questions. Beginning with open questions should elicit enough information to raise the possibility of pyelonephritis as an alternative diagnosis.

We shouldn't be defensive about our colleague's management in the previous consultation, nor should we be drawn into being critical of their care. Clinical presentations evolve, symptoms develop and conditions declare themselves, making the diagnosis more obvious over time. The patient is not upset about her management and the initial incorrect diagnosis is not an issue for her. Although the oral contraceptive is listed on her patient summary, the possibility of pregnancy should be specifically ruled out.

Hospitalising Hope, although unnecessary, would not result in a failure for the case providing the diagnosis is made correctly and appropriate treatment discussed. Similarly, a discussion about various strategies for preventing recurrent urinary tract infections is probably premature following her first episode.

References

1. Colgan, R, Williams, M & Johnson, J 2011, 'Diagnosis and treatment of acute pyelonephritis in women', *American Family Physician,* 1 September, vol. 84, no. 5, pp. 519-26.
2. Wagenlehner, FM, Lichtenstern, C & Rolfes, C 2013, 'Diagnosis and management for urosepsis', *International Journal of Urology,* vol. 20, no. 10, pp. 963-70.
3. Therapeutic Guidelines: Antibiotics 2019, 'Acute pyelonephritis in adults'. In: *eTG Complete* [Internet]. Available at: https://tgldcdp.tg.org.au/viewTopic?topicfile=acute-pyelonephritis-adults, accessed 23 May 2019.
4. Emergency Care Institute NSW 2017, 'Management of pyelonephritis', Available at: https://www.aci.health.nsw.gov.au/networks/eci/clinical/clinical-resources/clinical-tools/renal/pyelonephritis, accessed 23 May 2019.

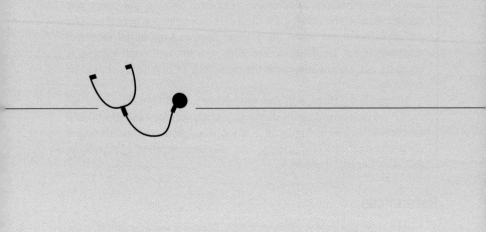

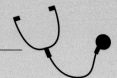

Section 6
Child health

Case 18
Kylie Chong

Instructions for the doctor

This is a short case.

Kylie does not attend this appointment. Please take a history from her mother, Ilana, and make suggestions for management. You are required to focus on the presenting complaint only.

> ### Scenario
>
> Kylie Chong is an 8-year-old girl who has seen you a few times for minor illnesses in childhood. Kylie's mum, Ilana, has booked to see you today because 'Kylie is out of control and won't do what she is told'. Ilana wants you to prescribe the drug that is used in attention deficit hyperactivity disorder (ADHD).

Instructions for Kylie's mother, Ilana Chong

You have three children and work part-time as a cleaner. You were brought up in Australia and so was your husband. His family migrated to Australia from China. Your husband and his family consider child rearing to be the mother's main responsibility. You are keen to have support and will be open to any suggestions from the doctor if you feel respected not blamed.

You had a normal pregnancy and birth. Kylie reached all her milestones.

Kylie is the middle child of the family. From the beginning she has been the most challenging but recently you feel things are out of your control. She is doing OK at school but her behaviour is very disruptive at home. It is so frustrating that the teachers report her to be good, while at home Kylie is disobedient and refuses to join in with the family. Getting her up to go to school in the mornings is a nightmare and at weekends all she does is watch TV and eat junk food. You have tried a strict diet free from preservatives but that made no difference. A recent hearing check was normal.

You have come to the doctor today because you have heard there is a drug for attention deficit hyperactivity disorder (ADHD) and you think it might be the answer for Kylie.

If the doctor asks about the three main symptoms of ADHD of inattention, hyperactivity and impulsiveness, you are to answer that Kylie does NOT have these symptoms.

Suggested approach to the case

Establish rapport
Open-ended questions to explore Kylie's mum's ideas, concerns and expectations.

Specific questions

Kylie's behaviour—define the issues
Pregnancy, birth and developmental history
Interests
Friendships
Relationship with siblings and family
Sleep
School performance, reports from teachers
General health, appetite, mood
Test against criteria expected in ADHD
    —Inattention
    —Hyperactivity
    —Impulsiveness.

Most likely diagnosis

Outline that ADHD doesn't seem likely
Sensitively suggest that it is a behavioural issue
Important to address the problem now
Praise Ilana for coming along now—lots of options for change.

Management

Outline available options
    —Positive parenting groups
    —Agreed family rules—reward appropriate behaviour, ignore
     undesirable behaviour

-Negotiate with whole family about the issue–involve Kylie's father
-Family therapy
-Offer online resources, e.g. https://raisingchildren.net.au
Assure of continued support.

 CASE COMMENTARY

Kylie is causing problems but the doctor needs to work out whether she has ADHD. This is characterised by inattention, hyperactivity and/or impulsiveness. This does not fit with Kylie's story of being able to concentrate on the TV for much of the day and her reasonable performance and behaviour at school.

The doctor will need to demonstrate empathy with Ilana about Kylie's problem and sensitively explain that the treatment for ADHD will not help, as it seems to be more of a behavioural issue. The doctor can then outline the options available to assist Ilana and her family. This could entail support and guidance from the GP, parenting courses or referral to more specialised children's services, depending on local availability and Ilana's choice.

Further reading

Feldman, HM & Reiff, MI 2014, 'Clinical practice. Attention deficit-hyperactivity disorder in children and adolescents', *New England Journal of Medicine,* vol. 370, pp. 838–46.

Furlong, M, McGilloway, S, Bywater, T, Hutchings, J, Smith, SM & Donnelly, M 2012, 'Behavioural and cognitive-behavioural group-based parenting programmes for early-onset conduct problems in children aged 3 to 12 years', *Cochrane Database of Systematic Reviews,* vol. 2:CD008225.

Jarman, R 2015, 'Finetuning behaviour management in young children', *Australian Family Physician,* vol. 44, no. 12, pp. 896–9

Halasz, G 2009, 'Attention deficit hyperactivity disorder: time to rethink', *Medical Journal of Australia,* vol. 190, pp. 32–3.

Case 19
Brandon Harkness

Instructions for the doctor

This is a short case.

You are expected to take a history from Brandon's mother, Julie. Results of the examination will be available from the facilitator. Outline your differential diagnosis to Julie and negotiate a management plan.

Scenario

Brandon is a lively two-year-old Caucasian boy. He has been a patient at the surgery since he was born and has attended only for coughs and colds, and immunisations. His growth has been along the 75th centile.

Four weeks ago, Julie brought Brandon in concerned that he had 'gastro'. He had vomited three times in the night and had profuse watery diarrhoea. He was not dehydrated. You advised fluids and expected that the illness would soon resolve. Today Julie has come to see you because Brandon's diarrhoea is continuing.

The following information is on Brandon's summary sheet:

Medication
Nil recorded
Allergies
Nil recorded
Immunisations
Fully immunised as per schedule.

Instructions for Brandon's mother, Julie Harkness

You work as a pharmacy assistant three days a week and spend the other days at home with your children. Your daughter, aged four, attends preschool and Brandon, your two-year-old, attends child care.

Four weeks ago, Brandon had 'gastro'. He was vomiting and had diarrhoea. The vomiting soon settled and, as advised, you continued with fluids and reintroduced solids when Brandon seemed hungry. He no longer has any fever.

Brandon is thriving with a good appetite and seems well but the diarrhoea has not stopped. He passes a light-coloured, loose, watery, foul-smelling stool about five times a day and you can see undigested food in it. Previously Brandon passed one to three stools per day. The situation is beginning to get you down because the staff at child care are worried about him and keep suggesting that he is not well enough to be there. When you talked with the pharmacist at work, she suggested you go back to the GP for a check-up.

The following information is on Brandon's medical record:

Medication
Nil recorded

Allergies
Nil recorded

Immunisations
Fully immunised as per schedule.

Information for the facilitator

Clinical examination findings

Clinical examination is entirely normal. Brandon's weight and height are on the 75th centile and tracking well.

Suggested approach to the case

Establish rapport
Open-ended questions to explore Julie's ideas, concerns and expectations.

Specific questions

Details about the episode of gastro
Details about the diarrhoea—frequency, smell, blood, colour, consistency, mucus
Systemic upset
Abdominal pain
Appetite and thirst
Current diet—any observed relationship between diet and diarrhoea
Consumption of fruit, fruit juice, milk
Medications used

Known allergies
Anyone else in family with diarrhoea
What else has Julie tried?
Any recent travel?
Request permission to examine.

Examination

Ask the facilitator for specific examination findings
Level of alertness, responsiveness and hydration
Weight and height plotted on centile chart (75th centile)
Pulse
Temperature
Ears, nose, throat
Absence of jaundice or rash
Abdominal examination
 —No tenderness elicited
 —No masses found
 —No organomegaly
 —No perianal rash or ulceration.

Differential diagnoses

Toddler's diarrhoea (also known as chronic non-specific diarrhoea)
Temporary lactose or other disaccharide intolerance
Worth excluding infectious cause, e.g. *Giardia.*

Management

Reassure
Regular weighing and follow-up
Check for pathogens—faecal MCS and PCR for enteric pathogens
Advise balanced diet, avoid snacks, reduce consumption of fruit juice
If not settling, consider further testing to include ESR, FBE, coeliac
    antibodies, stool pH (5.5 or less and sugars suggest carbohydrate
    intolerance).

 CASE COMMENTARY

The most important clinical feature is that Brandon is thriving. The
fact that he is still on the 75th centile excludes any potentially serious
cause of the diarrhoea and the doctor should emphasise this with Julie.

Brandon's symptoms are characteristic of toddler or chronic non-specific diarrhoea, the commonest cause of diarrhoea in children aged one to five years. Some speculate this is an iatrogenic problem that starts when parents are advised to push fluids, including fruit juices, and reduce fibre and fat intake, in children with gastroenteritis.[1] Children then enter a vicious cycle of diarrhoea and further dietary restrictions aimed at curing the diarrhoea. Treatment is rebalancing the 'four Fs'—Fat, Fibre, Fluid and Fruit juices—by reintroducing well-defined meals and snacks. Fruit juices, in particular clear apple juice, and other squashes should be limited. Toddler diarrhoea might be prevented by advising that children with acute diarrhoea require initial rehydration and then resumption of a normal feeding pattern as soon as it is tolerated.

Other common possible causes of Brandon's diarrhoea are residual infection (such as with *Giardia*), carbohydrate intolerance or temporary lactose intolerance.[2] Carbohydrate intolerance results in unabsorbed disaccharides in the stool which show positive on Clinitest or glucose testing strips.[3] Fermentation of unabsorbed sugars produces acids which yield a stool pH of <5.5. In temporary lactose intolerance, reduction of milk-based products is recommended for a short time. If the symptoms do not resolve in a week then this is not the cause of the problem and milk can be reintroduced. More complex changes to his diet would need supervision from a dietician to ensure any benefit in reducing the diarrhoea is not achieved at the expense of malnutrition.

The concern of the day care centre about Brandon's diarrhoea should be discussed. Once a stool test is confirmed as clear, Brandon can attend again and will not pose a risk to the health of the other children or the carers. The GP can offer to put this in writing to the day care centre.

References

1. Kneepkens, C & Hoekstra, J 1996, 'Chronic nonspecific diarrhea of childhood: pathophysiology and management', *Pediatric Clinics of North America,* vol. 43, pp. 375–90.
2. Zella, GC & Israel, EJ 2012, 'Chronic diarrhea in children', *Pediatrics in Review,* vol. 33, no. 5, pp. 207–17.
3. Klish, WJ 2006, 'Chronic non specific diarrhoea of childhood'. In: JA McMillan, RD Feigin & CD De Angelis et al. (eds), *Oski's Pediatrics Principles and Practice,* Lippincott Williams & Wilkins, pp. 1924–6.

Case 20
Natalie Jones

Instructions for the doctor

This is a short case.

Please conduct this consultation as you would in your clinical practice.

Scenario

Jacinta Jones comes in to see you to discuss Natalie, her six-year-old daughter. She had taken Natalie to a paediatrician because her asthma was not well controlled on her medication of prophylactic cromoglycate and salbutamol.

You have read the letter from the paediatrician suggesting that Natalie start on inhaled steroids. You are not quite sure why she has booked this appointment to see you today, particularly as she did not come to see you about Natalie before going to the paediatrician.

Instructions for Natalie's mother, Jacinta Jones

You are an articulate business executive in your late thirties. You live in a large house in a prestigious area of Sydney and travel a substantial amount for work. Natalie is your only child and you had her 'later on' so that you could establish your career first. Your husband is also in business and leaves the child care arrangements to you.

Natalie is six years old and has asthma. You are often up at night when she coughs and this is exhausting for both of you. Natalie uses a salbutamol inhaler and cromoglycate as a preventer. You recently took Natalie to see a private paediatrician about the asthma. You did not ask your GP for a referral and just paid the full price. You have precious little time for appointments and a friend's child sees a paediatrician for their asthma so you thought it would be best.

You are concerned that the paediatrician has decided to start Natalie on steroids. You know they are banned in athletes and do not understand why they are being given to Natalie. You have made an appointment to see the GP and have the following questions on your mind:

1. Why has Natalie been recommended steroids? How do they work?
2. Is there any alternative medication that could be tried?
3. How will the GP know if the medication is helping Natalie?
4. Are there any side effects to worry about?
5. The paediatrician gave you a spacer for helping Natalie use the medication. You didn't take in the instructions after a sleepless night and would like to be shown again.

Suggested approach to the case

Establish rapport
Open-ended questions to establish Jacinta's ideas, concerns and expectations about this consultation and Natalie's asthma
Answer Jacinta in terms that are understood, in a non-judgemental manner.

1. Explain that asthma is due to inflammation. Steroids are anti-inflammatory and will reduce the amount of wheezing and coughing and make it easier for Natalie to breathe.

   Explore why Jacinta is concerned about steroids: what has she heard about them and from whom? Tailor further answers about steroids to Jacinta's specific concerns.

   Jacinta has heard that steroids are banned in athletes. The doctor can reassure her that there are different types of steroids and that the body-building steroids abused by some athletes are different from the anti-inflammatory steroids used in asthma.

2. Explore with Jacinta what medication has already been tried. Outline the rationale for obtaining good asthma control and for helping Natalie to feel better. Natalie has previously tried regular cromoglycate as a preventer and uses salbutamol for symptom relief. She has not tried other medication. The next step according to current guidelines is to introduce inhaled corticosteroids.

3. Explain the role of monitoring Natalie's asthma symptoms. Asthma control is monitored by:
   - assessment of symptoms—cough, wheeze, nocturnal cough, shortness of breath, exercise tolerance
   - absence of signs—wheeze, peak expiratory flow rate, spirometry
   - function—can Natalie do all the sport and activities that she would like to or does her asthma stop her?

4. Side effects such as oral thrush and dysphonia are possible with inhaled corticosteroids. These can be reduced by using a spacer and rinsing the mouth after inhalation. Longer-term side effects include the development of cataracts, reduced bone density, depression of the hypothalamic–pituitary–adrenal axis and delay in growth. The list of potential problems from inhaled corticosteroids is long. The doctor needs to give a balanced description of the potential risks and benefits of this medication. The doctor can inform Jacinta that the lowest effective dose of inhaled steroids will be used and that Natalie's growth and general development will be monitored.

5. Demonstrate use of spacer device with advice regarding cleaning.

6. Suggest a written asthma management plan.

Any remaining time could be used to review preventive measures, such as encouraging exercise, and avoiding environmental triggers to Natalie's asthma, such as passive smoking.

 CASE COMMENTARY

This case tests the doctor's communication skills and understanding of the management of childhood asthma. Another twist is the potential for interprofessional issues to interfere with Natalie's care.

In the Australian health system, patients are referred to specialists by their GPs. However, many people are willing to pay for direct access to specialists. Natalie's asthma is not severe and would normally be dealt with by a GP. The GP may feel undermined that Jacinta has taken Natalie to a specialist.

Wounded professional pride is compounded by having to deal with Jacinta's response to the suggestions of inhaled corticosteroids. The GP should put aside their own reactions and approach Jacinta professionally and in Natalie's best interests.

The doctor needs to explore why Jacinta is concerned about giving Natalie steroids. While the doctor could guess at the causes for her concern from their general knowledge of patients' reactions, the reassurance will be more effective if it addresses Jacinta's particular fears.

Some doctors may feel threatened by Jacinta's questioning of medical advice. A good doctor will be able to discuss the issue with Jacinta as if in a partnership, whereas a poor doctor may show irritation and resort to medical dominance or cave in and, in an effort to appease her mum, deny Natalie the medication she needs.

Spacers come with simple written instructions. If you are not confident in using a spacer or in instructing others how to use one, ask a local pharmacist if you can look at one and read the instructions for use.

Further reading

National Asthma Council 2016, *Australian Asthma Handbook,* version 1.2, National Asthma Council, Melbourne, Vic. Available at: www.asthmahand book.org.au, accessed 19 February 2019.

Robinson, PD & Van Asperen, P 2009, 'Asthma in childhood', *Pediatric Clinics of North America,* vol. 56, no. 1, pp. 191–226.

Van Asperen, PP, Mellis, CM, Sly, PD & Robertson, CF 2011, 'Evidence-based asthma management in children—what's new?', *Medical Journal of Australia,* vol. 194, no. 8, pp. 383–4.

Zhang, L, Prietsch, S & Ducharme, F 2014, 'Inhaled corticosteroids in children with persistent asthma: effects on growth', *Cochrane Database of Systematic Reviews,* no. 7.

Case 21
Latu O'Donnell

Instructions for the doctor

This is a short case.

Please take a history from Latu's mother Mele. The findings of a relevant physical examination will be available from the facilitator. Negotiate a management plan with Mele. You are not required to take a history from Latu.

Scenario

Mele and her 11-year-old son Latu have been coming to your surgery since they moved to the area three years ago. Mele's ex-husband, Robert, moved interstate after their marriage ended. Mele is from Tonga and her parents live nearby. She works as a receptionist for the local council and has another part-time job as a cleaner. Latu has previously been healthy, presenting only for minor illnesses. Mele presents today to discuss her concerns about Latu's increasing weight and sedentary lifestyle.

The following information is on Latu's summary sheet:
Medication
Nil recorded
Allergies
Nil recorded
Immunisations
Up-to-date
Social history
Lives with his mother
Attends school.

Instructions for the patient's mother, Mele Kafoa

You and Latu have come to the doctor today to get some help with his weight. Latu is 11 and generally healthy, but since you moved to this area his weight has been steadily increasing. He is less physically active and you have talked to him several times about getting more exercise and eating better, but each time he reacts angrily and tells you to stop nagging him. What motivated you to bring him in was an episode last week when he was upset and told you about being bullied at school about his weight. Latu is naturally shy but increasingly he has been withdrawing into his computer gaming world, which seems to be the main place that he is happy and engaged.

Your break-up with Robert was very unpleasant and you were glad to make a new start with Latu when you moved back to the area where your parents live. Unfortunately, Latu hasn't really made good friends here, preferring to play online games with some of his previous friends. He goes to stay with Robert roughly one weekend a month and for some school holidays. From your point of view, Robert seeks to 'buy' Latu's love by giving him lots of presents (computer games, tablet, new phone) and basically letting him do what he wants when Latu is with him. You feel that this undermines your efforts to help him be healthier but haven't spoken to Robert about it. You would like to see Latu get outside more, play sport and be socially active but you're having trouble reaching him. You are conscious that this role would normally be performed by Latu's brothers or cousins, but in their absence you are doing the best you can.

You work hard both as a receptionist and a cleaner and are often not home until dinner time. You lack the energy to cook and often grab some takeaway on the way home. Both of you eat your dinner in front of the TV or the computer and most evenings you relax on the couch. You shop each Saturday and usually buy Latu some of his favourite foods (biscuits, chips, chocolates) for snacks and rewards. Working hard to pay the bills and keep the cupboard stocked takes all your energy—everything else feels overwhelming and tends to go into the 'too hard' basket. Your own weight has increased by several kilograms since moving. You put this down to not being physically active outside of work and to a habit of comfort eating (ice cream, chocolate) when you get down. You are close with your parents, who are a good support for you. Every Sunday after church they have you and Latu for lunch, which lasts for much of the day with lots of food. You have spoken to your mother about Latu's weight but she said, 'it is better to be bigger than skinny'. You are interested in the doctor's thoughts about whether you should be concerned about Latu and, if so, what practical steps you can take to help him.

The following information is on Latu's summary sheet:
Medication
Nil recorded
Allergies
Nil recorded
Immunisations
Up-to-date
Social history
Lives with his mother
Attends school.

Information for the facilitator

Clinical examination findings

General appearance: overweight boy sitting quietly in no distress
Height 141.5 cm (50th centile)
Weight 51 kg (96th centile)
BMI 26 kg/m^2 = 97th centile
Remainder of physical examination normal.

Suggested approach to the case

Open questions to explore Mele's concerns, without Latu present.

Specific questions for Mele

Latu's general health and co-morbidities
    —Sleep/snoring
    —Shortness of breath
    —Fatigue
    —Skin and musculoskeletal problems
Latu's psychosocial issues
    —Mood
    —Self-esteem
    —Body image
    —Disordered eating
    —Behavioural problems
    —Teasing and bullying
    —School avoidance
    —Social isolation

Family dynamics
  −Cultural beliefs about weight
  −Parenting difficulties
  −Parental coping
  −Social support
  −Financial difficulties
  −Parental motivation
The family's eating habits and food choices
Latu's physical activity and interests.

Examination

General appearance
BMI percentiles
Heart rate
Blood pressure
BSL
Urinalysis.

Management

Use a BMI chart to show Mele that Latu is bordering on obese.
Briefly outline the health consequences of obesity.
Affirm Mele's decision to present and existing positive aspects of her care, and build confidence in Latu's successful weight management.
Interventions with strong evidence in Latu's age group include limiting screen time, increasing water consumption, physical activity interventions with a home component and diet interventions with a community and home component.
Lifestyle interventions should ideally include the whole family. Mele has admitted to gaining weight herself so a program for her and Latu would be beneficial.
Ongoing follow-up with a health care team and monitoring weight and growth velocity will be important.

 CASE COMMENTARY

The prevalence of overweight and obesity in Australia is high and continues to increase. Obesity is particularly prevalent among those in the most disadvantaged socioeconomic groups, Aboriginal and Torres

Strait Islander peoples and many people born overseas. The prevalence is also higher in rural and remote areas compared to urban areas. Pacific Islanders rank among those with the highest rates of obesity. Culturally, large physical size is considered a mark of beauty and social status in many Pacific Island countries. There can be resistance to the view that obesity is a health problem. Childhood obesity is a sensitive issue—made even more complex by family and cultural factors, as in this case. The family doctor is well-placed to gently explore, educate and manage childhood obesity.

Due to the changes in body composition as children grow, single-point cut-offs are usually not suitable for establishing a child's weight status. BMI percentile curves specific for gender and age should be used. A BMI between the 85th and 95th percentile is considered to be overweight, and a BMI above the 95th percentile is considered obese. Weight maintenance as the child grows rather than weight loss is recommended for most children.

Generally, it is better to discuss a child's weight with parents when the child is not present, but from adolescence it is important to work primarily with the patient. Before this time, the GP has a key role to play in enhancing parental motivation, which is essential for effective weight management in children. Intervention is unlikely to be effective if parents are not motivated to change. Parents are more likely to be motivated to make changes to manage their child's weight when they have sufficient knowledge about children's weight and health, believe that their child's excess weight is important to control, believe that the required changes are worthwhile, and have confidence in their ability to make the necessary changes. Parents like Mele who have high levels of readiness for change can be offered specific and practical interventions.

Supporting Mele in an empathic and non-judgemental way will enhance her engagement, motivation and readiness for change. If we emphasise her family's strengths and avoid parent blame and criticism we can create an alliance that will combat the isolation generally felt by those caught between cultures and families. Respectful exploration of traditional beliefs and attitudes concerning weight will be needed and Mele will have to resolve how she is going to respond to these with her family.

COMMON PITFALLS

It is easy to fall into a dynamic where the doctor is suggesting strategies for change and the patient (in this case, the mother) is responding to each by explaining why they won't work. It has been shown that such a dynamic actually works against behavioural change and can be avoided by the application of motivational interviewing skills.

Further reading

Curtis, M 2004, 'The obesity epidemic in the Pacific Islands', *Journal of Development and Social Transformation,* vol. 1, November.

Kirk, SFL, Cockbain, AJ & Beazley, J 2008, 'Obesity in Tonga: a cross-sectional comparative study of perceptions of body size and beliefs about obesity in lay people and nurses', *Obesity Research & Clinical Practice,* vol. 2, no. 1, pp. 35–41.

Mavoa, HM & McCabe, M 2008, 'Sociocultural factors relating to Tongans, and Indigenous Fijians' patterns of eating, physical activity and body size', *Asia Pacific Journal of Clinical Nutrition,* vol. 17, no. 3, pp. 375–84.

Miller, WR & Rollnick, S 2002, *Motivational Interviewing: Preparing People for Change,* The Guilford Press, New York.

Mihrshahi, S, Gow, ML & Baur, LA 2018, 'Contemporary approaches to the prevention and management of paediatric obesity: an Australian focus', *Medical Journal of Australia,* vol. 209, no. 6, pp. 267–74.

National Health and Medical Research Council 2013, 'Clinical practice guidelines for the management of overweight and obesity in adults, Adolescents and Children in Australia', NHMRC, Melbourne, Vic. Available at: www.nhmrc.gov.au/_files_nhmrc/publications/attachments/n57_obesity_guidelines_130531.pdf, accessed 15 October 2014.

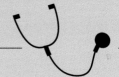

Section 7
Dermatology

Case 22
Sammy Burnside

Instructions for the doctor

This is a short case.

Please take a history from Jessica, Sammy's mum. A clinical photograph of Sammy's skin problem will be available for you on request. (Refer to Figure 2, centre insert page A.) Please discuss the diagnosis with Jessica and advise on the management of the condition.

Scenario

Sammy is a four-month-old boy who has an itchy rash.

The following information is on his summary sheet:

Past medical history
Normal vaginal delivery following uncomplicated pregnancy

Medication
Nil prescribed

Allergies
Nil known

Immunisations
Up-to-date

Family history
Mother asthmatic and allergic rhinitis
Father eczema as a baby.

Instructions for Sammy's mother, Jessica Burnside

You had a busy life as a teacher at the local preschool. You are on maternity leave following Sammy's birth but are soon due to return to work. Sammy has had an itchy rash on his face, arms, legs and trunk for a few weeks.

You've been using creams your Mum bought for you, plus tea-tree oil. You hate seeing your beautiful baby so distressed by the scratching and are worried about the thought of putting Sammy into child care when you return to work. You have asthma and allergic rhinitis and your partner had eczema as a baby.

The following information is on Sammy's medical record:
Past medical history
Normal vaginal delivery following uncomplicated pregnancy
Medication
Nil
Allergies
Nil known
Immunisations
Up-to-date
Family history
Mother asthmatic and allergic rhinitis
Father eczema as a baby.

Suggested approach to the case

Establish rapport
Explore Jessica's ideas, concerns and expectations.

Specific questions

Duration of the rash
Site of the rash
Scratching
Precipitating and relieving factors
Impact on Sammy and family
Previous treatment tried
Current treatment—including use of soaps
Request permission to examine.

Examination

Expose down to nappy
  —Dry skin with excoriations
  —Widespread patches of eczema
  —Exclude secondary infection.

Diagnosis

Eczema
Plus possible contact allergy to tea-tree oil.

Management

Discuss and explain the diagnosis of eczema
Explain that eczema can be controlled but not cured
Often improves as child grows up.

Prevention

Avoid heat
—Loose fitting, cotton clothing and bedding
—Tepid comfortable bath water preferred over hot water
Avoid prickle and irritants
—Wool, nylon, seams and clothing labels
—Chlorine, sand and grass
—Soaps and bubble baths, perfumed creams or other products
—Tea-tree oil is a common cause of contact allergy and should be
stopped
Avoid dryness
—Soap-free washes
—Regular emollient regime, e.g. 50% soft 50% liquid paraffin four
times per day
—Note that lotions are drying and are best avoided. Likewise,
sorbolene and aqueous cream can cause stinging and irritation and
are no longer recommended
Consider gloves to reduce scratching
Keep fingernails short.

Treat inflammation

Intermittent topical steroid to control flares
—For example, hydrocortisone 1% ointment bd to affected areas
—A more potent steroid for non-sensitive areas of the body may be
required to control more severe flares
—Provide guidance on how much to use, e.g. one fingertip unit covers
the area of two adult palms

—Topical steroids should be used until the skin is smooth and itch
and inflammation has settled
—Addressing any fear of topical steroid use is important to ensure
that adequate steroids are used to control the eczema
Treat infection if present
Plan follow-up
Consider referral if no improvement.

CASE COMMENTARY

The key issue in this case is to demonstrate competence in the management of a common skin condition. There are no hidden twists in this case. A good doctor will establish a good relationship with Jessica and explore the social and psychological impact of the problem as well as discuss medical management. For example, the doctor could allow Jessica to express her concerns about returning to work and having to ask staff at the childcare centre to put on creams. Or ask what impact is the problem having on her relationship with Sammy or her partner?

About 75% of children grow out of their eczema by the age of five, but the strong family history of atopy makes this less likely in Sammy's case. Regular use of emollients and intermittent topical steroids are the mainstay of therapy; severe eczema may need systemic immunomodulatory drugs, which require close monitoring by a doctor experienced in their use.

Eczema can be a challenging condition to manage well, and there are often multiple factors contributing to treatment failure. For example:

- inadequate topical steroid use (conflicting advice from medical practitioners, fear of side effects, lack of education/awareness of importance)
- failure to address preventative measures, e.g. avoiding soaps and other triggers
- recurrent infection and staphylococcal carriage
- allergies to dust mites or food allergens.

Bleach baths twice weekly have been shown to reduce severity of eczema in children with recurrent infections.

Food allergens may play a role in about 35 per cent of children with eczema, in particular milk, egg, wheat, soy and peanuts. However, rates of false positive allergen testing are high. Elimination diets and food challenges could be considered in difficult-to-control eczema, under the supervision of an allergy specialist and dietician.

COMMON PITFALLS

Pitfalls to avoid are the prescription of steroid creams without explanation regarding judicious use—avoiding both under-treatment and over-treatment—and the potential side effects, and failing to consider that the tea-tree oil is exacerbating the problem.

Further reading

Greenhawt, M 2010, 'The role of food allergy in atopic dermatitis', *Allergy and Asthma Proceedings,* vol. 31, no. 5, pp 392–7.

Katelaris, CH & Peake, JE 2006, 'Allergy and the skin: eczema and chronic urticaria', *Medical Journal of Australia,* vol. 185, no. 9, pp. 517–22.

McAleer, MA, Flohr, C & Irvine, AD 2012, 'Management of difficult and severe eczema in childhood', *British Medical Journal,* vol. 345, p. e4770.

Ross, T, Ross, G & Varigos, G 2005, 'Eczema: practical management issues', *Australian Family Physician,* vol. 34, no. 5, pp. 319–24.

Strathie Page, S, Weston, S & Loh, R 2016, 'Atopic dermatitis in children', *Australian Family Physician,* vol. 45, no. 5, pp. 293–6.

Therapeutic Guidelines Ltd 2018, 'Atopic dermatitis'. In: *eTG complete* [internet], Therapeutic Guidelines Ltd, Melbourne, Vic.

The Royal Children's Hospital Melbourne, 'Eczema', *Clinical Practice Guidelines.* Available at: www.rch.org.au/clinicalguide/guideline_index/eczema, accessed 15 August 2018.

Case 23
Robert Kerslake

Instructions for the doctor

This is a short case.

You are expected to take a brief history from Robert regarding a rash. A photograph of his rash will be available to you. There is no need to conduct any further examination. Outline to Robert your diagnosis and suggestions for management.

Scenario

Robert Kerslake is a 24-year-old chef with a rash on the outside of his right and left elbows. He has tried some 1% hydrocortisone cream purchased over the counter and it cleared the rash for a short time; however, it recurs each time he stops using it.

The following information is on his summary sheet:

Past medical history
Chickenpox aged eight
Medication
Nil recorded
Allergies
Nil known
Immunisations
Up-to-date
Social history
Lives alone
Smokes 10–20 cigarettes per day.

Instructions for the patient, Robert Kerslake

You are 24 years old and work as a chef. You work long hours and the kitchen is often very hot. A few months ago, you developed a rash on your elbows. You bought some hydrocortisone cream from a chemist and when you use it the rash goes; as soon as you stop using it, the rash reappears. The rash is only on your arms.

The rash is annoying you more and more and it is getting you down. Normally you like to socialise but the rash is making you stay home rather than going out with your mates and you are worried customers may think the rash is infectious.

You have no family history of skin disease and have no joint, hair or nail problems. You are keen to find out from the doctor what the rash is and what can be done about it.

When the doctor asks to look at the rash please show them the photograph. (Refer to Figure 3, centre insert page B.)

The following information is on your summary sheet:
Past medical history
Chickenpox aged eight
Medication
Nil recorded
Allergies
Nil known
Immunisations
Up-to-date
Social history
Lives alone
Smokes 10–20 cigarettes per day.

Suggested approach to the case

Establish rapport
Open-ended questions to explore Robert's concerns, ideas and expectations for the consultation.

Specific questions

Explore the symptoms of the rash and impact on his life
Ask about other involvement, e.g. joint pain, nails or hair
Ask about treatment so far
Observe clinical photograph.

Most likely diagnosis

Psoriasis.

Management

Confirm diagnosis of psoriasis
Education regarding psoriasis
   –Inform psoriasis is non-infectious
   –Treatment aimed at containment, not cure
   –Discuss impact of stress and smoking[1]
Initial topical treatments
   –Sunlight–improves psoriasis; balance sun exposure to help psoriasis
     while minimising risk of skin cancer
   –Emollients, e.g. liquid/soft paraffin
   –Salicylic acid + coal tar preparations
   –Intermittent use of corticosteroids for flares
   –Vitamin D analogues such as calcipotriol (usually in combination
     with corticosteroids)
Other topical therapies that can be considered
   –Dithranol
   –Topical retinoids, such as tazarotene
   –Calcineurin inhibitors, such as pimecrolimus (Elidel)
Systemic treatments may be required (under the direction of a dermatologist) for more severe or extensive psoriasis, or for psoriasis with systemic involvement, e.g. UV light therapy, systemic retinoids, methotrexate, cyclosporine or newer immunomodulatory drugs
Offer information about support groups, patient education leaflet
Opportunistic health promotion
   –Assess motivation to stop smoking
Arrange follow-up.

 CASE COMMENTARY

Psoriasis is an inflammatory immune-based disorder with a genetic predisposition:[2] activated T-lymphocytes release cytokines that cause keratinocyte proliferation.[3] Approximately 1.5% of the population are significantly affected by it and the overall incidence is up to 6%.[2] It should be appreciated that psoriasis is a systemic disease associated with increased risks of cardiovascular disease, diabetes and depression, as well as psoriatic arthritis.

The characteristic well-defined red plaques with adherent silvery scale make the diagnosis relatively easy.

The skill in this case, as in clinical practice, is tailoring the answer to the patient's circumstances. Robert's work as a chef means it is important to reassure him that the condition is not infectious; he can also be sensitively advised that stress and smoking can make psoriasis worse.

A significant range of treatments are available, but these can be messy. Topical agents and emollients are used initially: for example, regular moisturising plus corticosteroids and/or calcipotriol. Systemic treatment is reserved for when more than 20% of the skin is affected or when there are associated systemic problems.[1] It is not necessary to describe all available options during this initial consult. Doctors should focus on providing good education and reassurance regarding the diagnosis, and clear instructions regarding an initial treatment plan. Reviewing response to treatment is important and follow-up should be arranged.

Psoriasis has a high financial[4] and emotional cost.[5] A biopsychosocial framework will assist GPs to cover the important aspects of management, including the impact that the psoriasis has on Robert's self-image, relationships and his work.

References

1. Weigle, N & McBane, S 2013, 'Psoriasis', *American Family Physician,* vol. 87, no. 9, pp. 626–33.
2. Clarke, P 2011, 'Psoriasis', *Australian Family Physician,* vol. 40, no. 7, pp. 468–73.
3. Nestle, FO, Kaplan, DH & Barker, J 2009, 'Psoriasis', *New England Journal of Medicine,* vol. 361, pp. 496–509.
4. Jenner, N, Campbell, J, Plunkett, A & Marks, R 2002, 'Cost of psoriasis: a study on the morbidity and financial effects of having psoriasis in Australia', *Australasian Journal of Dermatology,* vol. 43, pp. 255–61.
5. Magin, PJ, Adams, J, Heading, GS & Pond, CD 2009, 'Patients with skin disease and their relationships with their doctors: a qualitative study of patients with acne, psoriasis and eczema', *Medical Journal of Australia,* vol. 190, pp. 62–4.

Case 24
Ken Anderson

Instructions for the doctor

This is a short case.

Please take a history from Ken Anderson, a 60-year-old Caucasian farmer. A clinical photograph of Ken's skin problem will be available to you on request. (Refer to Figure 4 on centre insert page B.) Please discuss with Ken the management of the condition.

Scenario

Ken Anderson is a 60-year-old sheep and cattle farmer who is a regular patient. He is usually healthy, but you have seen him for hypertension and hyperlipidaemia (both well-controlled), as well as for minor physical injuries.

The following information is on his summary sheet:

Past medical history
Hypertension
Hyperlipidaemia
Medication
Telmisartan 40 mg od
Rosuvastatin 10 mg od
Allergies
Nil known
Immunisations
Up-to-date
Social history
Married
Smokes 15 cigarettes per day.

Instructions for the patient, Ken Anderson

You've noticed a scaly lesion on your right cheek, which has been there for about six weeks. You have scratched it off a couple of times but it seems to come back. It is not painful, tender or itchy and does not bleed. It is pink or flesh-coloured, is slowly growing and is now about 3 mm in diameter. If asked you don't think you have had any previous skin lesions apart from the usual bumps, bruises and scratches that come with farming.

You are fair skinned but tend to tan rather than burn. You have spent your whole life in rural Australia and most of your days are in the sun. You wear a hat and usually long-sleeved clothes but don't use sun protection creams regularly. If asked, your father had a number of skin lesions removed by his doctor but you don't think any were melanomas.

You are fit and healthy and generally pretty cavalier about your health, although you are worried this spot might be a skin cancer.

The following information is on your summary sheet:

Past medical history
Hypertension
Hyperlipidaemia
Medication
Telmisartan 40 mg od
Rosuvastatin 10 mg od
Allergies
Nil known
Immunisations
Up-to-date
Social history
Smokes 15 cigarettes per day.

Suggested approach to the case

Establish rapport
Explore Ken's concerns about the lesion.

Specific questions

Duration of the lesion
Bleeding, itching or pain
Any treatment applied
Any previous lesions
Sun exposure

Skin type
Family history of skin conditions
General health
Request permission to examine.

Examination

Exposure—adequate lighting and magnification
Dermatoscopy
Check rest of skin for other lesions.

Diagnosis

Hyperkeratotic actinic keratosis
Background sun damage.

Management

Explanation of actinic (also called solar) keratosis and natural history
Outline treatment options—cryotherapy with liquid nitrogen as first-line
  management
Explain likely blister formation and aftercare required
Discussion about sun protection
Consider nicotinamide for prevention of further actinic keratoses
Advise regarding future skin checks.

CASE COMMENTARY

Australian rates of skin cancer rank among the highest in the world, and
farmers die from skin cancer at roughly twice the rate of other Australians
(65 years and over). This is a case to demonstrate the competent management of a very common condition. Actinic keratosis is a clinical diagnosis
that should be made with confidence. Ken needs advice about the natural
history of the lesion, which is likely to persist and slowly grow, and carries
a small risk of progression into a squamous cell carcinoma. Cryotherapy
with liquid nitrogen represents the simplest treatment option for a single
lesion, but the patient should be warned about likely blistering and its
management. Freezes of 20 seconds or longer are more likely to clear
the lesion, but risk of scarring and hypopigmentation increases as well.
The goal is to eradicate the lesion without scarring.

This is also an important opportunity to instruct Ken in ongoing sun protection and skin surveillance. In the future he will develop more lesions and will need further cryotherapy. Topical field treatments such as 5-fluorouracil, diclofenac or imiquimod are all possible future therapeutic options. Regular sunscreen application and nicotinamide (500 mg once or twice daily) have both been shown to reduce actinic keratosis burden.

 COMMON PITFALLS

It is always tempting to rush to look at skin lesions, but it is important to take a thorough history. Other common errors include neglecting to check the remainder of Ken's skin, as well as erring on the side of reassurance about a benign condition and missing a chance to educate and change Ken's behaviour with regard to sun protection.

Further reading

Australian Centre for Agricultural Health and Safety, *Farm Health and Safety Toolkit for Rural General Practices.* Available at: www.sydney.edu.au/medicine/ aghealth/uploaded/Health%20Workers/_gp_toolkit_booklet_lores.pdf, accessed 22 November 2018.

Sinclair, R 2012, 'Skin checks', *Australian Family Physician,* vol. 41, no. 7, pp. 464-9.

Uhlenhake, E 2013, 'Optimal treatment of actinic keratoses', *Clinical Interventions in Aging,* vol. 8, pp. 29-35.

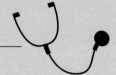

Section 8
Ear, nose and throat

Case 25
Ruby Chan

Instructions for the doctor

This is a short case.

Please take a history, conduct a focused examination and outline your diagnosis and management plan to the patient.

Scenario

Ruby Chan is 40 years old and works long hours at the local club. She has booked this appointment to see you because of facial pain.

You practise in a small rural town of 600 people. You are the only resident health professional.

The following information is on Ruby's summary sheet:

Past medical history
Two children
One termination of pregnancy aged 16

Medication
Nil

Allergies
Nil known

Immunisations
Nil known

Pap smear
Up-to-date

Social history
Works at the Memo Club
Non-smoker
Alcohol intake—special occasions only.

Instructions for the patient, Ruby Chan

You are a 40-year-old woman who has had facial pain for a few days. It is getting worse and it kept you awake last night. You have had a cold and are overdue for a check-up at the dentist. The nearest dentist is over 50 km away. The pain is worse when you chew food. You have a slight headache but this does not get worse on bending forwards or sneezing. Your sense of smell is undisturbed.

Your father died of cancer of the tongue. You have never been sure exactly what this is, but it does mean that you are more concerned than normal about your pain being something serious. You would like the doctor to find this out but will not reveal this unless asked appropriately.

Instructions for the facilitator

The candidate should perform a focused oral examination.

Clinical examination findings

Tapping of one of your molars gives you significant pain.

The following information is on your medical record:
Past medical history
Two children
One termination of pregnancy aged 16
Medication
Nil
Allergies
Nil known
Immunisations
Nil known
Pap smear
Up-to-date
Social history
Works at the Memo Club
Non-smoker
Alcohol intake—special occasions only.

Suggested approach to the case

Establish rapport
Open-ended questions to explore Ruby's ideas, concerns and expectations.

Specific questions

Ask about the pain, e.g. using **OLD CARTS** acronym
  —Onset
  —Location
  —Duration, diurnal variation
  —Characteristics—worse on chewing
  —Associated symptoms
  —Relieving factors
  —Treatment tried so far
  —Severity
Exclude systemic symptoms—weight changes, energy level, sleep disturbance
Request permission to examine.

Examination

Temperature
Inspect and/or palpate head and neck
Check teeth, lymph nodes, skin, eyes, salivary glands, temporomandibular
  joint, cervical spine, nose, mouth, pharynx and post-nasal space and
  sinuses.

Most likely diagnosis

Dental pain.

Management

Urgent dental consultation
Pain relief—aspirin or paracetamol, clove oil.

Extras for this case

Explore patient's concerns resulting from her father's cancer and previous
  occupational exposure to cigarette smoke
Explain need for patient to book another appointment to discuss
  vaccination status.

 CASE COMMENTARY

Ruby's pain is caused by a sore tooth. This will become obvious as the
doctor takes the history and taps the teeth.[1] After hours, and in rural
areas, GPs are often required to provide care for dental problems.[2]

Antibiotics are indicated if there is possible cellulitis secondary to an infected tooth. Dental abscesses require incision and drainage and root canal treatment or extraction.[3]

There is a long list of possible features to check in the face.[1] A good doctor can focus promptly on examination of the teeth, lymph nodes and temporomandibular joints. If tapping the teeth with a tongue depressor reproduces the pain there is no need to proceed with further examination. The time can then be spent explaining the diagnosis, planning management and exploring any particular concerns that Ruby has. A doctor who does a complete examination will not have time to explore the concerns about Ruby's father's tongue cancer or have time to discuss Ruby's vaccination status.

References

1. Quail, G 2015, 'Facial pain–a diagnostic challenge', *Australian Family Physician,* vol. 44, no. 12, pp. 901–4.
2. Wetherall, J, Richards, L, Sambrook, P & Townsend, G 2001, 'Management of acute dental pain: a practical approach for primary health care providers', *Australian Prescriber,* vol. 24, no. 6, pp. 144–8.
3. Beech, N, Goh, R & Lynham, A 2014, 'Management of dental infections by medical practitioners', *Australian Family Physician,* vol. 43, no. 5, pp. 289–91.

Further reading

Kingon, A 2009, 'Solving dental problems in general practice', *Australian Family Physician,* vol. 38, no. 4, pp. 211–6.

Case 26
Jane Matthews

Instructions for the doctor

This is a short case.

Please take a history and conduct an appropriate examination. Please tell the facilitator your findings and suspected diagnosis.

Scenario

Jane Matthews is a 31-year-old woman who is pregnant for the first time. She is coming to see you because she has noticed a slight swelling in her neck just below her Adam's apple.

The following information is on her summary sheet:

Past medical history
Nil significant. G1P0 18/40

Medication
Nil

Allergies
Nil known

Immunisations
Nil recorded

Cervical screening test
Normal this year

Family history
Nil significant

Social history
Married
Works as a hairdresser.

Instructions for the patient, Jane Matthews

You are a 31-year-old married hairdresser. You are excited about being pregnant for the first time. Everything has been going well. Last week you were on holiday and you have just been looking at the photos again. Your neck looked a bit odd in the photos and you have now had a closer look in the mirror. There is a smooth swelling in the middle below your Adam's apple.

You saw your GP last week about the pregnancy and the check-up was fine. You have booked today's appointment just to sort out the swelling. You are not particularly worried about it.

Clinical examination findings

You have a diffuse goitre but no other physical findings or symptoms.

The following information is on your summary sheet:
Past medical history
Nil significant. G1P0 18/40
Medication
Nil
Allergies
Nil known
Immunisations
Nil recorded
Pap smear
Normal this year
Family history
Nil significant
Social history
Married
Works as a hairdresser.

Suggested approach to the case

Establish rapport
Open-ended questions to explore patient's ideas, concerns and expectations.

Specific questions

Weight loss, appetite, vomiting, lumps elsewhere
Heat tolerance, energy levels, palpitations, tremor, and difficulty swallowing solids or liquids

Change in voice, change in skin or hair, sweating, sleep pattern
Previous thyroid dysfunction, medications (specifically amiodarone, lithium)
Family history: any family history of thyroid problems, diabetes
Request permission to examine.

Examination

Inspection of the swelling
Palpation
　　–Site
　　–Size
　　–Consistency
　　–Tenderness
Movement on swallowing
Percussion–not needed
Auscultation of swelling for bruits
Palpation of lymph nodes of the neck
Examination for thyroid signs
　　–Pulse
　　–Tremor
　　–Eyes–for proptosis
　　–Warmth of peripheries
　　–Reflexes
　　–General skin changes
There is minor diffuse thyroid swelling and no other abnormality.

 CASE COMMENTARY

Benign thyroid enlargement is the most likely cause of a midline neck swelling in a pregnant woman like Jane. A doctor should take a history about the swelling and any local symptoms and establish whether she is clinically hypothyroid or hyperthyroid.[1] The neck examination should reveal that the swelling moves on swallowing. Examination of the lymph nodes should show that the doctor knows the position of the lymph nodes and should be conducted from behind.

Routine biochemical screening for thyroid dysfunction is not recommended in pregnancy[2] but is indicated for symptomatic patients.[3] Traditional teaching is that any neck swelling or lump requires examination of the scalp, ears, skin, face, mouth and throat.[4] This is vital if the lump is an enlarged lymph node but is not needed in this case where the history and examination findings are so suggestive of a thyroid problem. This is an example of type 1 or pattern recognition rather than type 2 or hypothetico-deductive thinking. Experienced GPs use pattern recognition as a method of clinical reasoning because it is much quicker, in this case, allowing the doctor time to check on thyroid status as well as the swelling. Doctors who use the hypothetico-deductive method reasoning through this case will be safe but will have used valuable time on unnecessary issues.

The doctor is not expected to discuss management of the swelling.

References

1. Hughes, K & Eastman, C 2012, 'Goitre—causes, investigation and management', *Australian Family Physician,* vol. 41, pp. 572–6.
2. Royal Australian and New Zealand College of Obstetricians and Gynaecologists 2015, *Testing for hypothyroidism during pregnancy with serum TSH.* Available at: https://www.ranzcog.edu.au/RANZCOG_SITE/media/RANZCOG-MEDIA/Women's%20Health/Statement%20and%20guidelines/Clinical-Obstetrics/Testing-for-hypothyroidism-during-pregnancy-with-serum-TSH-(C-Obs-46)-Review-July-2015.pdf?ext=.pdf, accessed 19 February 2019.
3. Smith, A, Eccles-Smith, J, D'Emden, M & Lust, K 2017, 'Thyroid disease in pregnancy and postpartum', *Australian Prescriber,* vol. 40, pp. 214–9.
4. Roland, N & Bradley, PJ 2014, 'Neck swellings', *British Medical Journal* vol. 348, p. g1078.

Case 27
Pamela Taylor

Instructions for the doctor

This is a short case.

Please take a history, examine this patient appropriately and tell the examiner your diagnosis and management plan.

Scenario

You are asked to see Mrs Taylor, a 62-year-old tourist who has recently arrived in town. She is feeling dizzy.

Instructions for the patient, Pamela Taylor

You are a 62-year-old woman who is normally well. You are caravanning around Australia with your husband, and yesterday you were relieved to reach a town where you could finally get to a hairdresser.

This morning you woke up as normal, but when you turned your head to check the view from the caravan window, you suddenly experienced an overwhelming spinning sensation in your head and marked nausea. If you stay still you feel OK, but whenever you turn your head the spinning and nausea return. The symptoms last less than a minute. You have not had anything like this before.

Your opening line is, 'Doctor, I feel really dizzy'.

You have no tinnitus and your hearing is normal. You have no headache or any other neurological symptoms.

You regularly attend exercise classes in your home town, and your only medication is psyllium with ispaghula, one sachet once a day. In the past you have had surgery for a benign thyroid nodule.

You do not have any allergies, have never smoked and drink one to two standard alcoholic drinks at weekends.

Clinical examination findings

You will experience nausea when asked to move on and off the examination couch.

The candidate would observe nystagmus in your eyes during the Dix-Hallpike manoeuvre.

No other abnormalities are found on clinical examination.

Suggested approach to the case

Establish rapport

Open-ended questions to explore Pamela's ideas, concerns and expectations.

Specific questions

Dizziness—spinning feeling or as if about to faint, episodic or continuous
Vertigo—relationship to position
Nausea and vomiting, diarrhoea—exclude gastroenteritis
Tinnitus
Change in hearing
Visual symptoms
Previous history of similar episode
Exclude
    —Fits
    —Cardiac cause
    —Head injury
Past medical history
    —Medication including OTC and complementary or alternative
     medicines
    —Allergies
Request permission to examine.

Examination

Cardiovascular system
    —Pulse
    —BP lying and standing
    —Heart sounds
Neurological examination
    —Cognitive function—no apparent problem

—Cranial nerves

| III, IV, VI | eye movements, look for nystagmus |
| VIII | otoscope examination, hearing |

—Coordination—finger–nose or heel–toe test
—Gait
—Romberg's test
—Head-thrust test[1]
—Dix-Hallpike manoeuvre[1]

Neck
—Cervical spine movements.

Most likely diagnosis

Explain to the examiner that the most likely diagnosis is benign paroxysmal
positional vertigo (BPPV)
Reassurance—expect recovery.[2]

Management

Instruct patient on using the Epley manoeuvre or Brandt-Daroff exercises
to treat the condition by canalith repositioning[3, 4]
Limited role and efficacy for antihistamine and antiemetic agents
Arrange follow-up
Advise against driving
Investigate for alternative causes and consider specialist referral if symptoms
persist.

CASE COMMENTARY

Dizziness is a common presentation with multiple potential causes. The
history is essential to accurate diagnosis. The first step is to establish
that Mrs Taylor uses the term dizziness to describe a spinning sensation
(vertigo) and does not feel faint (suggests a cardiovascular cause).

The most likely cause in this case is benign paroxysmal positional
vertigo because the vertigo is exclusively related to changes in posture.
Being in a recumbent position for a prolonged time, as can occur at the
hairdresser, is a recognised precipitant of BPPV.

In vestibular neuronitis the symptoms are sustained but often worse on
movement, and there may have been a preceding viral upper-respiratory
infection. The head-thrust test would be abnormal. Menière's disease is

unlikely because there is no tinnitus or deafness. Stroke should be considered and is more likely if there are other new neurological symptoms and signs. Vestibular migraine is possible but would usually have an associated headache and, without any past history of migraine, would need investigation to exclude an underlying cause.

If the symptoms do not resolve with treatment, further investigation is needed to check for a cerebellar or cerebral lesion. Pamela will benefit from written advice to take with her on her travels.

References

1. Dommaraju, S & Perera, E 2016, 'An approach to vertigo in general practice', *Australian Family Physician,* vol. 45, pp. 190-4.
2. Kim, JS & Zee, DS 2014, 'Clinical practice. Benign paroxysmal positional vertigo', *New England Journal of Medicine,* vol. 370, pp. 1138-47.
3. Glasziou, P, Bennett, J, Greenberg, P et al. 2013, 'The Epley manoeuvre—for benign paroxysmal positional vertigo', *Australian Family Physician,* vol. 42, pp. 36-7.
4. Therapeutic Guidelines Ltd 2018, 'Brandt-Daroff exercises, patient handout'. In: *eTG complete* [Internet], Therapeutic Guidelines Ltd, Melbourne, Vic.

Case 28
Trevor Watts

Instructions for the doctor

This is a short case.

Please take a history from Trevor. You are not required to examine him. The results of an appropriate examination will be available from the facilitator on request. Outline the most likely diagnosis to the patient and initial suggestions for management.

Scenario

Trevor Watts is a 41-year-old man. For the last few months he has noticed a ringing sound in his right ear and sometimes there is ringing in his left ear. At first it did not bother him but now he is finding it very hard to live with. It is beginning to interfere with his sleep and it is getting him down.

He has no known deafness, balance problems or pain in his ears. He is otherwise well.

The following information is on his summary sheet:

Past medical history
Laceration left leg following motorcycle accident aged 20

Medication
Nil

Allergies
Nil known

Immunisations
Up-to-date. Last immunisation three years ago; ADT

Social history
Office manager.

Instructions for the patient, Trevor Watts

You are 41 years old and work as an office manager. For the last few months you have noticed a ringing sound in your right ear, and more recently an occasional ringing also in your left ear. At first it did not bother you but now you are finding it very hard to live with. It is beginning to interfere with your concentration and sleep and it is getting you down.

You have no known deafness, balance problems, vertigo or pain in your ears. You are otherwise well. You do not take any medication.

In your late teens and early twenties, you were a drummer in a successful rock and roll band. 'The louder the music the better' was your motto. You have always worked in an office environment in one capacity or another.

You live with your girlfriend and her two children from a previous relationship. You smoke 20 cigarettes a day and drink 10 stubbies of beer every Friday and Saturday night.

The following information is on your summary sheet:
Past medical history
Laceration left leg following motorcycle accident aged 20
Medication
Nil
Allergies
Nil known
Immunisations
Up-to-date. Last immunisation three years ago; ADT
Social history
Office manager.

Information for the facilitator

Clinical examination findings

Pulse 68 regular
BP 132/82 mmHg
No objective tinnitus
Inspection of the ears, including otoscopy: normal pinnas, external auditory canal and eardrums
Hearing—normal whisper test, normal Rinné and Weber tests
Balance—normal Romberg's test
Audiometry—bilateral sensorineural high frequency deafness
Cranial nerves normal.

Suggested approach to the case

Establish rapport
Open-ended questions to elicit Trevor's ideas, concerns and expectations.

Specific questions

Tinnitus—timeline, pitch, frequency, duration, character (pulsatile or not), continuous or intermittent
Deafness
Balance
Vertigo
Pain
Medication—exclude use of ototoxic drugs such as aspirin, loop diuretics
Past noise exposure—occupational or recreational
Past history of infections, surgery or trauma
Exclude depression with screening questions
Exclude serious neurological problem.

Ask for the examination findings

Pulse
BP
No objective tinnitus
Ear inspection with otoscope
Hearing—whisper test, Rinné and Weber
Balance—Romberg's test
Cranial nerves normal

Most likely diagnosis

Tinnitus—caused by noise exposure.

Investigations

BSL
Audiometry[1]—bilateral high frequency sensorineural deafness demonstrated.

Management[2, 3]

Reassure and explain nature of tinnitus
Aim for symptom control/habituation, cure unlikely
Suggest join support group

Tinnitus masker
Relaxation treatment
Cognitive behavioural therapy
Brief intervention regarding smoking and drinking
Arrange follow-up.

CASE COMMENTARY

Tinnitus is common and affects up to 10% of people in industrialised societies. Approximately 0.5% report that tinnitus has a severe effect on their daily life.[2] It is thought to originate from the central rather than peripheral auditory system. The number of years of work-related noise exposure correlates with increasing prevalence of tinnitus.

The doctor needs to take a history, to ask for the results of a focused examination and to establish that the most likely cause is noise exposure earlier in the patient's life. A vestibular schwannoma would need to be excluded if the tinnitus and deafness shown on audiometry was unilateral, otherwise further investigations or imaging is not indicated.[2]

Trevor needs reassurance that there is no underlying pathology to cause concern but the doctor should not dismiss the symptoms as insignificant or tell him glibly, 'Don't worry about it'. Tinnitus is a risk factor for suicide. It is important that the doctor accurately assess Trevor's psychological well-being and treat any associated anxiety or depression.[2] Management focuses on ways to habituate to the noises and using hearing protection to prevent exacerbation.[2, 3] Future options may include brain retraining, capitalising on brain plasticity.[4]

References

1. Rose, E 2011, 'Audiology', *Australian Family Physician,* vol. 40, no. 5, May, pp. 290-2.
2. Esmaili, A & Renton, J 2018, 'A review of tinnitus', *Australian Journal of General Practice,* vol. 474, pp. 205-8.
3. Flanagan, S 2013, 'How to treat: tinnitus', *Australian Doctor,* 5 July. Available at: www.ausdoc.com.au/therapy-update/treating-tinnitus, accessed 23 May 2019.
4. Lozano, AM 2011, 'Harnessing plasticity to reset dysfunctional neurons', *New England Journal of Medicine,* vol. 364, pp. 1367-8.

Case 29
Clayton Dixon

Instructions for the doctor

This is a short case.

Please take a history from Clayton's grandmother, Shirley Dixon. When you are ready, ask the facilitator to give you the results of an appropriate examination. No further investigations are available at this time.

Outline your differential diagnosis and management plan to the facilitator. The consultation takes place as a single session.

Scenario

Clayton Dixon is an 8-year-old Indigenous boy who lives with his grandmother, Shirley. They have been in the area for several years and often attend the accident and emergency department (ED) of the local hospital or a bulk-billing medical centre in town. You have some letters summarising his presentations to the ED but have no other notes. You have seen him for boils, scabies, chest infections and discharging ears, and he has been seen for similar presentations in the ED as well. Past medications include Flopen (flucloxacillin), Amoxil (amoxycillin), Kenacomb Otic (triamcinolone acetonide, neomycin, nystatin, gramicidin), Sofradex (dexamethasone, framycetin and gramicidin), Ascabiol (benzyl benzoate) and Lyclear (permethrin).

The following information is on his summary sheet:

Age
Eight
Past medical history
Chronic suppurative otitis media
Recurrent boils
Scabies

Upper and lower respiratory tract infections
Medication
No regular medications
Allergies
Nil known
Immunisations
Up-to-date
Social history
Lives with his grandmother, Shirley.

Instructions for the patient's grandmother, Shirley Dixon

You are Shirley Dixon, a 47-year-old married Indigenous woman who is bringing her 8-year-old grandson, Clayton, to the doctor because his ears are running again and you need more ear drops.

Clayton is assumed to be present.

Your opening line should be, 'I've got my grandson, Clayton, with me, Doctor. His ear is running again.'

You often look after Clayton and his little sister, Taneka, who is six years old. His mother struggles with alcohol and drugs and for the time being is living in another city. The authorities have never had any concerns about Clayton's welfare because you and your husband have stepped in whenever needed.

Clayton has always been thin. He has had recurrent boils, chesty coughs and runny ears. You have taken him to this clinic, another medical centre and the hospital emergency department. Currently his right ear has been running for the past two to three weeks. It's a thick, yellow discharge that comes out and stains his pillow and sheets. He says it sometimes hurts when he has infections, but he usually doesn't get a temperature.

If asked, Clayton's hearing hasn't been so good for the past few weeks. He does seem to get into trouble at school and has been suspended for poor behaviour a couple of times. He enjoys sport and playing outside with his friends but has never really liked school and doesn't do very well.

If asked, you have been using some ear drops you got from another doctor when his ears started running. You're not sure of the name but you think it is Keno-something. The bottle you had left over from a previous episode has just run out. You've had it lots of times in the past, as well as Sofra-something. Sometimes doctors give you an Amoxil mixture for Clayton to take as well, but you haven't got any at the moment. You use these drops when his ears run: two drops in the running ear, three or four times a day. Mostly you stop the drops when the ear stops running, but occasionally you have kept it going for a week or so to stop the infection coming back so quickly. You sometimes ring this clinic or the medical centre to get scripts for more ear drops without coming in. If asked, you've probably had one or two scripts for ear drops each month for the past six months.

If asked, Clayton has recently (for the last month or so) started complaining about ringing in his right ear and also some giddiness. You have noticed his balance isn't as good as it usually is.

If asked, you think his immunisations are up-to-date.

He has had a few chest infections, which have also required antibiotics. He's not on any other medications (apart from the drops you've been giving him) and has no allergies that you know of. You try to feed the children a healthy diet, but both Clayton and Taneka are very picky eaters, with a fondness for lollies. You sometimes suspect the healthy lunches you pack for school are traded for less healthy snacks.

At home with you, as well as Clayton and Taneka, is your husband, Gary. Your other children are grown and have left town—you see them for holidays.

If asked, neither you nor Gary are smokers and are both physically healthy.

The following information is on Clayton's summary sheet:

Age
Eight
Past medical history
Chronic suppurative otitis media
Recurrent boils
Scabies
Upper and lower respiratory tract infections
Medication
No regular medications
Allergies
Nil known
Immunisations
Up-to-date
Social history
Lives with his grandmother, Shirley.

Suggested approach to the case

Establish rapport
Open questions to explore Shirley's concerns.

Specific questions

History of the ear discharge
Pain
Hearing loss
Fever
Tinnitus/vertigo
Past (current) treatment
General health/diet
Social history
School performance (with respect to hearing loss)
Passive smoking
Medications/allergies.

Information for the facilitator

Clinical examination findings

General appearance: Indigenous male child of stated age in no distress
Height 135 cm (50th percentile)
Weight 27 kg (25th percentile)
BP 95/60 mmHg, no postural drop
Pulse 86/min regular
Temperature 37.4 tympanic (left ear)
ENT—throat normal, nose normal
External ear canals—right has purulent discharge; left normal
Tympanic membranes—right has suppurative otitis media with small inferior perforation; left is normal apart from some patches of tympanosclerosis
Cervical nodes normal
If asked, mastoid is normal
Gross hearing assessment indicates moderate hearing loss R > L
Chest/abdomen—NAD
Skin—several scars from previous infections, otherwise normal
Remainder of examination is normal.

Differential diagnoses

Chronic suppurative otitis media with perforation
Aminoglycoside ototoxicity
Possibility of cholesteatoma formation or suppurative labyrinthitis.

Management[1]

Cease aminoglycoside drops and caution against future use with signs of perforation

Regular ear toilet (Betadine 0.05% washes along with tissue ear spears)

Use of non-ototoxic fluoroquinolone drops (ciprofloxacin)

Oral antibiotics may benefit (amoxycillin)

Order appropriate investigations such as audiology, tympanometry

ENT referral

Scheduled GP follow-up

Encourage healthy diet.

CASE COMMENTARY

Chronic suppurative otitis media (CSOM) is a disease of poverty and represents a significant burden of disease for Indigenous Australians and refugee populations, with estimates of prevalence ranging from 15% to 80%. Complications include hearing loss, mastoiditis, cholesteatoma, facial nerve paralysis, meningitis, brain abscess and sigmoid sinus thrombosis. In children, hearing loss affects speech, language and intellectual, psychological and social development, as well as education.

Frequently, treatment is complicated by fragmented care, poor health literacy and issues with access to and cost of health care. In this case, Clayton is receiving treatment from a number of sources, including the local hospital and two different GP clinics. He has symptoms consistent with ototoxicity from repeated aminoglycoside ear drops in the presence of perforation. This is an uncommon but serious complication, and Australian recommendations include using non-ototoxic fluoroquinolone ear drops together with twice-daily ear cleaning, with weekly GP review and referral to ENT.[1]

Under the Pharmaceutical Benefits Scheme, ciprofloxacin ear drops are subsidised for Aboriginal and Torres Strait Islander people (aged one month or older).

Prevention principles include ensuring adequate nutrition, keeping immunisations up-to-date, encouraging nose blowing as well as breast-feeding of infants and avoiding passive smoking.

COMMON PITFALLS

It's easy to focus on treating the CSOM and perforation and to miss the subtle signs of ototoxicity. Instructing the carer in the techniques of ear cleaning is time consuming but important in Clayton's care. In a short case, reference could be made to the practice nurse instructing the grandmother how to use tissue ear spears and demonstrating the technique. Swabbing the discharge is unlikely to be helpful. We should be open about the iatrogenic complication of aminoglycoside ototoxicity, avoiding either a defensive or accusatory tone.

Reference

1. Indigenous and Rural Health Division 2015, 'Recommendations for clinical care guidelines on the management of Otitis Media in Aboriginal and Torres Strait Islander Populations', Department of Health, Canberra, ACT.

Further reading

Australian Institute of Health and Welfare 2018, '6.4 Ear health and hearing loss among Indigenous children', *Australia's Health 2018*. AIHW, Australia's health series no. 16, AUS 221, Canberra. Available at: www.aihw.gov.au/getmedia/12c11184-0c0a-43ad-8386-975c42c38105/aihw-aus-221-chapter-6-4.pdf.aspx, accessed 19 February 2019.

Closing the Gap Clearinghouse (AIHW & AIFS) 2014, 'Ear disease in Aboriginal and Torres Strait Islander children', resource sheet no. 35. Produced by the Closing the Gap Clearinghouse. Canberra: Australian Institute of Health and Welfare & Melbourne: Australian Institute of Family Studies.

Coates, H 2008, 'Ear drops and ototoxicity', *Australian Prescriber,* vol. 31, pp. 40–1.

'Deadly Ears, Queensland Health's Aboriginal and Torres Strait Islander Ear Health Program.' Available at: www.childrens.health.qld.gov.au/chq/our-services/community-health-services/deadly-ears/middle-ear-disease/, accessed 01 December 2018.

Hill, S 2012, 'Ear disease in Indigenous Australians: a literature review', *Australian Medical Student Journal,* vol. 3, no. 1, pp. 45–9.

Gunasekera, H, O'Connor, T, Vijayasekaran, S & Del Mar, C 2009, 'Primary care management of otitis media among Australian children', *Medical Journal of Australia,* vol. 191, no. 9, p. 55.

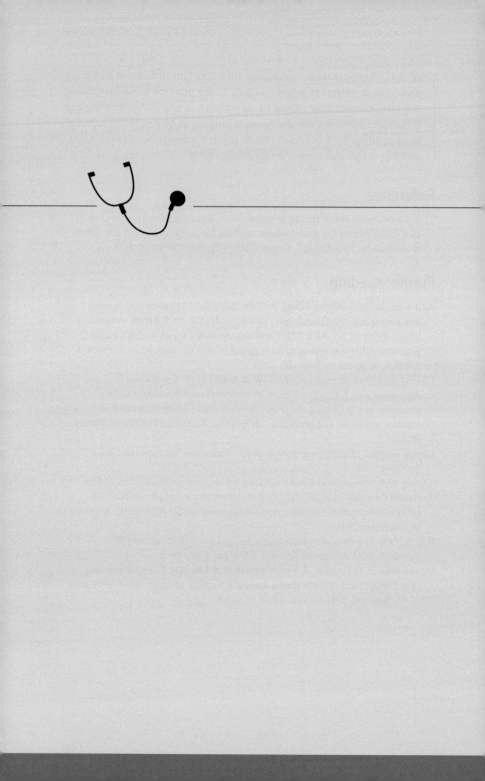

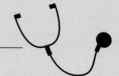

Section 9
Emergency medicine

Case 30
Catriona Chryssides

Instructions for the doctor

This is a short case about a new patient.

Please manage this medical emergency.

Scenario

Catriona Chryssides is a 29-year-old arts coordinator. You have been asked to see her as an emergency because of dizziness and palpitations on a Saturday morning.

You are doing a locum in a remote Aboriginal community. The clinic has a treatment room with emergency equipment and medication. The nearest hospital is 300 km away and patients requiring urgent hospital care are evacuated by the RFDS plane. Hospital specialists provide telephone advice if needed. An Aboriginal Health Practitioner is also working in the clinic.

The facilitator will give you the physical examination findings and the results of initial investigations when specifically requested.

Instructions for the patient, Catriona Chryssides

You have just moved to the area as an arts coordinator. You wanted a change of scene and to travel before your 30th birthday next month. It has been a major upheaval leaving your friends and family in the city. You are finding the work challenging and chaotic, and wonder if you will ever be able to make a worthwhile contribution.

It's Saturday morning. You started the day with a strong coffee and got up to go for a walk and felt fine. Suddenly you experienced a jolt in your heart and it feels as if it has gone haywire as it is pounding rapidly. You feel dizzy, unwell, a bit nauseated and frightened. You told your housemate how you felt and she promptly drove you down to the clinic.

You have never experienced anything like this before. You have no significant past medical history.

You smoke 10 cigarettes per day but do not consume alcohol or take recreational drugs.

Before leaving the city you made sure that you were up-to-date with your vaccinations and cervical screening test. You have a subcutaneous etonogestrel (Implanon) contraceptive implant.

You will suddenly feel well again when the doctor gives you the second injection.

Instructions for the facilitator

This scenario can be changed to assess the doctor's emergency skills in their own clinical setting, for example, the venue could be a small rural hospital or a suburban general practice.

The observations are:
- temperature normal (37.0°C)
- pulse 180 beats per minute, regularly regular rhythm by palpation
- 16 breaths a minute, no evidence of cyanosis
- BP 92/64 mmHg, sitting. JVP normal
- orientated to time, place and person.

Please show the candidate the ECG recording once the monitor is attached. (Refer to Figure 5, centre insert page C.) (Note: an ECG is given rather than just rhythm strip to enable the candidate to proceed with definitive treatment in the time available for the case.)

Ask the candidate for their diagnosis when they have looked at the ECG.

Sinus rhythm is restored after the second (12 mg) bolus of adenosine. When Catriona has returned to sinus rhythm ask the candidate to outline a future management plan.

Suggested approach to the case

Primary survey

DRABC

Danger—ensure safety of patient and personnel, move through to treatment room

Response—patient able to say name and describe symptoms of dizziness and 'heart racing'

Airway—patent as patient able to talk, no evidence of airway obstruction

Breathing—breathing regularly, no visible restriction to lung movement, give oxygen via mask

Circulation—pulse rapid

—Request Aboriginal Health Practitioner to check blood pressure; BP 92/64 mmHg

—Put on heart monitor and continue to monitor

—Request and interpret ECG

Patient assessed as having supraventricular tachycardia and is haemodynamically stable.

Focused history

Current symptoms—especially chest pain (nature of pain, radiation, etc.), shortness of breath, nature of palpitations (skipped beats, extra beats, etc.)

Risk factors for pulmonary embolism—recent travel, previous DVT

Any previous similar episodes of dizziness and chest discomfort and their treatment

Any family history of heart disease

Medication

Nil taken

Allergies

Nil known.

Treatment[1,2]

Valsalva manoeuvre and leg raise—no effect

Carotid sinus massage—no effect

Cold stimulus—not available

Insert IV cannula—take blood for FBC, UEC, troponin (TFTs can be delayed), magnesium, calcium

Intravenous adenosine as bolus of 6 mg, 12 mg, plus 20 mL saline flush (Note: if the candidate does not know the dose regime, it is acceptable for them to check this in a formulary)

Warning to patient of what to expect (sense of impending doom, or heart stopping)

Returns to sinus rhythm with resolution of symptoms after second bolus.

Further management

Finish secondary survey

Review history—history of palpitations

Explain what happened

Assess likely precipitants—caffeine intake, current stressors

Advice about manoeuvres to try if it recurs

Advise regarding work—unlikely to need time off

Driving—check in Austroads book/website[3]

ECG when in sinus rhythm to check for delta wave of
Wolf-Parkinson-White (WPW) syndrome.

Future management

Arrange follow-up and, if recurrent, other treatments available such as
medication or ablation

Health promotion—smoking cessation.

 CASE COMMENTARY

This scenario tests the doctor's ability to cope with an emergency situation. A logical and calm approach is needed and the doctor should proceed through DRABC in sequence. Some doctors who trialled this case argued that assessing Danger should not be needed when working in a clinic. They make a good point, but clinicians should consider staff and patient safety when responding to an emergency, especially as the realities of weekend on-call work when reduced staffing may mean omission of checks of emergency equipment.

This case also tests a doctor's ability to work well with the Aboriginal Health Practitioner and give clear instructions.

The doctor is expected to recognise the pattern of the SVT on the ECG and immediately commence vagal stimulation to try to revert the rhythm.[1] The order of pharmacological treatment is adenosine and then verapamil.[2] If these are ineffective, telephone advice should be sought about other options such as flecainide, sotalol or amiodarone[4] but availability of these drugs may be a problem. Not all clinics stock adenosine and so it is acceptable for a doctor to stabilise Catriona and arrange for the retrieval service to give adenosine on arrival.

DC reversion is reserved for patients who are haemodynamically unstable and require sedation. Longer-term recurrent SVT may be treated by ablation therapy.[5]

Once the emergency is under control, the doctor needs to consider other important aspects of care such as her fitness for work, driving, what to do if she has another episode and when she should be reviewed.

Doctors are not expected to remember the detail of the Austroads *Assessing Fitness to Drive* handbook[3] but must know to look at it for advice. Giving Catriona a copy of the arrhythmia captured on ECG is a practical tip that ensures it is available for health professionals in the future.[4]

References

1. Royal Australian College of General Practitioners 2018, 'Modified Valsalva manoeuvre for supraventricular tachycardia', *Handbook of Non-Drug Interventions* (HANDI), RACGP, Melbourne, Vic.
2. Medi, C, Kalman, JM & Freedman, SB 2009, 'Supraventricular tachycardia', *Medical Journal of Australia*, vol. 190, pp. 255–60.
3. Austroads and National Transport Commission 2017, *Assessing Fitness to Drive,* 5th ed, Sydney.
4. Whinnett, ZI, Sohaib, SM & Davies, DW 2012, 'Diagnosis and management of supraventricular tachycardia', *British Medical Journal,* vol. 345, p. e7769.
5. Lee, G, Sanders, P & Kalman, JM 2012, 'Catheter ablation of atrial arrhythmias: state of the art', *Lancet,* vol. 380, pp. 1509–19.

Case 31
Carrie Patterson

Instructions for the doctor

This is a short case.

Please manage this emergency.

Scenario

You are driving to work along the local high street. You see a cyclist swerve across the road and fall off her bicycle. You stop your car and grab your emergency equipment and drugs.

Instructions for the patient, Carrie Patterson

You are 28 years old and have had insulin-dependent diabetes for 15 years. You have just moved to this area for work as a barmaid. You enjoy the work but the late hours make it difficult to control your blood sugar.

You wear a medical alert bracelet on your wrist that says you are an insulin-dependent diabetic.

This morning you set off on your bike to do some shopping. You began to feel hypoglycaemic but did not have any snacks with you. One minute you were riding along, the next thing you know is that you're lying on the pavement next to your bicycle. This case begins with you lying beside your bicycle on the side of the road. A local GP comes up to you. You are able to say your name but mumble it slowly. If you are asked if you are diabetic, you can mumble 'Yes'.

You will recover quickly when the doctor gives you either:
- an injection of intravenous glucose
- an injection of glucagon IM, IV or SC, or
- oral/rectal glucose.

The following information is on your medical record at your own GP's surgery:

Past medical history

Insulin-dependent diabetes since age 13

Medication

Long-acting insulin glargine (Lantus 25 u at night)

Long-acting insulin mixed with short-acting insulin (Mixtard 30/70 42 u mane, 18 nocte)

Short-acting insulin (Novorapid 6–12 u before meals tds)

Allergies

Nil

Immunisations

Up-to-date

Social history

Employed as a barmaid.

Suggested approach to the case

Primary survey

DRABCDE

Danger—check for any danger at the scene, park car safely, use passers-by to divert traffic if repositioning the patient, make comment on spine precautions

Response—check for any response, person able to mumble their name

Airway—maintain cervical spine precautions

—Airway clear, as person able to mumble name

—Apply neck collar or manual in-line head and neck stabilisation

Breathing and ventilation—breathing regular and symmetrical with no added sounds

Circulation with haemorrhage control—ability to mumble name suggests brain perfusion

—No evidence of external haemorrhage

Disability—Glasgow Coma Scale 14

—Eye opening response—opens eyes spontaneously (4)

—Verbal response—says name, but not sure where they are and what happened (4)

—Motor response—does everything you ask (6)

Exposure/Environmental control

—Remove patient's clothes to enable a secondary survey, respecting their dignity

—Consider ambient temperature.

Secondary survey

History

AMPLE
A–no Allergies
M–Medication–insulin
P–Past history, injuries, hospital admissions
L–Last time ate or drank
E–Event
Top-to-toe examination including check for medical alert bracelet or identification
As soon as the doctor realises that the person is diabetic and on insulin, they should proceed with management of possible hypoglycaemia.

Treatment

- –Glucagon IV, IM or SC–adult dosage: 1 mg and/or
- –Glucose 50% IV at 3 mL/min via large vein–adult 20–50 mL depending on response
- –Offer slow-acting oral carbohydrate, such as bread, milk or fruit, once patient able to eat[1]

The scenario should finish with clearance from the scene and arrangement for transport to a hospital/clinic, preferably by ambulance
Full physical examination will be required in the hospital or clinic.

 CASE COMMENTARY

GPs should be equipped to cope with simple medical emergencies such as hypoglycaemia.[2] In urban areas, emergency care can often be provided more quickly by paramedics; in rural and remote Australia, the GP may be required to attend minor and major incidents at any time of night or day.[3] Tight glycaemic control reduces the long-term complications of diabetes but increases the risk of hypoglycaemia.[4]

 COMMON PITFALLS

Carrie's public hypoglycaemic episode means that emergency care needs to be given in a public space. However, the doctor needs to distinguish carefully between emergency care and routine ongoing care. The latter should be given by Carrie's GP of choice and in the privacy of the consulting room; this should include finding out reasons for the hypoglycaemic episode and assessing her fitness to drive[5] and work.

Apart from an imbalance between food intake and insulin dose, common causes of hypoglycaemia are unexpected extra exertion, alcohol and recreational drugs. Hypoglycaemia unawareness is more common in longer duration of diabetes, and in men and smokers.[1]

References

1. Craig, ME, Donaghue, KC, Cheung, NW, Cameron, FJ, Conn, J, Jenkins, AJ & Silink, M 2011, for the Australian Type 1 Diabetes Guidelines Expert Advisory Group. *National Evidence-Based Clinical Care Guidelines for Type 1 Diabetes for Children, Adolescents and Adults.* Australian Government Department of Health and Ageing, Canberra.
2. Baird, A 2008, 'Emergency drugs in general practice', *Australian Family Physician,* vol. 37, pp. 541–7.
3. The Royal Australian College of General Practitioners 2017, *Managing emergencies in general practice: A guide for preparation, response and recovery.* RACGP, East Melbourne, Vic, pp. 4–7.
4. Atkinson, MA, Eisenbarth, GS & Michels, AW 2014, 'Type 1 diabetes', *Lancet,* vol. 383, pp. 69–82.
5. National Diabetes Services Scheme 2011, *Diabetes and Driving,* Diabetes Australia.

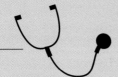

Section 10
Endocrinology

Case 32
Veronica Richards

Instructions for the doctor

This is a short case.

Please take a focused history from Veronica. Then ask the facilitator for the results of a relevant clinical examination and initial investigations.

Outline the diagnosis and your management plan to Veronica.

Scenario

Veronica Richards is 49 years old and has two teenage children. She grew up in the Philippines and has lived in Australia for the last 30 years. She came to you four weeks ago complaining of tiredness, at which time you provided some lifestyle advice.

The following information is on her summary sheet:

Past medical history
Two normal deliveries
Medication
Nil
Allergies
Nil
Immunisations
Up-to-date
Social history
Housewife, trained as a teacher
Non-smoker, no alcohol.

Instructions for the patient, Veronica Richards

You are 49 years old. You grew up in the Philippines and trained as a teacher. You have been in Australia for the past 30 years. You have two teenage children and are happily married. You are not depressed.

You saw your doctor four weeks ago complaining of tiredness, at which time your doctor suggested making some changes to diet and regular exercise. They suggested coming back for review if the tiredness continued, hence why you are here today—'I'm still tired, Doc'. You sleep well but don't have the energy you used to have. You have noticed the tiredness for about three months and it is getting worse.

Your periods are regular, not particularly heavy and you have no menopausal symptoms.

You eat a balanced diet, including red meat two or three times a week, and take your dog for a walk every day after the advice given last visit. You have put on a few kilos in the past year, including a further kilo since your last visit (despite eating healthier and exercising regularly). You have no night sweats or changes to your thirst, urine or bowel symptoms. If asked, you have noticed feeling the cold a little more than you usually would at this time of year.

The following information is on your summary sheet:

Past medical history
Two normal deliveries
Medication
Nil
Allergies
Nil
Immunisations
Up-to-date
Social history
Housewife, trained as a teacher
Non-smoker, no alcohol.

Instructions for the facilitator

Please give to the doctor on specific request.

Examination

Hydration good, no cyanosis, anaemia or jaundice
Weight 70.8 kg
Height 1.62 m
BMI 27 kg/m^2
Pulse 66 reg
BP 130/82 mmHg
No thyroid enlargement
No thyroid eye signs

Chest clear
Heart sounds normal
Abdomen soft, no masses, no organomegaly
Neurology—grossly normal, reflexes slow
Urine dipstick—negative.

Investigations

FBE, ESR or CRP—normal
UEC including calcium and magnesium—normal
LFTs—normal
Fasting blood sugar—normal
Urine for MCS—normal
Iron studies—normal
TSH   42.80 (0.3–4.0) mIU/L*
Free T$_4$ 8.0 (9.0–25.0) pmol/L*
Antithyroid peroxidase   345 (< 5.5) IU/mL*
Antithyroglobulin   23 (< 4.5) IU/mL*

Suggested approach to the case

Establish rapport.

History

Tiredness—character, duration
Exclude common/serious causes
    —Anaemia—diet, occult bleeding, heavy periods
    —Diabetes—excessive thirst, polyuria, nocturia
    —Menopause—skin changes, regularity of periods, flushing, sweats
    —Psychological—mood, affect, sleep, enjoyment of/satisfaction with
      life, relationships, stress
    —Thyroid—weight changes, skin changes, heat/cold intolerance, bowel
      changes
    —Occult malignancy—weight loss, cough, haemoptysis, date of last
      cervical screening test, breast symptoms, bowel changes, family
      history of cancer
Lifestyle factors
    —Ask about exercise, smoking, alcohol, drug use
Assess impact of tiredness on her, what treatments has she tried, is there
anything she is worried about?
Request permission to examine.

Examination

General appearance
Height/weight/BMI
BP and pulse
Thyroid examination
Cardiovascular and respiratory exam
Abdominal examination
Neurological exam
Urine dipstick.

Investigations

FBE, ESR or CRP
UEC including calcium and magnesium
LFTs
Fasting blood sugar
Urine for MCS
Iron studies
Thyroid function tests, request antibodies after abnormal thyroid function established.

Diagnosis

Hypothyroidism—auto-immune.

Management

Explain condition
Commence thyroxine
Need for regular blood tests and follow-up.

 CASE COMMENTARY

Tiredness is a common problem in general practice for which doctors need a system for assessment. This should be a stepped approach focusing on the common causes initially.[1] Australian research shows that testing is high[2] and few (3%) of patients have a significant clinical diagnosis based on an abnormal pathology test.[3] More elaborate tests risk false positives.[4] A watchful-waiting approach prior to ordering investigations is appropriate in the absence of red flags.[5]

Veronica has hypothyroidism. The doctor should explain that this is a common problem and can be treated with replacement thyroxine. Veronica will need ongoing follow-up to ensure that the correct dose is given. The most common cause of hypothyroidism in Australia is autoimmune chronic lymphocytic thyroiditis, characterised by raised circulating levels of thyroid peroxidase antibody.[6]

 COMMON PITFALLS

The doctor should avoid prematurely attributing the tiredness to Veronica's 'time of life'. Equally it is realistic to tell patients that the chance of finding treatable cause is low. This lays the foundation for taking a holistic approach to address psychological issues,[7] work/life balance and expectations, sleep, diet and exercise.[8]

References

1. Murtagh, J 2003, 'Fatigue: a general diagnostic approach', *Australian Family Physician,* vol. 32, no. 11, pp. 873–6.
2. Harrison, M 2008, 'Pathology testing in the tired patient: a rational approach', *Australian Family Physician,* vol. 37, no. 11, pp. 908–10.
3. Gialamas, A, Beilby, J & Pratt, NL et al. 2003, 'Investigating tiredness in Australian general practice. Do pathology tests help in diagnosis?' *Australian Family Physician,* vol. 32, no. 8, pp. 663–6.
4. Koch, H, van Bokhoven, MA et al. 2009, 'Ordering blood tests for patients with unexplained fatigue in general practice: what does it yield? Results of the VAMPIRE trial', *British Journal of General Practice,* vol. 59, no. 561, pp. e93–100.
5. Wilson, J, Morgan, S, Magin, PJ & van Driel, M 2014, 'Fatigue—a rational approach to investigation', *Australian Family Physician,* vol. 43, no. 7, pp. 457–61.
6. So, M, MacIsaac, RJ & Grossmann, M 2012, 'Hypothyroidism—investigation and management', *Australian Family Physician,* vol. 41, no. 8, pp. 556–62.
7. Dick, ML & Sundin, J 2003, 'Psychological and psychiatric causes of fatigue. Assessment and management', *Australian Family Physician,* vol. 32, no. 11, pp. 877–81.
8. Rosenthal, TC, Majeroni, BA, Pretorious, R & Malik K 2008, 'Fatigue: an overview', *American Family Physician,* vol. 78, no. 10, pp. 1173–9.

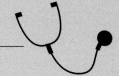

Section 11
Eyes

Case 33
Edward Galloway

Instructions for the doctor

This is a short case.

Please take a history from Edward, examine him and tell him the most likely diagnosis and your recommended management.

Scenario

Edward Galloway is a 66-year-old retired fireman. He spends much of his time fishing and playing golf and he has noticed increased watering of both eyes when he goes outside. He finds this frustrating and embarrassing and is thinking of stopping golf as sometimes it is so hard to see the ball.

He has decided to come to his usual GP for help.

The following information is on his summary sheet:

Past medical history

Transurethral resection of the prostate two years ago

Skin graft following extensive burn to left lower leg in a fire 10 years ago

Medication

Nil

Allergies

Nil

Immunisations

Up-to-date

Family history

Both parents died in their mid-80s

Mother had glaucoma

Social history

Retired fireman

Non-smoker, alcohol consumption unknown.

Instructions for the patient, Edward Galloway

You are a 66-year-old retired fireman. You spend much of your time fishing and playing golf and have noticed increased watering of both eyes when you go outside. You find this frustrating and embarrassing and are thinking of stopping golf as sometimes it is so hard to see the ball.

You decide to see your usual GP for help.

In the latter part of her life your mother was partially sighted due to glaucoma. You have heard that this runs in the family and are worried that this is what's causing the watering. You will only admit to this if the doctor is sensitive and empathic in their approach to you.

You have difficulty seeing at times because of the watering but your vision is 6/6 bilaterally when you wear your glasses.

The following information is on your summary sheet:

Past medical history

Transurethral resection of the prostate two years ago

Skin graft following extensive burn to left lower leg in a fire 10 years ago

Medication

Nil

Allergies

Nil

Immunisations

Up-to-date

Family history

Both parents died in their mid-80s

Mother had glaucoma

Social history

Retired fireman

Non-smoker, alcohol consumption unknown.

Suggested approach to the case

Introduction

Establish rapport

Open questions to allow Edward to tell his story.

Specific questions

Eyes watering—timing

Any discharge, eyes sticky or gritty in the morning

Exclude pain or visual disturbance

Treatments tried so far
Date of most recent optometry check-up—including screening for glaucoma
Confirm not on any medication, check OTC medications, e.g. decongestants
Request permission to examine.

Examination

Visual acuity and fields to confrontation
Conjunctivae and sclerae
Eyelids/lashes (exclude blepharitis), if lid eversion attempted facilitator to
    state this is normal and not necessary to perform
Pupil size, shape and reaction to light
Fluoroscein stain—need to ask to do but not expected to perform in the
    time available
Fundoscopy—need to ask to do but not expected to perform in the time
    available
All findings normal apart from mild conjunctival injection both eyes.

Most likely diagnosis

Dry eyes—age-related.

Management

Explain dry eyes[1]
Reassure unlikely to be glaucoma but still needs at least annual checks
    with optometrist
Recommend
    —Blink more
    —Trial of humidifiers
    —Regular use of tear ointment at night and drops during the day
    —Bathing of eyelid margins to encourage flow of oily tears
    —Arrange follow-up
    —Future options for severe symptoms could be discussed, e.g.
        tetracyclines, punctal plugs.[2]

 CASE COMMENTARY

> Dry eyes are a common problem in the elderly that can readily be
> diagnosed and treated in general practice. The GP will be able to get
> Edward back to regular golf and reassure him that these symptoms do

not indicate that he is getting glaucoma. However, Edward will require regular optometry checks on his eye pressure and visual fields.

As people age, less oily tears are produced. This reduced lubrication is felt particularly when outside, in arid areas and in air-conditioned rooms. The surface of the eye senses the dryness and reflex tearing (watery tears) occurs. Treatment is aimed at optimising the production of oily tears by bathing the eyelids, clearing any duct blockages and replacing the oily tears with artificial tears.

It is counter-intuitive to offer artificial tears to someone with watery eyes but is a simple way of improving someone's quality of life. Sometimes the preservatives in eye drops can irritate eyes further. If this is the case, or if frequent use is required, a preservative-free preparation should be recommended.[3]

 ## COMMON PITFALLS

Edward reports that he sometimes cannot see when he is playing golf. It is easy to assume that this is a problem with his visual acuity when in fact it is just that the excess watery tears reduce his vision. Careful questioning and assessment of visual acuity is needed to clarify the problem.

References

1. Hodge, C & Sutton, G 2003, 'Dry eyes: eye series 3', *Australian Family Physician,* vol. 32, no. 4, pp. 265–6.
2. Lemp, MA 2008, 'Advances in understanding and managing dry eye disease', *American Journal of Ophthalmology,* vol. 146, no. 3, pp. 350–6.
3. *British Medical Journal* 2016, 'The management of dry eye', vol. 353, pp. i2333.

Case 34
Henrik Schneider

Instructions for the doctor

This is a short case.

Please take a focused history from Henrik and look at a photograph of his eyes. (Refer to Figures 6 and 7, centre insert page D.) Please describe the eye signs on the photograph to the facilitator. You can ask the facilitator for other examination findings. You are expected to tell Henrik the most likely diagnosis and outline your initial management.

Scenario

You are working as a GP locum at a well-equipped clinic five hours drive away from the nearest base hospital. An Austrian tourist Henrik Schneider, aged 25, telephones you at 6.30 am saying he needs an urgent consultation for his painful, red, blurry right eye and you agree to see him. He is leaving in an hour for the town where the base hospital is located.

Henrik does not take any medication, has no known allergies and no significant past medical history.

Instructions for the patient, Henrik Schneider

You are a 25-year-old student backpacking around Australia. Yesterday your right eye became painful, the vision was a bit blurred and the eye looked red when you looked in the mirror at the hostel. You thought it might be due to your contact lenses, and so started to wear your glasses.

This morning you are due to travel five hours in a coach to the nearest town with a hospital. However, your eye is now more painful and the vision more blurred so you decide to see the resident GP as soon as possible. Bright lights make the eye more painful.

You have not had this eye problem before and have not injured the eye or got anything in it.

You do not take any medication, have no known allergies and have no significant past medical history.

Instructions for the facilitator

Clinical examination findings

When the doctor asks to examine the eye, please show them the photographs.
(Refer to Figures 6 and 7 (with fluorescein), centre insert page D.)
Visual acuity
—Left eye 6/12 uncorrected, 6/6 corrected through pinhole
—Right eye 6/18 uncorrected, 6/18 corrected through pinhole
Pupils—as per photograph, photophobia on examination
Eversion of lids: no foreign body.

Suggested approach to the case

Establish rapport
Open-ended questions to explore Henrik's ideas, concerns and expectations.

Specific questions

Pain
Vision
Redness
Photophobia
Exclude pus-like discharge
Exclude itching
Exclude foreign body or eye injury
Confirm normally wears contact lenses
Previous history of eye problems
Request permission to examine.

Examination

Visual acuity
Observe photograph, candidate should note
—Distribution of erythema—circumcorneal
—Anterior chamber clear/no hypopyon

–Cornea–no fluorescein uptake (excludes dendritic ulcer or corneal abrasion secondary to extruded foreign body or contact lens problem)

–Pupil size and reactions to light–pupil smaller on right and irregular

Check for foreign body, including everting upper lids

Check for photophobia.

Most likely diagnosis

Iritis (acute anterior uveitis) of right eye.

Management

Explain condition

Discuss with ophthalmologist at base hospital and arrange referral and review

Commence topical steroids if available

Not to wear contact lenses until ophthalmologist confirms it is safe to do so.

 CASE COMMENTARY

'Beware the unilateral red eye.' Most common eye problems in general practice affect both eyes so the history of a unilateral red eye is significant. Henrik also has the three sentinel warning signs of pain, photophobia and blurred vision. The presence of one or more of these symptoms should prompt urgent assessment. Misdiagnosis of anterior uveitis/iritis is common, and a delay of even a few days can lead to irreversible vision loss.

The doctor should ask about a history of a foreign body or eye injury. Contact lenses increase the risk of corneal ulcers, which can become infected.

A pinhole creates a very narrow light path that requires little focusing prior to hitting the retina and so demonstrates the potential corrected visual acuity. Henrik's reduced vision in the right eye is not corrected by using a pinhole. This shows the loss of vision in the right eye is not due to a refractive error, so the doctor must look carefully for an ocular problem.

Starting topical steroids in the eye is potentially dangerous and it is essential that the doctor excludes a herpetic cause of the problem before commencing treatment, specifically by looking for a dendritic ulcer on fluorescein staining. If possible discuss the case with a specialist ophthalmologist. However, the distance between the patient and the base hospital means that the GP needs to start steroids to prevent further exacerbation of the iritis.

Further reading

Cronau, H, Kankanala, RR & Mauger, T 2010, 'Diagnosis and management of red eye in primary care', *American Family Physician,* vol. 81, no. 2, pp. 137–44.

Durkin, SR & Casey, TM 2005, 'Beware of the unilateral red eye: don't miss blinding uveitis', *Medical Journal of Australia,* vol. 182, no. 6, pp. 296–7.

Statham, MO, Sharma, A & Pane, AR 2008, 'Misdiagnosis of acute eye diseases by primary health care providers: incidence and implications', *Medical Journal of Australia,* vol. 189, no. 7, pp. 402–4.

Case 35
Roger Chin

Instructions for the doctor

This is a short case.

Please take a focused history. Request the findings of an appropriate physical examination. Explain your management to Roger.

Scenario

Roger Chin is a 57-year-old financial planner who is a regular patient of the practice. He is generally healthy and is on perindopril (Coversyl) for hypertension. He is happily married with three grown children and two grandchildren. Along with most of his family he does get classic migraines but rarely in recent years. He called early this morning and asked to be seen urgently.

The following information is on his summary sheet:

Age
57
Past medical history
Hypertension
Migraine with aura
Medication
Perindopril 5 mg mane
Eletriptan (Relpax) 40 mg stat prn
Allergies
Nil known
Immunisations
Up-to-date

Social history
Married to Dorothy
Non-smoker
Occasional alcohol
Family history
Hypertension
Migraine.

Instructions for the patient, Roger Chin

Last night you noticed intermittent bright flashes in the temporal field of your left eye, 'a bit like lightning bolts'. It was provoked by moving your eye and was worse when you turned the light out. You were looking out the window and thought it was lightning but then noticed it inside the house as well.

The bright flashes have gone, but you now have a blurry floating opacity in the middle of your left eye's vision. It wafts around with the movement of your eye. You called the surgery for an urgent appointment as you were worried.

In answer to specific questioning:
There is no pain; no headache; you have not had this before. The only trouble you have had with your eyes is that you are short-sighted and wear glasses. They were last checked about 18 months ago and your prescription adjusted slightly. There has been no trauma or injury. Apart from your 'floater' you are not aware of any visual problem. Your migraine auras generally consist of bright zigzag lines in your vision that disappear after 10–15 minutes: they are unlike what you experienced last night.

If ophthalmological review is suggested, say something like: 'My office is really busy at the moment. Can it be delayed until next week?'

Ask what the doctor thinks is going on and (if referred) what the specialist will do. If surgery is mentioned, ask if you will need a general anaesthetic or, if not, whether it will hurt.

The following information is on your summary sheet:
Age
57
Past medical history
Hypertension
Classic migraine
Medication
Perindopril 5 mg mane
Eletriptan (Relpax) 40 mg stat prn

Allergies
Nil known
Immunisations
Up-to-date
Social history
Married to Dorothy
Non-smoker
Occasional safe alcohol
Family history
Hypertension
Migraine.

Suggested approach to the case

The key tasks are to take a focused history to separate the different causes of flashes and floaters, followed by a relevant physical examination, and a simple, clear explanation of the likely condition and its management for the patient. The most likely diagnosis in this setting is posterior vitreous detachment (PVD) with a possible retinal tear and associated vitreous haemorrhage. Prompt treatment is required to prevent progression to retinal detachment. Candidate's explanation should include the distinction between PVD and retinal detachment.

Roger's requests to defer because of a busy work schedule should be met with a clear explanation of the possible implications of deferring treatment. Points to address in the history include:
- details of the flashes and floater
- visual change especially field loss
- pain
- risk factors (myopia)
- brief general health screen.

Physical examination should include:
- general appearance
- vital signs
- visual acuity +/− glasses
- visual fields
- pupil response for relative afferent pupillary defect.

Management should include:
- explanation of the significance of his symptoms and the likely diagnosis i.e. PVD with vitreous haemorrhage and possible retinal tear. The risk and significance of retinal detachment should be discussed

- urgent referral (same day) to ophthalmologist
- an outline of the likely treatment i.e. retinal tear surrounded with laser burns to create a chorio-retinal scar that prevents fluid seeping into the sub-retinal space. This can be as an outpatient under topical anaesthesia and is relatively painless
- follow-up and safety netting.

Physical examination

General appearance: 'As you see him'
Vital signs
    −HR 70/min regular
    −BP 130/78 mmHg
    −Temp 36.1°C
    −BMI 26 kg/m^2
    −RR 12/min
Eye examination: (each item to be asked for individually)
Appearance: normal
Red reflex present bilaterally
Pupils equal, round and reactive to light and accommodation with no relative afferent pupil defect
Visual acuity
    −Uncorrected: L = R = both = 6/24
    −Corrected: L = 6/12; R = 6/7.5 both = 6/7.5
Visual fields by confrontation: normal
Fundoscopy (un-dilated pupil) is unremarkable
Cardiovascular exam: normal
Remainder of physical examination is normal
Surgery tests: BSL (random) 5.6 mmol/L
U/A: normal.

 CASE COMMENTARY

Acute onset of monocular floaters and/or flashes commonly present to GPs and the most likely diagnosis in this setting is posterior vitreous detachment (PVD). Although the majority of cases of PVD are benign, a significant proportion of patients with acute PVD develop an associated retinal tear that can lead to retinal detachment and permanent vision loss if left untreated. The sudden appearance of Roger's floater following immediately after his flashes is strongly suggestive of a retinal tear and associated vitreous haemorrhage. If retinal tears are not treated, one-third to one-half of cases will progress to retinal detachment, which can result in permanent visual loss.[1, 2]

The role of GPs is to make the diagnosis of probable PVD and to identify patients at increased risk of retinal tear and detachment based on history and physical examination to determine the urgency of ophthalmologic assessment.

As a minimum approach, candidates should take a history of change in vision, check visual acuity, and assess visual fields. Having recognised Roger's high-risk features for retinal tear he should have same-day assessment by an ophthalmologist. PVD is a common degenerative condition and should not be confused with retinal detachment. The explanation to Roger should demonstrate an understanding of the pathophysiology and difference between the two conditions. An intimate knowledge of the treatment of retinal tears is not required but Roger's simple questions about what is involved should be answered.

If Roger is subsequently found to have an uncomplicated PVD, he is at risk of subsequently developing a retinal tear and detachment over the next several weeks and requires follow-up.

One variation on the case would be to make it a long case and require candidates to conduct the clinical examination.

 ## COMMON PITFALLS

Eye symptoms may represent relatively benign conditions or serious conditions requiring urgent care. Taking a further history of eye complaints like flashes and floaters can help establish the diagnosis and therefore the urgency of further treatment if required. Not all floaters and/or flashes represent ocular problems, and non-ocular causes can usually be identified by taking a careful history. Roger's past history of migraine with aura represents a possible masquerade in this case and should be excluded based on the history.

Roger's normal visual acuity, fields and normal eye examination findings are consistent with PVD with associated vitreous haemorrhage and retinal tear, and should not delay urgent referral.

Many GPs are aware that there are serious conditions among these presentations and therefore are quick to refer without properly exploring the history or performing an appropriate physical examination. Patient explanation should clearly distinguish PVD from a retinal tear and retinal detachment.

References

1. Kahawita, S, Simon, S & Gilhotra, J 2014, 'Flashes and floaters. A practical approach to assessment and management', *Australian Family Physician,* April, vol. 43, no. 4, pp. 201-3. Available at: www.racgp.org.au/afp/2014/april/flashes-and-floaters/, accessed 25 February 2019.
2. Hollands, H, Johnson, D, Brox, AC, Almeida, D, Simel, DL & Sharma, S 2009, 'Acute-onset floaters and flashes: is this patient at risk for retinal detachment?', *Journal of the American Medical Association,* 25 November, vol. 302, no. 20, pp. 2243-9.

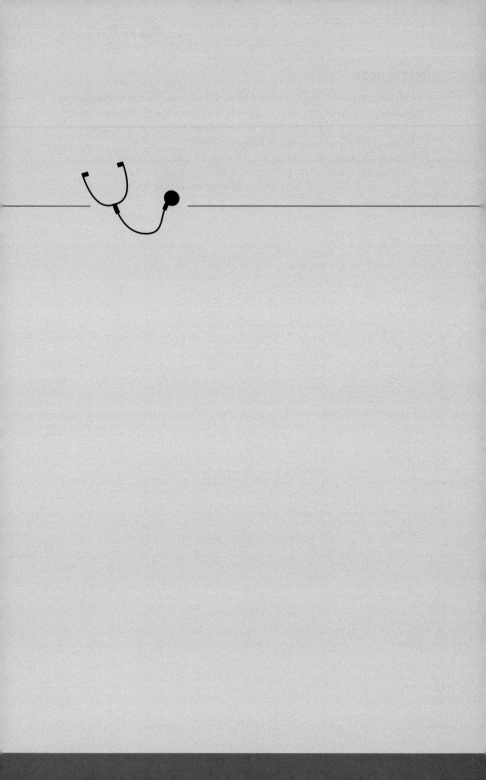

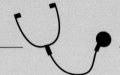

Section 12
Gastroenterology

Case 36
Jenna Banks

Instructions for the doctor

This is a short case.

Please take a history from Jenna and then ask the facilitator for the results of a focused examination. Tell Jenna the most likely diagnosis and your initial management plan.

Scenario

Jenna Banks is a 25-year-old tax manager studying for her chartered accountancy exams. You last saw her for contraception. She is coming to see you today because of recurrent abdominal pain and bloating.

The following information is on her summary sheet:

Past medical history
Fracture left humerus aged eight, from a rollerblading accident
Medication
On contraceptive pill
Levonorgestrel 150 mcg, ethinyloestradiol 30 mcg (Levlen ED)
Allergies
Nil known
Immunisations
Up-to-date
Cervical screen
Normal a few months ago
Family history
Parents both alive and well
Social history
Non-smoker
Alcohol—two standard drinks on two occasions per week.

Instructions for the patient, Jenna Banks

You are a 25-year-old tax manager studying for your chartered accountancy exams. Your abdominal pains started after you contracted traveller's diarrhoea during a trip to Bali six months ago. You saw a GP when your pain symptoms weren't improving and stool tests were negative for infection. Things have been worsening over the last few months as your stress regarding your accountancy exams has increased. Most days of the week you experience bouts of abdominal pain, bloating and flatus. The pain can be so severe that you need to lie down but mostly you can continue at work. The pain comes on at any time during the day, and is a squeezing, cramp-like pain, usually in the left or right side of your abdomen. The pain is sometimes relieved by defecating. You have never woken at night with symptoms.

You have not lost weight, been nauseated or vomited. Your bowel habit alternates between constipation (hard, rabbit-like pellets) and diarrhoea. You do not pass any blood or mucus rectally. You have not noticed any particular food triggers. You have tried some herbal remedies which did not improve your symptoms.

You are stressed and anxious regarding your exams, but are not depressed. You have no past history of anxiety or depression.

Your periods are regular on the contraceptive pill, and your bowel symptoms do not worsen with your menstrual cycle.

You want the doctor to make sure that you have nothing seriously wrong with you and to tell you what the problem is.

The following information is on your summary sheet:
Past medical history
Fracture left humerus aged eight, from a rollerblading accident
Medication
Levonorgestrel 150 mcg, ethinyloestradiol 30 mcg (Levlen ED)
Allergies
Nil known
Immunisations
Up-to-date
Cervical screen
Normal a few months ago
Family history
Parents both alive and well
Social history
Non-smoker
Alcohol—two standard drinks on two occasions per week.

185

Instructions for the facilitator

All physical examination findings are normal. Please give the following clinical examination findings on specific request:

- temperature, pulse, BP all normal
- looks well
- no hand or nail changes
- no jaundice or anaemia
- abdominal examination—no tenderness, no masses, normal rectal examination.

Suggested approach to the case

Establish rapport
Open questions to explore Jenna's ideas, concerns and expectations.

Specific questions

Pain
Bowel habit, including symptoms of urgency and faecal incontinence
Bloating
Exclude PR blood or mucus
Flatulence/belching
Nocturnal symptoms
Explore specific dietary triggers for symptoms, e.g. lactose, wheat/gluten, onions/garlic
Exclude other systemic symptoms including weight loss
Menstrual history—exclude relationship of symptoms to menstrual periods
Check current medication use, including over-the-counter and complementary medicines
Recent travel or gastroenteritis
Determine impact of symptoms on Jenna's life and impact of stress on symptoms
Exclude relevant family history, e.g. bowel cancer, inflammatory bowel disease
Request permission to examine.

Examination

Hands, face, mouth—normal
Abdominal and rectal examination—normal.

Most likely diagnosis

Irritable bowel syndrome.

Management

Provide explanation of the condition and reassurance, without minimising the impact of symptoms on quality of life

Targeted investigations: FBE, iron studies, ESR or CRP, coeliac serology including IgA

Suggestions for symptomatic management

–Modify diet–trial of increase in soluble fibre, trial of low FODMAPs diet

–Increase exercise

–Reduce volume of carbonated drinks

–Medication–antispasmodics (including peppermint oil or mebeverine), psyllium/ispaghula if constipation predominant, probiotics if diarrhoea or bloating predominant, tricyclic antidepressants[1]

–Psychological and behavioural therapy, such as cognitive behavioural therapy, relaxation therapy and mindfulness

Referral–consider referral to allied health professionals to help address above recommendations. Specialist gastroenterologist referral not required in the absence of red flags

Arrange follow-up.

 CASE COMMENTARY

Irritable bowel syndrome (IBS) is a common problem that accounts for 0.3 per 100 patient presentations in Australian general practice.[2] IBS is diagnosed using the Rome IV criteria, based on the clinical features of recurrent abdominal discomfort or pain related to defecation or associated with altered bowel habits. Symptoms must be chronic, occurring at least once per week, on average in the previous three months, with a duration of at least six months.[1]

The candidate should enable Jenna to tell her story about the symptoms, and check that there are no alarm symptoms, such as weight loss, nocturnal symptoms or rectal bleeding. The examination should focus only on a check of the hands, the face and the abdomen. Limited investigation to exclude relevant differential diagnoses (including coeliac disease) is appropriate. A poor candidate may initiate a large number of investigations or suggest early referral to a gastroenterologist.

Traditionally, IBS has been a diagnosis of exclusion, however current recommendations suggest that in a patient who has symptoms meeting

Rome IV criteria without alarm symptoms, a positive diagnosis should be made without resorting to a battery of tests.[2, 3] Early provision of a diagnosis which is clearly communicated is important to avoid a prolonged search for an alternative explanation and delay of effective management.[3]

The pathophysiology of IBS is complex and heterogeneous. Postulated mechanisms include disorders of the gut–brain axis; diet; genetic factors; infections and disturbances in the intestinal microbiota; low-grade mucosal inflammation, immune activation, and altered intestinal permeability; disordered bile salt metabolism; abnormalities in serotonin metabolism; and alterations in brain function.[4] While traditionally conceptualised as a brain–gut disorder due to the high association with coexisting psychological conditions and childhood trauma, it has now been shown that in at least a subset of patients the gastrointestinal changes happen prior to psychological distress developing later, suggesting the association happens both ways. Intestinal inflammation, the cytokine response and the microbiome have been suggested to precipitate such gut-to-brain changes in IBS.[1, 4]

The heterogeneity in both the pathogenesis and the symptomatology of IBS makes a 'one size fits all' approach to management difficult. A modified exclusion diet and stepwise reintroduction of foods containing gluten or fermentable dietary oligosaccharides, disaccharides, monosaccharides and polyols (FODMAPs) may be useful. This is best done under the guidance of a dietician.[5] Soluble fibre such as psyllium can help some patients (noting that insoluble fibres such as bran can exacerbate pain and bloating).[1] Antispasmodics (including peppermint oil and mebeverine), probiotics, tricylic antidepressants, exercise and psychological therapies can be effective in the treatment of IBS.[1, 3]

References

1. Ford, AC, Lacy, BE & Talley, NJ 2017, 'Irritable bowel syndrome', *New England Journal of Medicine,* vol. 376, pp. 2566–78.
2. Charles, J & Harrison, C 2006, 'Irritable bowel syndrome in Australian general practice', *Australian Family Physician,* vol. 35, pp. 840–1.
3. Linedale, EC & Andrews, JM 2017, 'Diagnosis and management of irritable bowel syndrome: a guide for the generalist', *Medical Journal of Australia,* vol. 207, pp. 309–15.
4. Holtmann, GJ, Ford, AC & Talley, NJ 2016, 'Pathophysiology of irritable bowel syndrome', *Lancet Gastroenterology & Hepatology,* vol. 1, pp. 133–46.
5. Bolin, T 2009, 'IBS or intolerance?', *Australian Family Physician,* vol. 38, pp. 962–5.

Case 37
Enrico Castallani

Instructions for the doctor

This is a long case.

Please take a history, conduct an appropriate examination and then outline your management plan to Mr Castallani.

Scenario

Enrico Castallani is the licensee of the local hotel. He rarely comes to the surgery, although you know that he has been in town for over two years now. Today he has asked for an urgent appointment because of bad abdominal pain. You agree to see him and note the following information on his medical records.

The following information is on his summary sheet:

Past medical history
MVA 2015—sustained no injuries, cause of accident unclear
Medications
Nil recorded
Allergies
Nil known
Immunisations
Nil known
Social history
Local hotelier
Lives with de facto partner.

Instructions for the patient, Enrico Castallani

You have been the licensee of a hotel for the last two years. You rarely see the doctor. Today you have asked for an urgent appointment because of bad abdominal pain.

For the last 24 hours you have experienced constant severe abdominal pain, which radiates through to your back. The pain has been so bad that you can't work or walk. You have come today because your partner has persuaded you. You have been vomiting and are off your food. You cannot get comfortable, and you are sweating and feel generally weak.

You have not vomited blood and have no symptoms or signs of liver failure. You are very sensitive about your alcohol problem and will only open up about this if the doctor approaches the issue in a non-judgemental manner.

You have a long-term drinking problem. Both your parents were alcoholics and although you saw the impact of alcohol on them, you started drinking at a young age. You have had a series of jobs working in the hospitality industry. You left your last job in a hurry as you had a car accident while drunk. No one was injured in the crash, but there was significant damage to the car and public property; the police were never able to establish a cause, but you left the town to escape suspicion.

For the past few months you have switched to drinking port rather than wine. You have about a cask a day.

The following information is on your summary sheet:

Past medical history
MVA 2015—sustained no injuries, cause of accident unclear

Medication
Nil recorded

Allergies
Nil known

Immunisations
Nil known

Social history
Local hotelier
Lives with de facto partner.

Instructions for the facilitator

This is a case of acute pancreatitis. Please give the candidate the following examination findings on specific request.

Clinical examination findings

Temperature 38.0°C, sweating
Pulse 110 regular
BP 116/80 mmHg
Abdomen—guarded, with tenderness maximal in periumbilical region.

Suggested approach to the case

Establish rapport
Open questions about abdominal pain.

Specific questions

Nature of pain and radiation
Absence of haematemesis
Vomiting and nausea—present
Absence of melaena or blood in stool or change in bowel habit
Absence of symptoms of liver disease—no jaundice
Absence of symptoms of gallstones
Explore alcohol consumption and motivation for change—negotiate a
    follow-up plan
Discuss need for overall health check at some stage
Request permission to examine.

Examination

Temperature 38.0°C, sweating
BP 116/80 mmHg
Pulse 110
Height 1.78 m
Weight 92 kg
BMI 29 kg/m^2
Hands normal, no liver flap, no jaundice
Examination of abdomen
    —Severe abdominal pain with guarding, rebound and rigidity
    —Pain hypogastrium
    —Absence of ascites, hepatomegaly
    —Bowel sounds—reduced
Lungs clear
BSL 4.5 mmol/L
Urine—NAD.

Management

Arrange analgesia
Nil by mouth
Admission to hospital—transfer by ambulance essential
Commence intravenous fluids
Give oxygen
Explain to patient procedure for admission and rationale.

Initial investigations

Lipase levels; complete blood count with differential; biochemistry (blood urea, creatinine, glucose, liver function tests and calcium levels); triglyceride level; urinalysis; and arterial blood gases and imaging (ultrasound scan +/− CT/MRI)[1, 2]

Explore social impact of admission—who will run the pub?

CASE COMMENTARY

The doctor is expected to make the provisional diagnosis of pancreatitis and arrange for urgent admission to hospital via ambulance. A useful acronym for possible causes of pancreatitis is **GET SMASHED**.[3]

Gallstones

Ethanol

Trauma

Steroids

Mumps

Auto-immune

Scorpion venom

Hyperlipidaemia, hypothermia, hypercalcaemia

ERCP (endoscopic retrograde cholangiopancreatography) and emboli

Drugs, e.g. azathioprine

The commonest causes in the Australian population are alcohol and gallstones.

A good doctor will establish rapport with Mr Castallani and explore his alcohol consumption in a non-judgemental manner. The **CAGE** questionnaire is a useful tool for diagnosing alcoholism. The questions focus on **C**utting down, **A**nnoyance by criticism, **G**uilty feeling and **E**ye-openers.[4] Arrangements for another appointment should be suggested to discuss Mr Castallani's drinking. Even if the admission shows that the pancreatitis was due to another cause, such as gallstones, this level of drinking is harmful.

References

1. Basnayake, C & Ratnam, D 2015, 'Blood tests for acute pancreatitis', *Australian Prescriber,* vol. 38, no. 4, pp. 128–30.
2. Nesvaderani, M, Eslick, G & Cox, M 2015, 'Acute pancreatitis: update on management', *Medical Journal of Australia,* vol. 202, no. 8, pp. 420–3.
3. Wilkinson, I, Raine, T, Wiles, K, Goodhart, A, Hall, C & O'Neill, H 2017, *Oxford Handbook of Clinical Medicine,* 10th ed, University Press, Oxford.
4. Ewing, J 1984, 'Detecting alcoholism: the CAGE questionnaire', *Journal of the American Medical Association,* vol. 252, pp. 1905–7.

Case 38
Kirrilee DeMarco

Instructions for the doctor

This is a long case.

Please take a history and conduct an appropriate examination. The observing examiner will give you specific examination findings and the results of your initial investigations on request.

Discuss your differential diagnosis and negotiate a management plan with Kirrilee.

Scenario

Kirrilee is a 23-year-old fashion designer. She presents to you with a three-week story of abdominal pain.

She is a new patient at the practice and so no past medical history is available.

Instructions for the patient, Kirrilee DeMarco

You are a 23-year-old fashion designer. You live with your female partner, Natalie, who is a nurse.

In the last three weeks you have had abdominal pain. At times the pain is severe. Since the pain started, you have needed to rush to the toilet, and have been passing loose bowel motions at least three times a day. On a couple of occasions, you have been woken from sleep with pain and a need to pass bowel motions. Last week you noticed some blood mixed in with the stool and that was when you decided to make a doctor's appointment.

You feel the pain in your right iliac fossa. It is worse after you eat.

You are nauseated but have not vomited. You have lost your appetite and have two painful ulcers in your mouth. You have lost 2 kg in weight and feel weak. You have not had fevers.

Your periods are generally regular and non-painful. Your last period was last week and normal. There is no vaginal discharge. You have no dysuria, frequency or haematuria. You have no history of any eye issues or joint pains.

You work in the city as a fashion designer. You and Natalie have been together since you met at university.

You have never smoked. Most Saturday nights you drink four to five glasses of wine.

You recently visited your brother on the central New South Wales coast but have not travelled overseas.

Medication

Nil prescribed

A friend gave you ginger tablets from the herbal shop but they had no effect, nor did the ranitidine or antacids that you bought from the chemist

Allergies

You have no allergies

Family history

Both your parents are alive and well

Clinical examination findings

Tenderness without guarding to be demonstrated in the right iliac fossa.

Instructions for the facilitator

Clinical examination findings

To be given if requested/examination demonstrated:

Temperature 37.0°C

Hands normal

BP 114/80 mmHg

Pulse 64

Height 171 cm

Weight 76 kg

BMI 26 kg/m^2

No jaundice or pallor

Mouth ulcers × two

Examination of chest and cardiovascular system—normal

Examination of abdomen

    —Abdominal pain without guarding in right iliac fossa

    —Bowel sounds—normal

    —Rectal examination and proctoscopy—normal

Urine dipstick—NAD.

Investigations

To be given to the candidate on specific request by the observing examiner.

Full blood count

Haemoglobin	116 (115−155) g/L	
MCV	85 (82−99) fL	
RDW	14 (<16) %	
Platelets	311 (150−400) × 10^9/L	
White cells	10.3 (4.0−11) × 10^9/L	
Neut	70% 7.2	(1.8−7.5) × 10^9/L
Lymph	22% 2.27	(1.0−4.0) × 10^9/L
Mono	6% 0.41	(0.1−1.2) × 10^9/L
Eosin	2% 0.2	(<0.7) × 10^9/L
ESR	43 mm/hr	
CRP	19 (<10) mg/L	

Electrolytes/liver function tests

Na	136 (134−146) mmol/L
K	4.2 (3.4−5.5) mmol/L
Cl	106 (95−108) mmol/L
HCO3	24 (22−32) mmol/L
Urea	4.9 (3.0−8.0) μmol/L
Creatinine	54 (30−100) μmol/L
Bilirubin	11 (<16) μmol/L
ALP	42 (20−105) μmol/L
GGT*	49 (<36) μmol/L
ALT	15 (<31) μmol/L
Albumin	42 (38−50) g/L
Total protein	74 (65−85) g/L

Ironstudies

Iron	9 (9−30) umol/L
Transferrin	3.2 (2.0−3.6) g/L
T. saturation*	11 (15−45) %
Ferritin*	240 (10−80) ug/L

Coeliac serology
   −Deamidated gliadin IgG/tissue transglutaminase IgA both negative, normal IgA level
Stool tests
   −Microscopy—semi-formed faecal matter
   −Normal faecal bacterial growth, pcr negative

—No ova, cysts or parasites
—Viral pcr negative
—Clostridium difficile toxin negative.

Suggested approach to the case

Establish rapport
Open questions about abdominal pain
Closed questions to determine cause and exclude differentials
    —Nature of pain, relieving and alleviating factors
    —Appetite–decreased
    —Nausea–present, but no vomiting
    —No haematemesis
    —Blood in stool and change in bowel habit
    —Nocturnal symptoms
    —Weight loss, fevers
    —Absence of symptoms of liver disease–no jaundice
Absence of symptoms of gallstones
Genitourinary symptoms–no dysuria, no haematuria, no frequency, no discharge
LMP last week, female partner, pregnancy not possible
No history of painful or heavy periods
Travel–nil relevant
Medication–has tried ranitidine and antacids and ginger tablets
Allergies–nil known
Family history–nil known.

Examination

Vital signs including temperature, BP/pulse
Height, weight and BMI
General inspection for pallor and jaundice
Hand signs
Cardiovascular/respiratory examination
Examination of abdomen
    —Palpation, auscultation, percussion
    —Ask to do rectal examination and proctoscopy
Urine dipstick.

Initial investigations

FBC
ESR or CRP

UEC
LFTs
Iron studies
Coeliac serology
Stool for MCS/pcr, ocp, viral pcr and clostridium difficile toxin.

Summary of key findings

Abdominal pain, nausea, reduced appetite, weight loss, mouth ulcers, rectal bleeding
Results—confirm inflammation, no infectious cause
No features of severe acute disease such as hypotension, tachycardia or fever.

Differential diagnosis

Crohn's disease
Ulcerative colitis
Appendicitis—much less likely given symptom duration
Irritable bowel syndrome—in the presence of alarm symptoms the above differentials need exclusion prior to making this diagnosis.

Management

Explanation of possible cause and plan of investigation
Recommend referral for colonoscopy
Phone contact with a gastroenterologist may be appropriate to ensure early review
Arrange follow-up—with result of colonoscopy
Discuss safety-netting to ensure early review if symptoms worsen
Discuss impact of illness on ability to work, assess need for medical certificate
High alcohol intake at weekends, raised GGT—motivational interviewing regarding willingness/ability to consider change.

 CASE COMMENTARY

Abdominal pain is a common problem with a wide differential diagnosis. A thorough history and examination in this case should give the doctor the clues needed to consider Crohn's disease in the differential diagnosis. More common causes of pain and bleeding, such as infection, need to be excluded, prior to referral for endoscopy.

It is estimated that over 75 000 people are living with inflammatory bowel disease in Australia, with over 1622 new cases being diagnosed every year. Inflammatory bowel disease occurs at any age, with a typical age of onset in the twenties. It is a chronic disease with a high degree of morbidity and commonly affects young people at a time when they are trying to establish careers and relationships. Psychological co-morbidity is common, and it is important to consider the impact of this diagnosis on Kirrilee at future follow-up consultations.

 COMMON PITFALLS

Pregnancy should be considered in the differential diagnosis but can be discounted when Kirrilee states she has a female partner and has never had heterosexual intercourse.

Faecal calprotectin may be considered by some candidates as part of investigations. Faecal calprotectin is a useful test due to its high negative predictive value in the absence of alarm symptoms. In this case, Kirrilee has alarm symptoms including PR bleeding, weight loss and nocturnal symptoms, which necessitate endoscopy irrespective of this result. It is worth noting that faecal calprotectin does not have a Medicare rebate, leading to a cost to the patient if this is requested.

Likewise, faecal occult blood testing is useful as a screening test for asymptomatic patients and is inappropriate in a presentation of overt PR bleeding, as a negative or positive result will not change management.

Further reading

Alex, G, Andrews, JM, Bell, S, Connor, S, Moore, G, Ward, M & van Langenberg, D 2018, 'Clinical update for general practitioners and physicians: inflammatory bowel disease', Gastroenterological Society of Australia, Melbourne. Available at: www.gesa.org.au/resources/clinical-guidelines-and-updates/inflammatory-bowel-disease, accessed 9 December 2018.

Knight, A 2008, 'I've been bleeding from the bowel', *Australian Family Physician,* vol. 37, no. 11, pp. 918–21.

Morrison, G, Headon, B & Gibson, P 2009, 'Update in inflammatory bowel disease', *Australian Family Physician,* vol. 38, no. 12, pp. 956–61.

Mozdiak, E, O'Malley, J & Arasaradnam, R 2015, 'Inflammatory bowel disease,' *British Medical Journal,* vol. 351, p. h4416.

Case 39
Mohammed Noor

Instructions for the doctor

This is a long case.

Please take a history and conduct an appropriate physical examination. The facilitator will give you the results of initial tests on request. Outline the most likely and differential diagnoses to Mohammed and negotiate a management plan with him.

Scenario

Mohammed Noor is a 23-year-old student studying business at university. He presents today complaining of epigastric burning.

The following information is on his summary sheet:

Past medical history
Nil recorded
Medication
Nil recorded
Allergies
Nil known
Immunisations
Up-to-date
Social history
Lives with mother and five younger siblings
Studying business
Rohingya refugee born in Burma, spent two years in refugee camp in Bangladesh, arrived in Australia 10 years ago
Alcohol—nil
Non-smoker

Family history
Mother—migraines
Father killed in Burma prior to rest of family fleeing to Bangladesh.

Instructions for the patient, Mohammed Noor

You are 23 years old and are studying a business degree at university. You are a Rohingya refugee and arrived in Australia 10 years ago. You speak English very well. You completed high school here, achieving good marks, and have almost finished your university studies. Over the past month or so, you have noticed some indigestion after meals. Particularly after spicy foods, you notice burning pain in your upper abdomen. It seems to be worse on university days when you drink three cups of coffee and feel more stressed. Indigestion tablets that you bought from the pharmacy have helped a little to relieve the symptoms. You have felt a little nausea but have not vomited. You have noticed a need to burp associated with times you are feeling pain, which is embarrassing when in a group.

Your bowels are unchanged and there is no rectal bleeding or black motions. You have no trouble swallowing and no sensation of reflux or bitter taste in your mouth. You have not lost any weight (and in fact have probably gained a few kilos over the last couple of years due to eating at the university cafeteria). You do not take any over-the-counter medications other than the indigestion tablets (including no anti-inflammatories).

You are fit and active, playing soccer twice per week with no shortness of breath or chest pain. Your diet consists of traditional food at home (often heavy on the chilli which you grow in your garden) and fast food from the university cafeteria.

You are worried as a friend's mother just passed away from stomach cancer, which has shocked your small community as she was relatively young. You remember her always complaining of symptoms after eating spicy foods, like yourself. You have no personal family history of gastric cancer.

The following information is on your medical record:
Past medical history
Nil recorded
Medication
Nil recorded
Allergies
Nil known
Immunisations
Up-to-date

Social history
Lives with mother and five younger siblings
Studying business
Rohingya refugee from Burma, two years in refugee camp in
Bangladesh, arrived in Australia 10 years ago
Alcohol—nil
Non-smoker
Family history
Mother—migraines
Father killed in Burma prior to rest of family fleeing to Bangladesh.

Examination

You display epigastric tenderness on examination of the abdomen. Physical
examination is otherwise normal.

Instructions for the facilitator

Examination

BP 123/74 mm Hg
P 65 bpm
Height 165 cm
Weight 78 kg
BMI 28.7 kg/m^2
The patient should demonstrate epigastric tenderness. Physical examination
  is otherwise normal.

Results of tests

Blood tests must be requested item per item; do not give a result unless it
has been requested
FBC confirms a normal Hb 131 g/L, and normal white cell count
CRP normal
Iron studies: ferritin 44 μg/dL (normal 20–150 μg/dL)
Helicobacter pylori (*H. pylori*) serology positive, urea breath test positive,
  stool antigen positive
UEC, LFTs and all other tests normal.

Suggested approach to the case

Establish rapport
Open questions to explore patient's ideas, concerns and expectations.

Specific questions

Gastrointestinal
- —Clarify nature, frequency, severity and duration of symptoms
- —Relationship to meals, identification of specific triggers (spicy foods, caffeine, alcohol, smoking, fatty foods, stress)
- —Relieving factors
- —Acid reflux or waterbrash
- —Nausea or vomiting
- —Early satiety, bloating, belching
- —Changes in bowels

Exclude alarm features
- —PR bleeding, melaena/haematemesis
- —Dysphagia or odynophagia
- —Unintentional weight loss
- —Family history of gastrointestinal malignancy

Discuss the impact of symptoms on day-to-day life
Brief systems review
Past medical history
Drugs—NSAIDs, prescribed medication, OTC, recreational/illicit
Allergies
Family history
Social history—alcohol consumption, smoking
Request permission to examine.

Examination

Pulse, BP
BMI
Check for: jaundice, pallor
Abdominal examination
- —Inspection
- —Palpation
- —Examine for liver, spleen, kidneys
- —Percussion
- —Auscultation.

Investigations

Request results from the facilitator
FBC
CRP
UEC

LFTs

Iron studies

H. pylori serology (useful only if negative)

Urea breath test (gold standard, can be requested instead of serology) or stool antigen test if serology positive.

Most likely diagnosis

H. pylori-associated dyspepsia (gastritis +/− peptic ulcer disease).

Differential diagnoses

Malignancy unlikely in the absence of alarm features.

Management

Explain most likely diagnosis

Discuss general measures–avoiding triggers (spicy food, caffeine etc.); smaller, more frequent meals; weight reduction; over-the-counter antacid or alginate medications

Commence triple therapy for *H. pylori*

Plan review, repeat *H. pylori* testing after six weeks to ensure eradication

If symptoms persist after eradication, consider acid-suppression therapy

Sensitively address and reassure patient regarding fear of malignancy.

 CASE COMMENTARY

H. pylori infection is a major cause of morbidity and mortality worldwide. Differences in prevalence exist within and between countries, with higher prevalence among people with lower socioeconomic status. Mohammed was born overseas in a country with likely higher prevalence and has also grown up in a large family and spent time in a refugee camp (which frequently have issues with overcrowding and poor sanitation), increasing his risk of having contracted *H. pylori.*

In those under 55 years old, a 'test and treat' policy (in the absence of alarm symptoms such as dysphagia, haematemesis or weight loss) is considered safe practice because of the high effectiveness of *H. pylori* treatment plus the low yield for upper GI malignancy on scoping.

Arrangements for a follow-up are essential to ensure that persisting dyspepsia despite eradication and adequate acid-suppression trial is investigated with endoscopy. Mohammed has likely experienced some trauma in his childhood, leading to a higher likelihood of persisting symptoms and a diagnosis of functional dyspepsia.

Further reading

Duggan, AE 2007, 'The management of upper gastrointestinal symptoms: is endoscopy indicated?' *Medical Journal of Australia,* vol. 186, pp. 166–7.

Mitchell, H & Katelaris, P 2016, 'Epidemiology, clinical impacts and current clinical management of Helicobacter pylori infection', *Medical Journal of Australia,* vol. 204, pp. 376–80.

Talley, NJ 2017, 'Functional dyspepsia: advances in diagnosis and therapy', *Gut and Liver,* vol. 11, pp. 349–57.

Yaxley, J & Chakravarty, B 2014, '*Helicobacter pylori* eradication—an update on the latest therapies', *Australian Family Physician,* vol. 43, pp. 301–5.

Case 40
Annie Nguyen

Instructions for the doctor

This is a short case.

Please take a history from Annie. Then outline to the facilitator what examination and investigations you would normally do in your clinical practice and indicate the most likely diagnosis.

Scenario

Annie Nguyen is 19 years old and in her first year at university. She has not been to the clinic before. She has made the appointment because she has been nauseated for the past three days.

While waiting to see the doctor she completed a new patient questionnaire in which she gave the following information:

Past medical history
Glandular fever Year 12 of high school

Medication
Nil

Allergies
Nil known

Immunisations
Fully immunised

Family history
Nil relevant

Social history
Lives on campus in hall of residence
Non-smoker
Alcohol—three standard drinks per week.

Instructions for the patient, Annie Nguyen

You are 19 years old and in your first year at university. You have not been to this GP before. You have been nauseated for the past three days but have not vomited. You had diarrhoea for the first two days but this has now settled. You do not feel like eating. You experienced colicky abdominal pain just before each episode of diarrhoea.

Your last menstrual period was one week ago. You have no other symptoms. You are not currently sexually active.

You have filled out the new patient questionnaire as follows:

Past medical history
Glandular fever Year 12 of high school
Medication
Nil
Allergies
Nil known
Immunisations
Fully immunised
Family history
Nil relevant
Social history
Lives on campus in hall of residence
Non-smoker
Alcohol—three standard drinks per week.

Suggested approach to the case

Establish rapport
Open-ended questions to explore Annie's ideas, concerns and expectations.

Specific questions

Gastrointestinal
   —Anorexia
   —Nausea and vomiting
   —Haematemesis
   —Suspect food prior to onset of symptoms
   —Abdominal pain
   —Diarrhoea/constipation
   —Blood or melaena pr
Associated features, such as headache

Systems review—fever, energy level
Genitourinary
   —Frequency, haematuria, discharge
   —Menstrual cycle, LMP, risk of pregnancy
Infectious contacts—are any other students or staff at hall of residence unwell? Potential public health issues may need consideration if history suggests others with similar symptoms
History of recent travel
Substances—medication prescribed elsewhere, OTC, alcohol, drugs of abuse
Request permission to examine.

Examination

Pulse
Temperature
Hydration
Jaundice
Abdominal examination—for tenderness, masses or organomegaly
Urine specimen dipstick.

Most likely diagnosis

Gastroenteritis.

Investigations

Nil needed.

CASE COMMENTARY

Nausea is a common presenting symptom in general practice and the list of potential causes is extensive. This case tests the doctor's ability to adopt a systematic approach to the diagnosis and follow the dictum that 'common things are common'. It is essential to explore Annie's risk of pregnancy.

The question asks the doctor to tell the facilitator what physical examination and investigations they would normally do in their clinical practice. The history is strongly suggestive of gastroenteritis and there are no alarming symptoms so a rectal examination and investigations are not needed at this consultation.

Further reading

Anderson 3rd, WD & Strayer, SM 2013, 'Evaluation of nausea and vomiting: a case-based approach', *American Family Physician,* vol. 88, pp. 371–9.

Murtagh J 2018, 'Nausea and vomiting'. In: Murtagh, J, Rosenblatt, J, Coleman, J & Murtagh, C (eds), *Murtagh's General Practice*, 7th ed, McGraw-Hill, Sydney, pp. 685–9.

Case 41
Kathy Jones

Instructions for the doctor

This is a long case.

Please take a history from your patient, Kathy Jones, and request the findings of an appropriate physical examination. The facilitator will give you the results of any relevant investigations on request. Then negotiate a management plan with Kathy.

Scenario

Kathy Jones is a 55-year-old woman who has been attending your practice for several years. She is mostly healthy but has hypertension and dyslipidaemia, which are well-controlled with telmisartan and atorvastatin. She is married with three grown children and works as a school librarian. She went through menopause about five years ago and found some relief from her hot flushes with some over-the-counter natural remedies. She is quite health conscious, enjoys a good diet and remains physically active.

The following information is on her summary sheet:

Past medical history
Hypertension
Dyslipidaemia

Medication
Telmisartan 40 mg od
Atorvastatin 20 mg od

Allergies
Nil known

Immunisations
Up-to-date

Social history
Lives with husband
Non-smoker
Alcohol—one to two units on rare special occasions.

Instructions for the patient, Kathy Jones

You are coming to the doctor because of three to four months of tiredness. Your fitness is OK and your interest is fine; you just feel lethargic. Your mood is good and you remain active in your work and various interests. You've never felt like this before and have no idea what could be going on. You have not had any cold or flu symptoms apart from some vague aching of your joints—mainly the hands and wrists—over the past couple of months. You have taken some paracetamol when your joints have been sore. None of your joints are red, swollen or tender. You've not had a temperature, your appetite is good and your weight is stable. You sleep well and you don't snore.

You are happily married with three grown children and four grandchildren, who are all healthy. You took some over-the-counter natural remedies for hot flushes when you went through menopause about five years ago. You still have some issues with vaginal dryness and your libido has been low in recent months.

You've been on medication for blood pressure and to lower cholesterol for several years and you are extremely conscientious in taking these. You have no known allergies, have never smoked and are not aware of any significant family history.

Your cervical screening test, mammogram and FOBT are all up-to-date.

The following information is on your summary sheet:
Past medical history
Hypertension
Dyslipidaemia
Medication
Telmisartan 40 mg od
Atorvastatin 20 mg od
Allergies
Nil known
Immunisations
Up-to-date
Social history
Lives with husband
Non-smoker
Alcohol—one to two units on rare special occasions.

Information for the facilitator

Clinical examination findings

Please give the candidate the following examination findings on specific request.

General appearance: well-dressed woman in no distress
BMI 22 kg/m^2
Pulse 70/min
Temperature 36.5°C
BP 124/82 mmHg
BSL 5.5 mmol/L (random)
Urinalysis—normal
All physical examination findings are normal.

Investigation results

Please give the candidate the following investigation results on specific request.
FBC, ESR—normal
EUC—normal
LFTs—normal
TSH—normal

Iron	Transferrin	TIBC	Transferrin saturation	Ferritin
(9–31 μmol/L)	(2.0–3.7 g/L)	(45–80 μmol/L)	(16–60%)	(30–300 μg/L)
40.6*	2.8	46	90*	920*

HFE gene—C282Y homozygous (only to be given if candidate has requested)
Fasting BSL—normal
Fasting lipids—normal
MSU—normal.

Suggested approach to the case

Establish rapport
Open questions to explore fatigue, how she experiences it and the impact on her function.

Specific questions

Exclude cardiac symptoms (no SOB, palpitations, etc.)
Mood/energy/appetite/sleep/libido

Weight loss
Fevers/night sweats
Medications, including over-the-counter
Allergies
Systems review—should elicit arthralgia
Social history—alcohol, drugs
Occupational history
Family history
Preventative health, e.g. cervical, breast and bowel cancer screening.

Examination

Request permission to examine
General appearance (no jaundice, pallor or pigmentation)
Vital signs
Cardiovascular and respiratory examination
Thyroid examination
Check lymph nodes
Abdominal examination
Examination of hands/wrists
Urine dipstick
BSL.

Investigations

FBC
EUC
LFTs
TSH
ESR/CRP
Ferritin/iron studies
HFE gene test.

Management

Explanation of hereditary haemochromatosis
Commence therapeutic venesection—initially weekly, then maintenance
    schedule to keep ferritin within normal range
Avoid vitamin C (and iron) supplements
Avoid alcohol until iron stores are normalised
Will need regular monitoring of iron studies and venesections to maintain
    normal indices
Screening of adult family members.

CASE COMMENTARY

Fatigue is a common presentation in general practice and is a good test of our ability to sort out all the possible causes with a thorough history, appropriate examination and rational investigation. Kathy is over 50, previously well, and gives a history of new-onset fatigue and arthralgia—this warrants the initial investigations listed above.

Hereditary haemochromatosis is the most common genetic condition of Caucasian populations, with more than one in 200 individuals at genetic risk of having this disease. Importantly, early diagnosis and treatment of hereditary haemochromatosis prevents complications and results in a normal life expectancy. Being able to interpret iron studies is an important skill for GPs to have. The transferrin saturation (ratio of serum iron and iron binding capacity) reflects increased absorption of iron, which is the underlying biological defect in hereditary haemochromatosis. In very early disease, transferrin saturation may be elevated before a rise in ferritin. A fasting transferrin saturation >45% is the most sensitive test for detecting early iron overload, but a raised fasting transferrin saturation or ferritin is not diagnostic of hereditary haemochromatosis. Hereditary haemochromatosis is unlikely if the ferritin is high and the transferrin saturation is normal. An elevated serum ferritin reflects an increase in body iron stores but is also an acute phase reactant and can be elevated non-specifically in the presence of alcohol consumption, infection or inflammation, as well as some malignancies.

Kathy presents with the classic triad of fatigue, arthralgia and low libido at a typical age for women to present with hereditary haemochromatosis. Before menopause, physiological blood loss from menstruation and pregnancy provides a degree of protection from clinical disease. With a ferritin below 1000 μg/L, Kathy does not require a liver biopsy and should proceed to venesection, which can be expected to improve her tiredness but possibly not her arthralgia or libido. She should be cautioned about avoiding vitamin C supplements, which increase absorption of dietary iron and also facilitate release of iron from storage.

There is some controversy regarding the ideal target range for ferritin from venesection therapy. Previous guidelines have suggested that venesection should continue until ferritin is <50 μg/L. However, with genetic testing and less severe disease on presentation as a result of earlier detection, some experts now recommend normalisation of ferritin to <300 μg/L for men and postmenopausal women, and <200 μg/L for pre-menopausal women. More aggressive management may be required for those presenting with more severe iron overload and ferritin >1000 μg/L, when the risk of cirrhosis is higher and the aim is to iron deplete extrahepatic organs in addition to the liver to minimise risk of haemochromatosis.

Hereditary haemochromatosis is unusual in that treatment by venesection helps other patients who require blood transfusions.

Further reading

Allen, K 2010, 'Hereditary haemochromatosis: diagnosis and management', *Australian Family Physician,* vol. 39, no. 12, pp. 938-41.

Delatycki, M & Allen, K 2013, 'Hereditary haemochromatosis: how to treat', *Australian Doctor,* vol. 12, April.

Goot, K, Hazeldine S, Bentley, P, Olynyk, J & Crawford, D 2012, 'Elevated serum ferritin: what should GPs know?' *Australian Family Physician,* vol. 41, no. 12, pp. 945-49.

Wilson, J, Morgan, S, Magin, P & van Driel, M 2014, 'Fatigue—a rational approach to investigation', *Australian Family Physician,* vol. 43, no. 7, pp. 457-61.

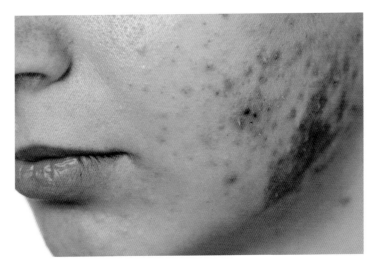

Figure 1 Teenage acne (see page 14).

Photo courtesy of iStockphoto

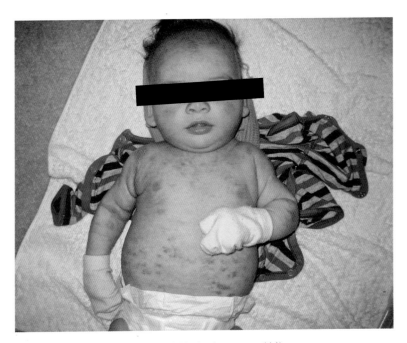

Figure 2 Rash on four-month-old baby (see page 114).

Photo courtesy of the Eczema Association of Australasia Inc.

A

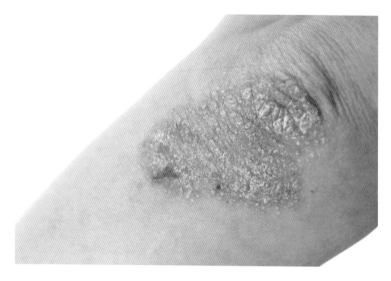

Figure 3 Rash on outside of left elbow (see page 120).
Photo courtesy of iStockphoto

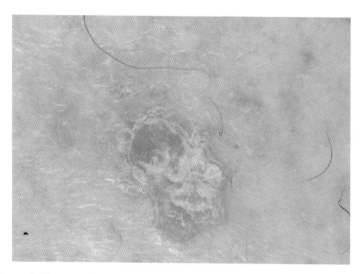

Figure 4 Close up of Ken's lesion (see page 123).
Photo courtesy of Dr Andrew Moreton

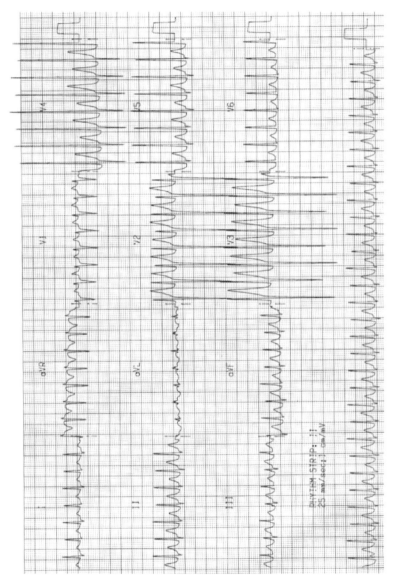

Figure 5 ECG courtesy of Dr Brendan Bell (see page 153).

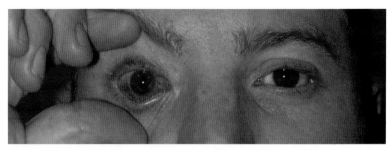

Figure 6 Painful, red blurry right eye (see page 172).
Photo courtesy of Dr Andrew Moreton

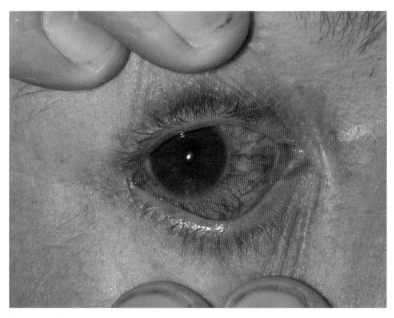

Figure 7 Close-up of painful, red blurry right eye (see page 172).
Photo courtesy of Dr Andrew Moreton

Case 42
Jack Kingsley

Instructions for the doctor

Please take a focused history from Jack and answer his questions.

Scenario

Jack is a 43-year-old man whose wife Julie and two children attend the practice. He saw you last week for a full check-up, including a physical examination, which was normal. He feels he can trust you and so made another booking to discuss something else.

The following is on his summary sheet:

Past medical history
Nil recorded

Medications
Nil

Immunisations
ADT 2019 after stepping on a nail last week
Unsure about childhood immunisations

Family history
Brother died MVA aged 35
Mother died of cirrhosis aged 57

Social history
Lives with his wife Julie and two children
Works as a manager at an electrical store
Non-smoker
Drinks four to six full-strength beers at the weekend

Instructions for the patient Jack Kingsley

You have known you were hepatitis C positive since 2001 when you were diagnosed. You injected drugs in your twenties so think this is when you became infected.

Julie and the children know about your diagnosis. You take precautions around them and they have never had any exposure to your blood. Julie is your only sexual partner since diagnosis and you no longer use drugs.

You were diagnosed when in prison for car theft and were commenced on interferon. You only had about four weeks of treatment as it made you unwell and after leaving prison you wanted to get your life together and leave your past behind.

The treatment didn't work and you accepted that you would live with hepatitis C until it killed you as it did your mum. One of your friends from your drug days recently died of liver cancer. At his funeral another friend told you of his cure on a new treatment.

You had a difficult childhood and ended up in foster care. As a young adult you were homeless and used IV drugs.

You know you should have seen a doctor regularly but you have lived in fear of your past coming back to haunt you and just preferred to get on with your life. But now, with talk of a new treatment, you think it's worth investigating the options and you want to ask the doctor about it.

You feel fit and run three times a week and ride 10 km to work and back five times a week. You don't smoke. You drink four to six stubbies of full-strength beer on the weekends.

You have avoided your favourite sport of AFL due to the risk of injury and blood exposure for your teammates but would love to play again.

You don't take any other drugs and vow never to do that again.

You are very careful with any blood exposure and would never dream of getting a tattoo or anything similar.

If there is a new treatment you are happy to undergo any testing the doctor suggests.

If the treatment sounds like the interferon treatment you are more reluctant as you remember how bad it made you feel.

If the doctor asks about mood, you are in good spirits. The trauma of your childhood will never go away but most days you feel lucky to be part of a loving family, have a good job and a safe home. You do have your moments, but you had counselling in prison, which gave you some strategies to deal with nightmares and jumpy moments. You have no thoughts of hurting yourself.

Suggested approach to the case

History

Re-establish rapport
Elicit patient's concerns
Explore diagnosis and possible cause
Ask about past treatment attempts
Approach in a sensitive, non-judgemental manner
Reassure and encourage his newly proactive approach
Brief screen for symptoms of depression and recognise that there is a risk of co-morbid depression/post-traumatic stress disorder
Check for possible exposures for family members
Brief history regarding any ongoing high-risk activities—tattoos, IV drug use, sexual partners
SNAP—smoking, nutrition, alcohol, physical activity assessment.

Management

Pre-treatment work-up for hepatitis C treatment
  −FBC, EUC, INR
  −Liver biochemistry
  −Blood glucose
  −HCV RNA and genotype
  −Upper abdominal ultrasound
  −Serology for HIV, hepatitis A virus and hepatitis B virus
For immunisation if not immune to hepatitis A and/or B
Treatment can be commenced by GPs unless there is cirrhosis (needs gastroenterologist referral)
Offer a GP management plan (prefilled plan available on ASHM website)
Advise to reduce alcohol intake and warn that if there is evidence of cirrhosis alcohol should stop completely
Ensure understanding of the need for compliance
Reassure patient about improved side effect profile and efficacy of treatment compared with interferon.

Follow-up

Follow-up to discuss results and decide on best course of treatment
Discuss further exploration of mental health at next visit.

CASE COMMENTARY

In Australia there are approximately 230 000 people affected by chronic hepatitis C (HCV) and it is the most common disease requiring liver transplant. Recent advances in treatment mean that HCV is curable, whereas treatment with interferon was poorly tolerated and had limited efficacy. Direct antiviral agents have minimal side effects and up to 95% cure rate after 12–24 week treatment courses. They can be initiated by GPs if there is no cirrhosis or other complications. Those with cirrhosis have the most to gain from treatment and should be referred to a hepatologist/gastroenterologist for treatment.

75% of acute HCV infections will become chronic, leading to increased risk of liver failure, cirrhosis and hepatocellular carcinoma. 20–30% of people will develop cirrhosis generally 20–30 years after infection.

All Australians living with HCV should be considered for treatment, so it is important for GPs to know about the treatment and the pre-treatment work-up.

COMMON PITFALLS

Jack has not had adequate medical care for his chronic HCV. However, he is now motivated. Discussing the care he has not received will threaten the therapeutic relationship; focusing on his new proactive approach is preferable.

Jack may already have cirrhosis or possibly hepatocellular carcinoma. At this visit it is important to think about these complications when ordering investigations, but there is cause for optimism with the new direct antiviral agents even if his test results show elements of cirrhosis. Candidates are not expected to know the details of the medications but should be able to describe that they are oral for a 12–24 week course and have a high chance of cure.

Further reading

Khoo, A & Tse, E 2016, 'A practical overview of the treatment of chronic hepatitis C virus infection', *Australian Family Physician*, vol. 45, no. 10, pp. 718–20.

Strasser, S 2017, 'Managing hepatitis C in general practice', *Australian Prescriber*, vol. 40, no. 2, pp. 64–9.

Therapeutic Guidelines Ltd 2017, 'Hepatitis C'. In: *eTG complete* [Internet]. Therapeutic Guidelines Ltd, Melbourne.

Hepatitis C Management and Treatment. Available at: www.ashm.org.au/HCV/management-hepc/, accessed 26 February 2019.

Hepatitis C Virus Infection Consensus Statement Working Group 2017, Australian recommendations for the management of hepatitis C virus infection: a consensus statement, August. Gastroenterological Society of Australia, Melbourne, Vic.

Case 43
Neil Dawson

Instructions for the doctor

This is a short case.

Please read the following scenario. No further history or examination are required. Please discuss the results of your initial investigations with the patient and negotiate a management plan with him.

Scenario

Neil Dawson is a 61-year-old insurance broker who has spent most of his life avoiding doctors. His wife, worried about him, finally convinced him to come and see you last week for his first doctor appointment in at least a decade. She was worried about his increasing fatigue and his ankles that sometimes swell.

Your further history and systems review elicited no alarm symptoms. You established that Neil has had some psychosocial stressors (caring for his mother with dementia who passed away 12 months ago, plus some financial concerns regarding his home business), but has no signs of depression or anxiety.

You ascertained that Neil is not particularly bothered by his swollen ankles, but that he thought this was a sign that it was time to come to get things checked up.

You collected the below information:
Past medical history
Bilateral inguinal hernia repairs aged 45

Medications
Nil
Allergies
Nil known
Family history
Mother—deceased (dementia, aged 85)
Father—deceased (bowel cancer, aged 79)
Social history
Lives with wife
Owns insurance brokerage business
Preventative health
Non-smoker
Alcohol—four to six full-strength beers most nights
Nutrition—typical daily intake consists of three slices of toast with jam plus a glass of orange juice for breakfast, a pie and a can of coke for lunch, half a packet of biscuits and cheese with a few beers after work, meat/potatoes/beans/carrots for dinner and a large bowl of ice-cream while watching TV at night
Physical activity—mows the lawn fortnightly, sedentary job
Bowel cancer screening—non-participant.

Examination

BP 138/85, pulse 80 and regular
Weight 132 kg
Height 177 cm
BMI 42.1
Chest clear, good air entry
Heart sounds dual, nil added
JVP not elevated
Mild peripheral oedema to ankles
Respiratory examination normal
Thyroid examination normal
No lymphadenopathy
Abdominal exam difficult due to body habitus, some distension, shifting dullness
Few spider naevi upper chest
Palmar erythema noted
You arranged for some initial blood tests and asked Neil to return for a follow-up appointment.

Initial investigations

Full blood count

Haemoglobin	142 (130–170) g/L		
MCV	98 (82–99) fL		
Platelets*	132 (150–400) × 10⁹/L		
White cells	10.3 (4.0–11) × 10⁹/L		
Neutrophils	70%	7.2	(1.8–7.5) × 10⁹/L
Lymphocytes	22%	2.27	(1.0–4.0) × 10⁹/L
Monocytes	6%	0.41	(0.1–1.2) × 10⁹/L
Eosinophils	2%	0.2	(<0.7) × 10⁹/L

Electrolytes and liver function tests

Na	134 (134–146) mmol/L
K	4.2 (3.4–5.5) mmol/L
Cl	106 (95–108) mmol/L
HCO$_3$	24 (22–32) mmol/L
Urea	4.9 (3.0–8.0) μmol/L
Creatinine	77 (30–100) μmol/L
Bilirubin (total)*	36 (<16) μmol/L
ALP*	117 (20–105) U/L
GGT*	92 (<36) U/L
ALT*	109 (<40) U/L
AST*	198 (<35) U/L
Albumin*	30 (38–50) g/L
Total protein*	60 (65–85) g/L

Iron studies

Iron	15 (9–30) umol/L
Transferrin	2.8 (2.0–3.6) g/L
Transferrin saturation	30 (15–45) %
Ferritin*	180 (10–80) ug/L

HbA1c, thyroid function tests, CRP and B12 are normal.

Information for the patient

You are a 61-year-old insurance broker and have spent most of your life avoiding doctors. Your wife booked your initial appointment last week as she was worried about your increasing fatigue over the last six months and had noticed that your ankles are sometimes a bit swollen. This was your first doctor appointment in at least a decade.

You are otherwise well and have not noticed any other symptoms. Your mum passed away from dementia 12 months ago, and prior to this you had a very stressful couple of years caring for her in your house. Your business suffered over this time and is still recovering, but you are feeling alright about this now, and are not depressed.

You are not overly bothered by the swollen ankles, but wished you had some more energy. You agreed with your wife that it was time to get a check-up and are a little apprehensive about the results.

The following information is on your medical record:

Past medical history
Bilateral inguinal hernia repairs age 45

Medications
Nil

Allergies
Nil known

Family history
Mother—deceased (dementia, aged 85)
Father—deceased (bowel cancer, aged 79)

Social history
Lives with wife
Owns insurance brokerage business

Preventative health
Non-smoker
Alcohol—four to six full-strength beers most nights
Nutrition—typical daily intake consists of three slices of toast with jam plus a glass of orange juice for breakfast, a pie and a can of coke for lunch, half a packet of biscuits and cheese with a few beers after work, meat/potatoes/beans/carrots for dinner and a large bowl of ice-cream while watching TV at night
Physical activity—mows the lawn fortnightly, sedentary job
Bowel cancer screening—non-participant.

Suggested approach to the case

Establish rapport
Explore patient's ideas, concerns and expectations regarding this consultation
Explain results clearly and sensitively

Discuss that results are highly suggestive of liver failure/liver cirrhosis, and explain what this is

Arrange further investigations to confirm diagnosis and rule out other causes

- Ultrasound of liver and abdomen
- INR
- Liver screen including hepatitis B serology (surface antibody, surface antigen and core antibody) and hepatitis C serology
- Check immunity to hepatitis A
- Check AFP

Hepatology referral once above investigations are complete

Discuss likely aetiology of alcohol and obesity to liver disease

Address alcohol—abstinence recommended given there is evidence of liver failure

Address nutrition and physical activity

Arrange follow-up

Consider GP management plan and allied health referral including dietician and exercise physiologist

Extras for the case, most likely in future consultations—other preventative health including bowel cancer screening, check of fasting lipids and absolute cardiovascular risk assessment, look for and address other complications of obesity (e.g. obstructive sleep apnoea), immunisations.

 ## CASE COMMENTARY

There is a lot of written information to take in during the three-minute reading time. Try not to be flustered by this; it is OK to take a few short moments while in the exam room to gather your thoughts if necessary. This is a management case that requires candidates to accurately interpret results, convey a new diagnosis of a chronic disease in a sensitive and informative manner, and provide motivational interviewing to initiate lifestyle changes essential for the management of this condition.

Cirrhosis and chronic liver failure are common causes of morbidity and mortality and are in most cases preventable. They are often diagnosed at a late stage, as patients remain asymptomatic until the occurrence of decompensation. Non-alcoholic fatty liver disease (NAFLD) and alcohol are becoming an increasingly important cause of cirrhosis (especially as incidence of hepatitis C–related cirrhosis is expected to reduce). Management of NAFLD predominantly involves addressing lifestyle factors, including nutrition, alcohol and physical activity, something we as general practitioners are well-placed to achieve.

Further reading

Duggan, AE & Duggan, JM 2011, 'Alcoholic liver disease: assessment and management', *Australian Family Physician,* vol. 40, pp. 590–3.

Heidelbaugh, JJ & Bruderly, M 2006, 'Cirrhosis and chronic liver failure: part I. Diagnosis and evaluation', *American Family Physician,* vol. 74, pp. 756–62.

Iser, D & Ryan, M 2013, 'Fatty liver disease: a practical guide for GPs', *Australian Family Physician,* vol. 42, pp. 444–7.

MacDonald, G 2009, 'Nonalcoholic fatty liver disease', *Medicine Today,* vol. 10, pp. 68–9.

Pattullo, V & Strasser, SI 2017, 'Managing the rising burden of chronic liver disease: nonalcoholic fatty liver disease and alcoholic liver disease', *Medicine Today,* vol. 18, pp. 28–35.

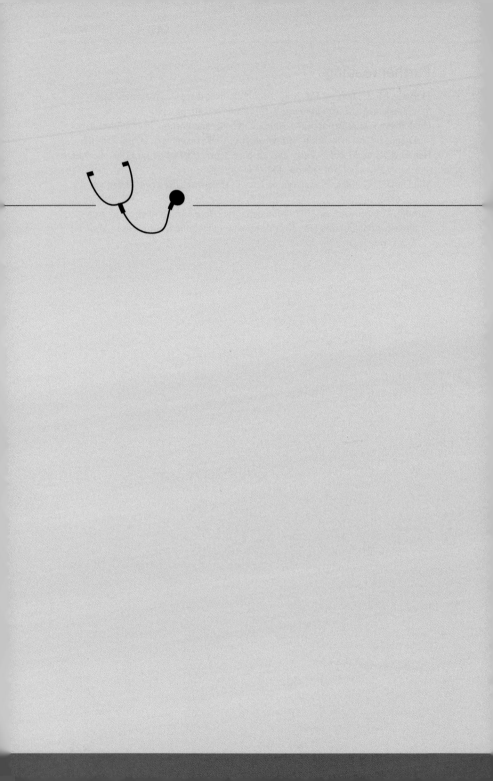

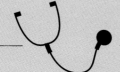

Section 13
Men's health

Case 44
Kim Hosking

Instructions for the doctor

This is a short case.

Please take a history. The facilitator will give you the results of the examination on request. Outline the most likely diagnosis to the patient and negotiate a management plan with him.

Scenario

Kim Hosking is a 70-year-old retired architect. He comes to see you every few months for a blood pressure check. At the last check Kim mentioned that he was having 'waterworks trouble' and you suggested he make an appointment to discuss this further.

The following information is on his summary sheet:

Past medical history
Hypertension—diagnosed 2009
Medication
Perindopril 5 mg od
Allergies
Nil
Immunisations
Up-to-date, including influenza
Social history
Married
Three children, now grown-up
Ex-smoker.

Instructions for the patient, Kim Hosking

You are a 70-year-old retired architect. Over the past few years your urine stream has become weaker. You pass urine more often and now have to get up about three times each night. You get frustrated that, having got out of bed, you then have to wait a while before the stream starts. It embarrasses you that you often dribble after passing urine, which wets your clothes.

Your blood pressure is currently well-controlled and except for the urinary symptoms, you enjoy being retired. Two weeks ago, at your blood pressure check, you mentioned to your GP that you had 'waterworks trouble'. The GP suggested that you make an appointment to discuss this, which is why you are here.

The following information is on your summary sheet:

Past medical history
Hypertension—diagnosed 2009

Medication
Perindopril 5 mg od

Allergies
Nil

Immunisations
Up-to-date, including influenza

Social history
Married
Three children, now grown-up
Ex-smoker.

Information for the facilitator

Clinical examination findings

Temperature, pulse and blood pressure are within normal limits
Abdominal examination is normal
Rectal examination reveals a smooth, non-tender, symmetrically enlarged prostate.

Suggested approach to the case

Establish rapport
Open-ended questions to gain understanding of Kim's ideas, concerns and expectations.

Specific questions

Details—urinary frequency, hesitancy, stream, nocturia, incomplete
    emptying, incontinence, terminal dribbling
Pain or dysuria
Haematuria
Fever
Systemic malaise, weight loss
Sexual function
Urethral discharge.

Ask for the examination findings

Temperature
Pulse
BP
Abdominal examination
    —Inspection
    —Palpation—exclude palpable bladder
Genitalia
Rectal examination to assess the prostate.

Most likely diagnosis

Obstructive lower urinary tract symptoms due to benign prostatic
    hypertrophy.

Investigations

Bladder diary
Urine for MCS
UEC, BSL
PSA—needs informed consent.

Management

Modify caffeine and fluid intake if excessive
Encourage bladder training
For benign prostatic hypertrophy, alpha-adrenoreceptor antagonists or
    5-alpha-reductase inhibitors or phosphodiesterase inhibitors (private
    script), or refer for surgery (transurethral resection or minimally invasive)
Arrange follow-up.

Extras for this case

Discuss alcohol consumption.

CASE COMMENTARY

Kim has obstructive lower urinary tract symptoms, a common problem for older men. The doctor will need to take a history of these symptoms and must not be too embarrassed to ask about sexual function. The most likely cause is benign prostatic hypertrophy, but the doctor needs to ask about haematuria, weight loss, fatigue and bone pain, which would suggest malignancy.

The examination will focus on the abdomen, including a rectal examination, and exclude an enlarged bladder. Practise rectal examinations on a simulated model if you can.

Testing for prostatic specific antigen (PSA) is controversial in asymptomatic men. In Kim's case, PSA testing might reveal an advanced prostate cancer, or might be useful in deciding on and monitoring treatment with 5-alpha-reductase inhibitors.

Kim's history of hypertension increases the risk of renal failure, so it is reasonable for doctors to check his renal function tests. Because of the nocturia and frequency, Kim needs a fasting BSL to exclude diabetes. An alpha-blocker relieves symptoms straight away but also has a hypotensive effect. Kim's blood pressure will need monitoring for hypotension and a reduction or cessation of the perindopril dose may be indicated. 5–alpha-reductase inhibitors, such as finasteride, can take up to six months to work. Longer acting phosphodiesterase type 5 inhibitors, for example, tadalafil, may be effective for lower urinary tract symptoms but are only available on a private script. Patients can purchase saw palmetto from health food shops, but a Cochrane review[2] has not confirmed any superiority over a placebo.

Renal ultrasound is only indicated in patients with moderate-to-severe symptoms, or an abnormal serum creatinine, to assess bladder capacity, post-void urine residual volume, prostate volume and exclude hydronephrosis.[1]

References

1. Jiwrajka, M, Yaxley, W, Perera, M, Roberts, M, Dunglison, N, Yaxley, J & Esler, R 2018, 'Review and update of benign prostatic hyperplasia in general practice', *Australian Journal of General Practice*, vol. 47, no. 7, pp 471–5.

2. Cochrane Complementary Medicine, Prostate Enlargement, Cochrane Collaboration. Available at: https://cam.cochrane.org/prostate-enlargement#sawpalmetto_prostate, accessed 20 February 2019.

Further reading

Arianayagam, M, Arianayagam, R & Rashid, P 2011, 'Lower urinary tract symptoms. Current management in older men', *Australian Family Physician,* vol. 40, pp. 758-67.

Woo, HH, Gillman, MP, Gardiner, R, Marshall, V & Lynch, WJ 2011, 'A practical approach to the management of lower urinary tract symptoms among men', *Medical Journal of Australia,* vol. 195, pp. 34-9.

Case 45
Jock Palmer

Instructions for the doctor

This is a short case.

Provide and explain the appropriate information to Jock and answer any questions he has. You do not need to take any history or examine Jock.

Scenario

Jock Palmer is a 52-year-old executive whose employer offers annual screening tests to their employees. This year they have included the prostate specific antigen (PSA) test. The company sent round an information letter but this left Jock confused. Jock trusts you as his GP and wants your opinion as to whether he should have this PSA test. Please discuss this with Jock.

The following information is on his summary sheet:

Past medical history
Nil significant
Medication
Nil
Allergies
Nil
Immunisations
Up-to-date
Family history
Nil significant
Social history
Business executive
Divorced
Non-smoker
Alcohol—six standard drinks per week.

Instructions for the patient, Jock Palmer

You are a 52-year-old executive. Your employer offers you annual screening tests. This year you received a letter informing you that the tests would include the prostate specific antigen (PSA). The company sent round an information letter but this left you confused. You trust your GP and want the GP's opinion as to whether you should have this PSA test. You have made this appointment with your GP to discuss the PSA test.

You are well and have no urinary symptoms.

During the consultation you will ask the following questions:
1. What is the PSA test?
2. What are the advantages of having the test?
3. Is there any reason not to have the test done?
4. If the test is high, does that mean that I have cancer?
5. What would happen if the result was high?
6. Should I have the test?

The following information is on your summary sheet:
Past medical history
Nil significant
Medication
Nil
Allergies
Nil
Immunisations
Up-to-date
Family history
Nil significant
Social history
Business executive
Divorced
Non-smoker
Alcohol—six standard drinks per week.

Suggested approach to the case

Re-establish rapport
Acknowledge that this is a complex and controversial issue
Question Jock about his understanding of PSA tests
Question Jock about his general health—exclude weight loss, fatigue, fever, bone pain, family history of prostate cancer

Specific questions

To exclude urinary symptoms
- –Frequency
- –Stream
- –Nocturia
- –Haematuria
- –Dysuria

Tailor explanation of PSA test to address Jock's concerns
- –PSA comes from the prostate
- –Test has limited accuracy and can be affected by a number of conditions/scenarios
- –Low result does not mean that there is no cancer
- –Raised result does not mean that there is cancer
- –Trend of results provides some clinical information

If PSA is raised Jock will need to have further tests with a specialist, including prostatic biopsies

Early treatment of prostate cancer has not consistently been proved to increase life expectancy, and there are expected harms of false-positives, overdiagnosis and overtreatment[1]

PSA testing does not fulfil criteria for a screening test, and there is no national screening program in Australia.[2] The Royal Australian College of General Practitioners[3] does not recommend screening for prostate cancer unless the man specifically asks for it and he is fully counselled on the pros and cons.

 CASE COMMENTARY

This case tests the doctor's ability to advise patients on a controversial topic. The hope was that PSA testing would enable early detection of prostate cancer and, by allowing early treatment, improve prognosis. The evidence is that prostate cancer screening can reduce risk of death from prostate cancer but the absolute benefit is small, and the chance of prostate cancer being diagnosed and treated (even if biologically unimportant) is increased by a much larger amount.[1] Jock's confusion at the information that he was given is not surprising and the doctor needs to try to explain the principles of screening, the concepts of false-negatives and false-positives and enable Jock to make the right decision for himself.

The doctor needs to have a clear understanding of the criteria for a useful screening test. The WHO[4] defined these as follows:

1. The condition should be an important health problem
2. The natural history of the condition should be understood
3. There should be a recognisable latent or early symptomatic stage
4. There should be a test that is easy to perform and interpret, acceptable, accurate, reliable, sensitive and specific
5. There should be an accepted treatment recognised for the disease
6. Treatment should be more effective if started early
7. There should be a policy on who should be treated
8. Diagnosis and treatment should be cost-effective
9. Case finding should be a continuous process.

The National Health and Medical Research Council Information for Health Practitioners summarises the evidence that shows why PSA test does not fulfil these criteria, as follows:

Possible benefit of PSA testing[5]
- For every 1000 men tested, two men will avoid death from prostate cancer before 85 years of age because of PSA testing. This benefit might be greater for men at high risk of prostate cancer, such as those with a strong family history of the disease.
- For every 1000 men tested, two men will avoid metastatic prostate cancer before 85 years of age because of PSA testing.

Expected harms of PSA testing
False-positive results:
- For every 1000 men tested:
  - 87 men who do not have prostate cancer will have a false positive PSA test that will lead to a biopsy
  - 28 men will experience a side effect from the biopsy that they consider to be a moderate/major problem that may require healthcare, and one will require hospitalisation.

Overdiagnosis:
- For every 1000 men tested, 28 men will have prostate cancer diagnosed as a result of the PSA test, many of whom would have remained asymptomatic for life (i.e. are overdiagnosed).

Overtreatment:
- For every 1000 men tested:
  - 25 men will choose to undergo treatment (surgery or radiation) because of uncertainty about which cancers need to be treated, many of whom would do well without treatment (i.e. are overtreated)

- 7–10 of these 25 men will develop persistent impotence and/or urinary incontinence, and some will develop persistent bowel problems, due to treatment.
- For every 2000 men tested, one man will experience a serious cardiovascular event, such as myocardial infarction, due to treatment.[1]

(One option for running this case is to provide candidates with a copy of the NHMRC four-page summary of information for health professionals[1] or the RACGP patient information sheet.[5] This would test the candidate's ability to interpret medical information for patients, rather than test their memory on the outcomes of PSA testing.)

References

1. National Health and Medical Research Council 2014, *PSA Testing for Prostate Cancer in Asymptomatic Men. Information for Health Practitioners.* Available at: https://nhmrc.gov.au/sites/default/files/documents/reports/ clinical%20guidelines/men4d-psa-testing-asymptomatic.pdf, accessed 20 February 2019.
2. Cancer Council Australia 2018, 'Prostate Cancer Detection'. Available at: www.cancer.org.au/about-cancer/early-detection/prostate-cancer-screening. html, accessed 1 December 2018.
3. Royal Australian College of General Practitioners 2018, 'Guidelines for preventative activities in general practice, Prostate Cancer', RACGP, Melbourne, Vic. Available at: https://www.racgp.org.au/clinical-resources/ clinical-guidelines/key-racgp-guidelines/view-all-racgp-guidelines/red-book/ early-detection-of-cancers/prostate-cancer, accessed 20 February 2019.
4. Wilson, J & Junger, G 1968, 'The Principles and Practice of Screening for Disease', World Health Organization, Geneva.
5. Royal Australian College of General Practitioners 2015, *Should I have prostate cancer screening?* RACGP, Melbourne, Vic. Available at: https://www. racgp.org.au/download/Documents/Guidelines/prostate-cancer-screening- infosheetpdf.pdf, accessed 1 December 2018.

Further reading

Prostate Cancer Foundation of Australia and Cancer Council Australia PSA Testing Guidelines Expert Advisory Panel 2016, 'Draft clinical practice guidelines for PSA testing and early management of test-detected prostate cancer', Prostate Cancer Foundation of Australia and Cancer Council Australia, Sydney.

237

Case 46
Costa Rinaldi

Instructions for the doctor

This is a long case.

Please take a history. The facilitator will give you the results of the examination on request. Then negotiate a management plan with the patient.

Scenario

Costa Rinaldi is a 36-year-old man. He rarely comes to see the GP but has booked an appointment today because his girlfriend sent him. They want a family but have not achieved a pregnancy after a year without using contraception. Costa's girlfriend has a child from a previous relationship.

The following information is on his summary sheet:

Past medical history
Chickenpox aged 11
Medication
Nil
Allergies
Nil
Immunisation
Nil recorded
Social history
Works as an engineer.

Instructions for the patient, Costa Rinaldi

You are 36 years old and work hard as an engineer. Over the last few years you have put on weight and now have a BMI of 35.5 kg/m². You have always been keen to have a family and were delighted to meet Brenda. You want to start a family with her.

You have a great sex life but it is getting you down that Brenda is not pregnant. You have not used contraception for a year. You have a constant reminder that the lack of pregnancy is probably your problem, as Brenda's 6-year-old daughter from a previous relationship lives with you.

This problem is beginning to affect your work and your relationship with Brenda. You do not smoke and you drink at least five bottles of wine a week. You have heard that some childhood infections can cause infertility and you are worried that the chickenpox is to blame. Brenda has sent you to this appointment.

You have no genitourinary symptoms.

The following information is on your summary sheet:

Past medical history
Chickenpox aged 11
Medication
Nil, no supplements
Allergies
Nil
Immunisation
Nil recorded
Social history
Works as an engineer.

Instructions for the facilitator

Clinical examination findings

On specific request please give the doctor the following results:
Pulse 74
BP 136/82 mmHg
Height 1.75 m
Weight 108.8 kg
BMI 35.5 kg/m^2
No gynaecomastia
Abdominal examination—normal
Hair distribution—normal
Genitalia—normal testicular and penile examination; no varicocele.

Suggested approach to the case

Establish rapport

Open-ended questions to explore Costa's ideas, concerns and expectations about the problem and the consultation.

Specific questions[1]

General health–fever, systemic malaise, weight loss
Sexual function/genitalia
 –Frequency of coitus
 –Libido, exclude erectile dysfunction, ejaculatory failure, retrograde ejaculation
 –Urethral discharge.

Past medical history

History of undescended testes, trauma, orchitis
History of mumps, other infections–STIs, TB
Chemotherapy/radiotherapy.

Drugs

Prescribed, OTC, drugs of abuse (e.g. anabolic steroids).

Social history

Alcohol consumption, smoking, recreational drugs.

Occupational history

Impact of current issue on relationship and self-esteem
Seek permission to examine.

Ask for the examination findings

Pulse
BP
BMI
Gynaecomastia
Hair distribution
Abdominal examination
Genitalia, in particular size of testes (Klinefelter's syndrome), varicocele.

Most likely diagnosis

Subfertility.

Differential diagnosis

Female subfertility
—Cannot assume that it is a male problem
—Need to address the issue as a couple.

Investigations[1]

Sperm count × two—ideally fresh specimen after three days abstinence, two to three weeks apart
LH, FSH and morning testosterone[1] +/− total testosterone, prolactin
Screening for STI and HIV.

Advice

Discuss impact on relationship and consider need for relationship counselling
Reassurance subfertility not caused by chickenpox
Reduction in weight and alcohol consumption needed
Timing of intercourse
Plans for follow-up with partner.

Extra for this case

Check smoking status.

CASE COMMENTARY

Infertility affects 15–20% of couples, with up to 50% having male contributing factors; 5% of male infertility is potentially correctable. It is unrealistic in a single consultation to find the cause of the problem but Costa needs to leave this consult sensing that he is supported and that the doctor has set up a management plan.

It is important for the doctor to reassure Costa that chickenpox has not caused infertility. He is confusing chickenpox with mumps.

Hormone measurements can help determine whether Costa has gonadotropin deficiency (low testosterone and low or inappropriately normal LH and FSH), primary testicular failure (low testosterone, elevated LH and FSH), spermatogenic failure (normal testosterone and LH, elevated FSH), or androgen resistance (high testosterone, elevated LH). A majority of infertile men have normal testosterone, LH and FSH levels. Obstruction should be ruled out in azoospermic men with normal testosterone, LH and FSH levels. Yq microdeletions, specifically in the azoospermia factor (AZF) region, are the most prevalent cause of spermatogenic failure in men with azoospermia or severe oligozoospermia. Infertile men with azoospermia or severe oligozoospermia should be referred to male fertility specialists for further investigations such as karyotyping and testing for Yq microdeletions.[1]

 COMMON PITFALLS

A pitfall to avoid is agreeing with Costa that he is without doubt the cause of the problem. Brenda's previous pregnancy is not proof of current fertility. Joint consultations with the GP emphasise that this is an issue for Brenda and Costa as a couple, not just for one partner. This can be suggested for the future. The opportunities in this consultation are to conduct a physical examination, discuss Costa's drinking (alcohol can suppress spermatogenesis) and obesity, and recommend increased physical activity and arrange follow-up.

Reference

1. Katz, D, Teloken, P & Shoshany, O 2017, 'Male infertility—the other side of the equation', *Australian Family Physician,* vol. 46, no. 9, pp. 641–6.

Further reading

Hirsh, A 2003, 'Male subfertility: ABC of subfertility', *British Medical Journal,* vol. 327, pp. 669–73.

Cissen, M, Bensdorp, A, Cohlen, BJ, Repping, S, de Bruin, J & van Wely, M 2016, 'Treatments for male subfertility', Cochrane Collaboration, 26 February.

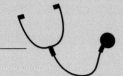

Section 14
Mental health

Case 47
Phyllis Brown

Instructions for the doctor

This is a short case.

Please take a history from Phyllis and outline to her the most likely diagnosis. Negotiate an initial management plan with Phyllis.

Scenario

You have been called to see Phyllis Brown, aged 74, at home. She has not attended the practice since her husband, Ernie, died two years ago. Ernie and Phyllis were very close and did everything together. They were involved in the local bowling club and seemed to almost live there.

Ernie died suddenly of a heart attack at the club one day and Phyllis took it badly. She now relies on most of her shopping being delivered or done by her daughter. The daughter has asked for this visit as she feels that her mother needs a good check-up.

The following information is on her summary sheet:

Past medical history

Cholecystectomy 1994

Medication

Nil

Allergies

Nil known

Immunisations

Nil known

Social history

Widowed

Non-smoker.

Instructions for the patient, Phyllis Brown

You are 74 years old and were widowed two years ago. You and Ernie had a good marriage and you find it hard without him. Most of the time you manage at home on your own but going out is impossible. As soon as you know you have to go out, you get anxious. Your heart races and you get diarrhoea. You start to shake and feel a lump in your throat. At times it even becomes difficult to breathe. As soon as you decide not to go out, everything calms down and you feel much better.

As a result you are staying home more and more. Life is just easier when you don't try to go out. You have adapted by using the phone to pay bills and your daughter has been good about helping with the shopping. Your daughter is concerned that you have not had a check-up with the doctor and so has persuaded the GP to do a home visit.

You would like to go out as you miss your friends but feel helpless and do not know how to get over your problems.

The following information is on your medical record:
Past medical history
Cholecystectomy 1994
Medication
Nil
Allergies
Nil known
Immunisations
Nil known
Social history
Widowed
Non-smoker.

Suggested approach to the case

Introduction, establish rapport
Open-ended questions to explore Phyllis's concerns about her situation.

Specific questions

Establish history of agoraphobia (anxiety regarding public places)
Explore bereavement and possible prolonged grief reaction
Exclude depression
Confirm diagnosis and possible link to grief.

Suggestions for therapy

Psychological—grief counselling, relaxation techniques, anxiety management, cognitive behavioural therapy, graded exposure

Medication—beta-blockers, selective serotonin reuptake inhibitors (SSRIs)

Referral to local mental health team

Mental health care plan

Plan follow-up to include review of physical health.

 CASE COMMENTARY

Agoraphobia is a disabling condition that GPs may have limited experience of—the illness itself prevents sufferers from attending for help. The illness can be improved with treatment. Initially home visits may be the only way to provide assistance for the agoraphobia, preventive health care and the management of other acute or chronic problems.

In this case, it is important for the doctor to establish rapport with Phyllis and demonstrate empathy for her problem.

Cognitive behavioural therapy (CBT) is more effective—and more cost-effective—than medication. Phyllis may be able to access CBT via a mental health care plan. Free online access to CBT training is another option, for example, MoodGYM (http://moodgym.anu.edu.au) or www.emhprac.org.au. Developing new skills such as mindfulness meditation can help.

SSRIs and TCAs are equal in efficacy with SSRIs and are more often used because of their relative lower side effect profile and safety in overdose. Benzodiazepines are not recommended first line due to side effect profile and the risk of dependence. However, they are as effective as SSRIs and may have a place in specific situations, such as enabling Phyllis to leave the house for an important event.

 COMMON PITFALLS

A doctor who is not able to establish rapport with Phyllis will fail to elicit the full list of symptoms from her. This most often occurs when doctors bombard patients with questions rather than listening carefully to their story. Another pitfall is telling Phyllis that she must come to the surgery for check-ups soon. This fails to recognise her illness and risks making her feel worse. Similarly, advising that she should pull herself together or that a cure is guaranteed are unrealistic and unhelpful.

Note: in the time available for a short case the doctor is unlikely to be able to give details of the treatment options as detailed above. It would be sufficient to mention referral, medication and psychological assistance.

Further reading

Andrews, G et al. 2018, 'Royal Australian and New Zealand College of Psychiatrists clinical practice guidelines for the treatment of panic disorder, social anxiety disorder and generalised anxiety disorder', *Australian and New Zealand Journal of Psychiatry,* vol. 52, no. 12, pp. 1109–72.

Lampe, L 2013, 'Drug treatment for anxiety', *Australian Prescriber,* vol. 36, no. 6, pp. 186–9.

Taylor, CB 2006, 'Panic disorder', *British Medical Journal,* vol. 332, pp. 951–5.

Case 48
Shirley Hill

Instructions for the doctor

This is a long case.

Please take a history from Shirley. You are expected to tell her your diagnosis and negotiate a management plan with her.

Scenario

A young mum, Shirley Hill, has arranged for a neighbour to look after her children so she can see a GP. She has been feeling tired all the time since the birth of her second child. She has just moved to the area. Just before she moved she went to her previous GP who did the following tests for tiredness which were all normal: FBC, ESR, UEC, TFTs, BSL, iron studies and urine for MCS.

The following information is on her summary sheet, which she brought from her previous GP:

Past medical history
First child, two years ago
Second child, six months ago
Medication
Nil
Allergies
Nil known
Immunisations
Up-to-date
Cervical screening test
Normal this year
Social history
Ex-nurse

Husband—Bill, a businessman, travels interstate regularly
Non-smoker
Alcohol intake—30 standard drinks per week recorded three years ago.

Instructions for the patient, Shirley Hill

You used to work as a nurse. You enjoyed your work as a clinical nurse consultant at a major teaching hospital. You met Bill when he was just starting up his own business. You brought in the regular income so he could spend time promoting the company before it became profitable. Over the last few years the business has thrived but has taken up more and more of his time. Because he is away so much you have had to give up your casual shifts at the local hospital.

Since the birth of your second child you have been feeling exhausted. You are getting some sleep but not as much as you need. You fall asleep as soon as your head hits the pillow. You are not refreshed when you wake up. You often get up around 3–4 am, sometimes it's for a breastfeed, but lately your baby is sleeping through and you're still waking up. It's difficult to get to sleep after this. You are finding it difficult to concentrate and have forgotten to pay a phone bill and power bill lately, which is really out of character.

You always wanted to be a mum, but it feels like more of a chore at present, which you feel guilty about. Other mums seem to have it all together. You don't want to admit it, but often you shout at the children and spend hours wondering what's gone wrong in life. You have a beautiful home and wonderful children but feel miserable and resentful and just can't be bothered any more.

You don't have much of an appetite lately and are still losing your baby weight.

You have no friends to share child care with as you did before. Your relationship with Bill is almost non-existent because he is away so much. If asked sensitively you will admit that you have thought that the children would be better off without you but have not made any suicide attempts or plans.

If the doctor asks you if you could get extra help, you think maybe your Mum would come from interstate for a while but you haven't really considered anyone helping. You also have enough money to get some paid help.

You'd be keen to try medication if this is suggested by the doctor.

The following information is on your medical record, which you brought from your previous GP:

Past medical history
First child, two years ago
Second child, six months ago

Medication
Nil
Allergies
Nil known
Immunisations
Up-to-date
Cervical screening test
Normal this year
Social history
Ex-nurse
Husband—Bill, a businessman, travels interstate regularly
Non-smoker
Alcohol intake—30 standard drinks per week recorded three years ago.

Instructions for the facilitator

Explain full physical examination is normal and ask the doctor to continue
with the scenario
Edinburgh Postnatal Depression Score—16 (high likelihood of depression)
If asked for a different tool give findings 'high likelihood of depression'.

Suggested approach to the case

Establish rapport
Open questions to explore Shirley's ideas, concerns and expectations.

Specific questions

Mood
Tearfulness
Function and energy
Sleep—terminal insomnia present
Appetite
Interest in life
Relationships
Libido
Social concerns—money, social supports
History of abuse
Use of drugs or alcohol
Brief systems review—weight changes, thirst, fever
Question about delivery, feeding and current health of baby

Risk assessment—suicidal ideation
Ask about and assess the safety of the children
Past or family history of depression.

Ask for the examination findings

All normal
EPDS or other depression scale.

Management

Explain most likely diagnosis—postnatal depression
Investigations—no more needed than as above
Psychoeducation regarding diagnosis
Options for treatment
—Counselling, support groups, online resources
—Greater interaction with community, e.g. mothers' group,
playgroups etc.
—Mobilising social/family support in the short term
—Drug therapy—SSRIs first line (fluoxetine and paroxetine best
avoided in the peripartum period)
—Cognitive behavioural therapy with psychologist
—Regular exercise
Discuss situation with Bill
Consider referral to psychiatrist if not improving
Offer mental health plan
Arrange early review.

CASE COMMENTARY

The doctor needs to diagnose and assess the severity of Shirley's depression, consider her safety and that of her children. Next is negotiation with Shirley regarding the different management options and exploring supports that Shirley can access. The doctor can be optimistic that the situation will improve but must be realistic that it will take time.

Studies in Australia show one in ten women experience depression during pregnancy and one in seven during the year after pregnancy. Mental health conditions in the perinatal period often go undiagnosed and can have deleterious effects on both the Mum, baby and family unit. Screening of all pregnant and post-partum women will help increase rates of diagnosis, using screening tools such as the Edinburgh Post

Natal Depression Scale (EPDS). Women scoring 13 or higher on the EPDS require further assessment. Consider more culturally appropriate tools where available, such as the Kimberley Mum's Mood scale, a tool validated for use with Aboriginal women in the Kimberley region of Western Australia.

 ## COMMON PITFALLS

A poor or inexperienced doctor will miss that this is postnatal depression and organise further tests or a specialist referral to chase a physical cause for the tiredness. This is an inappropriate use of resources and denies Shirley access to the assistance she needs to improve her mental health and the short-term and long-term health of her children.

Further reading

Austin, M-P, Highet, N & the Expert Working Group 2017, 'Mental health care in the perinatal period: Australian clinical practice guideline', Centre of Perinatal Excellence, Melbourne.

Goldin Evans, M, Phillippi, S & Gee RE 2015, 'Examining the screening practices of physicians for postpartum depression: implications for improving health outcomes', *Women's Health Issues,* vol. 25, no. 6, pp. 703–10.

Marley, JV, Kotz, J, Engelke, C, Williams, M, Stephen, D, Coutinho, S, et al. 2017, 'Validity and acceptability of Kimberley mum's mood scale to screen for perinatal anxiety and depression in remote Aboriginal health care settings', *PLoS ONE* vol. 12, no. 1, pp. e0168969. http://doi:10.1371/journal. pone.0168969.

Therapeutic Guidelines Ltd 2014, 'Psychiatric conditions in pregnancy and the postpartum'. In *eTG Complete.* Available at: http://online.tg.org.au.

Case 49
Monica Middlethorpe

Instructions for the doctor

This is a short case.
Please take a history and suggest your management plan to Monica.
You are Monica's usual GP.

Scenario

Monica Middlethorpe is 36 years old and comes to see you for assistance
with claustrophobia. She is planning a trip to Europe and is worried
about the flight.

The following information is on her medical record:
Past medical history
Asthma
Medication
Fluticasone/salmeterol 250 mcg/25 mcg per dose (Seretide) inhaler
1 puff twice daily
Salbutamol 100 mcg/dose (Ventolin) inhaler 2 puffs as required
Allergies
Nil
Immunisations
Nil recorded
Family history
Nil recorded
Social history
Administrative assistant (ex-tour guide)
Non-smoker.

Instructions for the patient, Monica Middlethorpe

You are 36 years old. You work as an administrative assistant and used to be a tour guide.

You now get anxious when in enclosed spaces. It starts with butterflies in your stomach, then your chest feels tight, your heart races, you feel frightened and you have a strong urge to run out into an open space. You recently flew interstate and your husband was quite upset with you when you almost didn't get on the plane home. You drank a couple of glasses of wine in the bar before take-off and somehow managed to fly.

You are planning a trip to Europe in six weeks and are worried about the flight. You have come to see your usual GP for help.

If the doctor asks sensitively, you will reveal that three years ago you had an asthma attack when leading a tour group in a cave. You did not have any salbutamol with you and became unwell and anxious. You had to change jobs because it was so awful. Since then you have been afraid of closed spaces and realised, when planning this trip, how much it is affecting your life.

The following information is on your medical record:

Past medical history

Asthma

Medication

Fluticasone/salmeterol 250 mcg/25 mcg per dose (Seretide) inhaler 1 puff twice daily

Salbutamol 100 mcg/dose (Ventolin) inhaler 2 puffs as required

Allergies

Nil

Immunisations

Nil recorded

Family history

Nil recorded

Social history

Administrative assistant (ex-tour guide)

Non-smoker.

Suggested approach to the case

Establish rapport

Explore Monica's ideas, concerns and expectations.

Assessment of the problem

Ask about recent event on flight

Sensitively probe for possible precipitating event
Explain correlation between significant event and current symptoms
Exclude underlying generalised anxiety or depression or substance misuse.

Management

Psychoeducation and reassurance that help is available
Short term—can use benzodiazepines for specific situations but risk of
addiction, not suitable for long-term use
Longer term—cognitive behavioural therapy (CBT)
Offer online resources available via online portal
www.mindhealthconnect.org.au
Review or arrange for review of chronic disease
—Asthma control, inhaler technique
—Need for flu vaccine.

 CASE COMMENTARY

Monica describes anxiety attacks when in confined spaces (claustrophobia) that started when she was underground and had an asthma attack
without having her inhaler nearby. Since that incident she has changed
jobs and avoided closed spaces whenever possible. However, she now
has the chance to travel and does not want to miss out.

In the short-term, benzodiazepines are effective anxiolytic drugs.
However, patients can become reliant on them, so alternative ways to
manage the anxiety in the long-term are preferred.

CBT is first-line treatment in anxiety disorders and can be delivered
in a variety of ways, depending on Monica's preference. A GP Mental
Health Care Plan would assist with the cost of face-to-face CBT with a
psychologist, and online programs or telephone CBT have been proven
effective also.

Anxiety is common and disabling with an estimated 1.6 million
presentations to Australian GPs per year. It is important for the doctor
to establish that Monica's anxiety is specific to a situation and is not
part of a more pervasive mental health problem. Strategies used to cope
with anxiety include 'self-medicating' with alcohol or illegal drugs, such
as marijuana, or avoidance of likely precipitating events or functions.
It is worth checking that Monica's couple of drinks prior to her most
recent plane trip was a one-off, not a routine part of life, and assessing
how much she has altered her life to avoid an anxiety attack.

255

COMMON PITFALLS

Beta-blockers can be effective in reducing the physical symptoms of anxiety and are a useful first-line therapy EXCEPT in asthmatics like Monica, for whom they can cause fatal bronchoconstriction.

Further reading

Andrews, G, et al. 2018, 'Royal Australian and New Zealand College of Psychiatrists clinical practice guidelines for the treatment of panic disorder, social anxiety disorder and generalised anxiety disorder', *Australian and New Zealand Journal of Psychiatry*, vol. 52, no. 12, pp. 1109–72.

Bassilios, B, Pirkis, J, King, K, Fletcher, J, Blashki, G & Burgess, P 2014, 'Evaluation of an Australian primary care telephone cognitive behavioural therapy pilot', *Australian Journal of Primary Health*, vol. 20, no. 1, pp. 62–73.

Handbook of Non Drug Intervention (HANDI) Project Team 2013, 'Internet-based cognitive behaviour therapy for depression and anxiety', *Australian Family Physician*, vol. 42, no. 11, pp. 803–4.

Lampe, L 2013, 'Drug treatment for anxiety', *Australian Prescriber*, vol. 36, no. 6, pp. 186–9.

Orman, J, O'Dea, B, Shand, F, Berk, M, Proudfoot, J & Christensen, H 2014, 'e-Mental health for mood and anxiety disorders in general practice', *Australian Family Physician*, vol. 43, no. 12, pp. 833–7.

Case 50
Tom Newton

Instructions for the doctor

This is a short case.

Please read the scenario below. Ann Newton has made an appointment with you to discuss her son's recent hospital admission. Please respond to Ann's questions as you would in clinical practice.

Scenario

Last week you were on call and admitted Tom Newton to the local mental health unit. Tom is 19, lives with his parents and is in second year, studying engineering at university.

Tom's parents called you as his behaviour was markedly disturbed; they suspect Tom has been using illicit drugs. For the last week the television had been telling Tom that it was his role to save the world from itself. When Tom said that the TV had told him that he had to die to save the world, his parents sought help.

The hospital has told Tom's parents that he has had an acute psychosis. Tom's mother, Ann, has made this appointment to talk with you about psychosis; she has heard from a friend that Tom is at risk of schizophrenia.

Instructions for Tom's mother, Ann Newton

You are nearly 60 years old and about to retire from your position as a school secretary. When you retire you are planning to travel around Australia.

Your eldest daughter is married and lives nearby. Tom, your son, is 19 and still at home. He is in his second year of an engineering degree. Some of Tom's university friends seem weird to you and you suspect Tom has been trying illicit drugs.

Over the past few weeks Tom's behaviour had become increasingly worrying—he was saying that the television wanted him to save the world.

When Tom announced that the TV had told him that he had to die to save the world, you and your husband decided to take Tom to the local GP.

Tom was admitted to the mental health unit at the hospital. The psychiatrist has said that Tom has had an acute psychosis. A friend told you that acute psychosis can lead to schizophrenia. You have made this appointment with the GP to find out more about this illness. You would like to know the answers to the following questions:

1. What is an acute psychosis?
2. What is schizophrenia?
3. Can it be cured?
4. What causes it?
5. Was it my fault?
6. What will happen to Tom now?
7. Will I still be able to travel around Australia as planned?

Suggested approach to the case

Establish rapport

Enquire about Tom's mother's ideas, concerns and expectations regarding acute psychosis and schizophrenia

No clear diagnosis yet—one psychotic episode is not diagnostic of schizophrenia, but acknowledge that Tom is at risk of schizophrenia

Explain that you can only talk in general terms, not specifically about Tom, because of confidentiality requirements

Target answers to Ann's concerns
   —Dispel myths, e.g. not split personality

Diagnostic features
   —Gradual change (prodrome usually about two years)
   —Changes in thinking, mood and behaviour

Positive symptoms
   —Hearing voices or seeing things that are not there (hallucinations)
   —Feeling controlled by someone or something else (passivity phenomena)
   —Believing things to be true that are not (delusions)
   —Thought disorders

Negative symptoms
   —Abnormal affect
   —Talking less (poverty of speech and poverty of content of speech)
   —Reduced motivation
   —Social withdrawal

Causes
- —Multifactorial, combination of genetic susceptibility and environmental factors
- —Link with illicit drugs such as cannabis and amphetamines

Advise of improved outcomes with early intervention

Advise of current therapies

Treatment
- —Aim to reduce symptoms, prevent relapse, early intervention of relapse
- —Antipsychotics
- —Family support
- —Community mental health team

Acknowledge any emotional response, e.g. shock and sadness

Assure Ann of your ongoing interest and support, and support groups for families caring for the mentally ill

Acknowledge planned trip around Australia, too early to make definite decision, continue to make plans to go.

 CASE COMMENTARY

Acute psychosis is frightening for all involved. Tom's and his family's world has suddenly changed; his mother, Ann, needs support and space to express her concerns and adjust to the new situation. Ann also needs help trying to decide what to do about her plans for travelling around Australia after retirement.

Without Tom's permission the GP cannot give specific information to Ann but instead has to give general advice. Evidence-based guidelines on early psychosis suggest supporting the family with information about psychotic disorders and recovery.[1]

A single episode of psychosis does not necessarily lead to schizophrenia. Early intervention can help people maintain cognitive and social function.[2] Relapse prevention includes stopping illicit drug use[3] and promoting a healthy lifestyle through social support, physical care and vocational rehabilitation.[4]

 COMMON PITFALLS

In practice, especially when as a GP you care for whole families, it can be hard to remember who has given permission for you to say what to whom.

259

Things can never be 'unsaid' so, if anything, it is wise to be cautious rather than overly open. Conversely, saying nothing at all is unhelpful, as evidence suggests that Tom will benefit from his family's support.[1, 3]

References

1. Early Psychosis Guidelines Writing Group and EPPIC National Support Program 2016, *Australian Clinical Guidelines for Early Psychosis,* 2nd ed, update, Orygen, The National Centre of Excellence in Youth Mental Health, Melbourne, Vic.

2. Stafford, MR, Jackson, H, Mayo-Wilson, E, Morrison, AP & Kendall, T 2013, 'Early interventions to prevent psychosis: systematic review and meta-analysis', *British Medical Journal,* vol. 346, p. f185.

3. Lee, HE & Jureidini, J 2013, 'Emerging psychosis in adolescents—a practical guide', *Australian Family Physician,* vol. 42, pp. 624-7.

4. Fraser, R, Berger, G, Killackey, E & McGorry, P 2006, 'Emerging psychosis in young people: Part 3—key issues for prolonged recovery', *Australian Family Physician,* vol. 35, pp. 329-33.

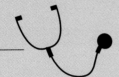

Section 15
Musculoskeletal medicine

Case 51
Anthony Campbell

Instructions for the doctor

This is a short case.

Please take a history from Anthony and conduct a focused examination. Outline the most likely diagnosis and your proposed management to the observing examiner.

Scenario

Anthony Campbell is a 46-year-old Aboriginal man who is complaining of pain in his right foot. He sprained his ankle when he was leaving a council meeting a few months ago. For the last few weeks he has experienced pain first thing in the morning, and after standing or walking for a period of time.

The following information is on Anthony's summary sheet at your suburban general practice:

Past medical history
Hypertension

Medication
Ramipril 5 mg od

Allergies
Nil known

Immunisations
Nil recorded

Family history
Nil known

Social history
Married
Works as a finance officer for the local town council
Non-smoker
Infrequent alcohol consumption.

Instructions for the patient, Anthony Campbell

You are a 46-year-old Aboriginal man. You work as a finance officer for the local council. You have come to see the GP today because of a pain in your right heel. You experience sharp intense pain when you put your heel down first thing in the morning or after sitting.

The pain eases after you have been up for a while, but it gets worse after walking any distance. It is worse when you walk around barefoot.

The pain is getting worse, not better. You first noticed it a few weeks ago.

A few months ago, you sprained your ankle when coming out of a council meeting late at night. Your ankle discomfort had seemed to have completely resolved, but you wonder if the two problems are connected (they turn out not to be).

The following information is on your medical record:

Past medical history
Hypertension
Medication
Ramipril 5 mg once a day
Allergies
Nil known
Immunisations
Nil recorded
Family history
Nil known
Social history
Married
Works as a finance officer for the local town council
Non-smoker
Infrequent alcohol consumption.

Suggested approach to the case

Introduction
Establish rapport.

History

Use open questions to explore Anthony's ideas, concerns and expectations.

Specific questions[1]

Location of the pain—plantar fascia insertion right foot
Duration of the pain

Timing

What's been tried so far?

Injury to ankle—sprain after council meeting, location of current pain suggests no connection

Exclude other musculoskeletal/systemic symptoms[1]

Request permission to examine.

Examination

Height 1.85 m

Weight 99 kg

BMI 29 kg/m^2

Expose both feet and ankles to the knees

Look

    —Alignment and range of movement normal

    —No scars or skin changes

    —Observe gait—some pain on putting down right heel

Feel

    —Acutely tender right calcaneum at insertion of plantar fascia, no lateral/medial calcaneal tenderness

    —No other tenderness or increased temperature

Move

    —Normal foot and ankle movements

    —No excess joint laxity.

Most likely diagnosis

Plantar fasciitis.

Management

Explanation

Reassurance not caused by ankle injury

Treatment

    —Stretching exercises—of plantar fascia and Achilles tendon[2]

    —Arch supports and heel cushions

    —Ice

    —Non-steroidal anti-inflammatory medication, if needed, but caution because on Ramipril for hypertension

    —Avoid walking barefoot or wearing flat shoes

If not settling, consider referral/steroid injection or trial of custom-made night splints.

CASE COMMENTARY

It is important to take the history of the recent fall but to realise that this is not the actual cause of the problem and explain this to Anthony. Diagnosis of plantar fasciitis is primarily based on history and physical examination.[3] The presence or absence of heel spurs is not helpful in diagnosing plantar fasciitis; imaging is needed only if other diagnoses seem more likely.

Most patients with plantar fasciitis improve with conservative or no therapy. Anthony can try rest, shoe inserts, ice massage and techniques that stretch the plantar fascia. His higher risk of renal disease suggests caution with non-steroidal anti-inflammatories and there is limited evidence of their effectiveness with the condition.[4] Custom-made orthotics and night splints can be useful, as may shock therapy and steroid injections, although these may risk longer-term tendon rupture and pain relief may only last four weeks.[5] Failed initial treatment is an indication for specialist surgical referral. Some cases persist despite surgery.

Anthony may benefit from encouragement regarding activity modification and suggestions on exercise he can do that will not exacerbate his heel pain, such as cycling or swimming. Losing weight will reduce the load on the ankle and can help. A thorough candidate will arrange a follow-up to check Anthony's blood pressure, BMI, other cardiac risk factors, kidney function and immunisation status.

References

1. Rio, E, Mayes, S & Cook, J 2015, 'Heel pain: a practical approach', *Australian Family Physician,* vol. 44, no. 3, pp. 96–101.
2. The Royal Australian College of General Practitioners 2018, 'Stretching exercises for plantar fasciitis', *Handbook of Non-Drug Interventions (HANDI),* RACGP, Melbourne, Vic.
3. Goff, JD & Crawford, R 2011, 'Diagnosis and treatment of plantar fasciitis', *American Family Physician,* vol. 84, no. 6, pp. 676–82.
4. Covey, CJ & Mulder, MD 2013, 'Plantar fasciitis: how best to treat?' *Journal of Family Practice,* vol. 62, no. 9, pp. 466–71.
5. McMillan, AM, Landorf, KB, Gilheany, MF, Bird, AR, Morrow, AD & Menz, HB 2012, 'Ultrasound guided corticosteroid injection for plantar fasciitis: randomised controlled trial', *British Medical Journal,* vol. 344, p. e3260.

Case 52
Martin Chatterjee

Instructions for the doctor

This is a short case.

Please do a focused clinical examination. You are not required to take any further history. Tell the examiner your examination findings, your differential diagnosis and initial plans for management.

Scenario

Martin Chatterjee is a 48-year-old office manager who does little regular exercise. Last week he played Masters' cricket and scored a career best of 32 runs. He does not recall specifically injuring his shoulder, but has since had pain in his left (non-dominant) shoulder. He is finding it difficult to move his left arm and to sleep, as the pain wakes him up whenever he tries to move. He has applied ice and is taking paracetamol at night. This is his first experience with a shoulder problem.

The following information is in Martin's medical record:

Medical history
Type 2 diabetes diagnosed two years ago
Height 1.85 m
Weight 106 kg
BMI 31 kg/m^2
Waist circumference 95 cm
Medication
Metformin 500 mg bd
Paracetamol 500 mg 2 nocte prn
Allergies
Nil

Social history
Office manager
Stopped smoking two years ago.

Instructions for the patient, Martin Chatterjee

You are a 48-year-old office manager who does little regular exercise. Last week you played Masters' cricket and scored a career best of 32 runs. Since then you have had pain in your left (non-dominant) shoulder. It is difficult to move your left arm and to sleep as the pain wakes you up whenever you try to move. You have applied ice and are taking paracetamol at night. This is your first experience with a shoulder problem.

The following information is on your medical record:
Medical history
Type 2 diabetes diagnosed two years ago
Height 1.85 m
Weight 106 kg
BMI 31 kg/m^2
Waist circumference 95 cm
Medication
Metformin 500 mg bd
Paracetamol 500 mg 2 nocte prn
Allergies
Nil
Social history
Office manager
Stopped smoking two years ago.

Please wear a shirt that buttons all the way down the front. You have no difficulty unbuttoning the shirt but struggle to take your shirt off (removing your arms from the sleeves) because of the pain in your left shoulder.

You have no bony tenderness. You have difficulty abducting your left shoulder. When the doctor gets your shoulder beyond the 120° angle you can then raise your arm and the pain eases.

All other shoulder movements are normal.

Instructions for the facilitator

Please report to the doctor that neck/back movements and axillae are normal when they start to examine these. This is to save time.

Suggested approach to the case

Introduction

Brief summary of the case by the candidate leading to request to examine the patient.

Examination[1]

Ask patient to remove shirt completely and observe for pain and restricted movement.

Look

Inspect anterior and posterior for
- —Asymmetry—expect non-dominant shoulder to be higher than dominant
- —Bruising
- —Scars
- —Muscle wasting.

Feel

Bones and joints
- —Sternoclavicular joint
- —Clavicle
- —Acromioclavicular joint
- —Glenohumeral junction
- —Humerus
- —Scapula.

Muscles and tendons
- —Subscapularis muscle, teres minor muscle
- —Supraspinatus and infraspinatus muscles
- —Long head of biceps
- —Pectoralis muscle
- —Deltoid muscle.

Move

Active and passive examination
- —Forward flexion
- —Extension

—Abduction—difficult to initiate abduction, painful arc between 60°
   and 120°
—Adduction
—Internal rotation
—External rotation
—Circumduction—limitation at lateral arc
—Neck/back movements and axillae (facilitator, report to doctor
   results are normal to save time).
Repeat with movement resisted
—Finding: pain on resisted abduction suggesting supraspinatus
   problem
—Test supraspinatus—resist abduction with thumb pointing upwards
—Test infraspinatus—resist abduction with thumb pointing
   downwards.

Apprehension test

Patient lying down, supine, arm externally rotated with elbow flexed to 90°.

Differential diagnosis

Most likely diagnosis—supraspinatus tendinopathy causing impingement
   (candidate will still pass if says rotator cuff inflammation/tendinopathy)
Consider rotator cuff tear or adhesive capsulitis
Ex-smoker—consider risk of lung tumour.

Management

Continue rest, ice
Analgesia
Explain—inflammation should settle and resolve
Physiotherapy[2]
Prevent frozen shoulder (more common in diabetics and 40–60 year olds)[2]
Discuss safety driving
Need for certification for work
No indication for other investigations at this stage, do CXR if pain persists/
   worsens
Follow-up, encourage continued fitness and weight loss and monitor
   diabetes
Consider subacromial corticosteroid injection if symptoms persist.[3]

CASE COMMENTARY

Shoulder pain is a common presentation in general practice. Most often the pain is musculoskeletal in origin but it can also signify serious visceral pathology. General practitioners must be able to conduct a thorough shoulder examination, report their findings clearly and synthesise the information from the history and examination to form a differential diagnosis.[1, 2]

COMMON PITFALLS

Finding pathology on ultrasound is common and does not necessarily correlate well with the clinical picture. Research suggests that GPs are over-reliant on shoulder imaging.[4] In many cases a focused but thorough history and examination provide sufficient information to form a differential diagnosis and a management plan.[5]

References

1. Brun, S 2012 'Initial assessment of the injured shoulder', *Australian Family Physician,* vol. 41, no. 4, pp. 217–20.
2. Masters, S 2007, 'Shoulder pain', *Australian Family Physician,* vol. 36, no. 6, pp. 414–20.
3. Arroll, B & Goodyear-Smith, F 2005, 'Corticosteroid injections for painful shoulder: a meta-analysis', *British Journal of General Practice,* vol. 55, no. 512, pp. 224–8.
4. Awerbuch, MS 2008, 'The clinical utility of ultrasonography for rotator cuff disease, shoulder impingement syndrome and subacromial bursitis', *Medical Journal of Australia,* vol. 188, no. 1, pp. 50–3.
5. Johal, P, Martin, D & Broadhurst, N 2008, 'Managing shoulder pain in general practice: assessment, imaging and referral', *Australian Family Physician,* vol. 37, no. 4, pp. 263–5.

Case 53
Sarah Cosgrove

Instructions for the doctor

This is a short case.

Please examine Mrs Cosgrove, who presents with hip pain. You are not required to take any further history. Please tell the examiner your examination findings, your differential diagnosis and initial plans for management.

Scenario

Sarah Cosgrove is 71 years old and has come to see you complaining of pain in her right hip. This pain has been gradually getting worse over the past few years. The pain is beginning to interfere with her daily activities and she gets some stiffness after she has rested. She still cycles to do her shopping.

Mrs Cosgrove has pain in both first metacarpophalangeal joints, both knees and her neck.

The following information is on her summary sheet:

Past medical history
Appendicectomy as a child
Medication
Nil
Allergies
Nil
Immunisations
Up-to-date
Cervical screening test and breast screen
Normal one year ago
Social history
Married
Two children, one overseas

Alcohol—two standard drinks per week
Non-smoker.

Instructions for the patient, Sarah Cosgrove

You are a 71-year-old retired personal assistant. You have always been active and still cycle to do your shopping. You have come to see the GP today because of pain in your right hip. This pain has been gradually getting worse over the past few years. Your symptoms now interfere with your daily activities and you experience some stiffness after resting.

You also have pain in both first metacarpophalangeal joints, both knees and your neck.

Both your older brothers have had hip replacements because of osteoarthritis. You suspect this is what you have but you are concerned about possible surgery because one brother had serious postoperative complications and nearly died.

Clinical examination findings

On examination you will indicate that the pain is felt centrally in the right inguinal canal. Please demonstrate minimal tenderness on palpation over the greater trochanter of the right hip and reduced hip movement on abduction, internal rotation and extension. When the doctor asks to examine your back, other hip and knees please report that this is not necessary.

The following information is on your medical record:
Past medical history
Appendicectomy as a child
Medication
Nil
Allergies
Nil
Immunisations
Up-to-date
Cervical screen test and breast screen
Normal one year ago
Social history
Married
Two children, one overseas
Alcohol—two standard drinks per week
Non-smoker.

Information for the facilitator

Alternative scenario

The doctor is told that Mrs Cosgrove has osteoarthritis of the right hip. They are required to focus on management. The emphasis would be on ensuring Mrs Cosgrove understands the problem and chooses with the doctor the options for treatment. The doctor should notice hesitation when surgery is discussed and explore the rationale for her concern.

Suggested approach to the case

Introduction
Request permission to examine.

Examination

161cm, 68 kg
BMI 26 kg/m^2
Timed Up and Go[1]
Gait
Posture, look for Trendelenburg's sign

Hip and knee

Look—scars, swelling, deformity
Feel—temperature, crepitus, effusion
Move
  —Active then passive
  —Rotation internal and external
  —Flexion/extension
  —Abduction/adduction.

Most likely diagnosis

Osteoarthritis of hip.

Management[2]

Aim to minimise pain and maintain function
Maintain fitness and exercise
Symptomatic treatment
  —Analgesia: paracetamol as first line, NSAIDs as second line
Physiotherapy, hydrotherapy, walking stick
Referral for joint replacement when pain is intractable
Arrange follow-up.

CASE COMMENTARY

The doctor needs to establish a rapport with Mrs Cosgrove and request permission to examine her. Some doctors I've watched have achieved this by briefly summarising the story to show Mrs Cosgrove that they understand what the issues are.

The doctor must conduct the examination efficiently, moving with ease from one aspect to the next and not cause unnecessary pain. The examination should appear as a well-rehearsed routine; it is obvious to observers when doctors are thinking what to do next rather than being able to focus on the findings and their interpretation.

The most likely diagnosis is osteoarthritis of the right hip, which does not need further investigations at this stage. The doctor should suggest a range of non-pharmaceutical, pharmaceutical and surgical options for treatment.[2, 3] Strengthening and flexibility exercises can reduce pain and maintain function.[4] Glucosamine and acupuncture[2] may not be more effective than a placebo, and there is evidence that the small-to-moderate beneficial effects of non-tramadol opioids are outweighed by large increases in the risk of adverse events.[5]

References

1. Waldron, N, Hill, A & Barker, A 2012, 'Falls prevention in older adults. Assessment and management', *Australian Family Physician,* vol. 41, no. 12, pp. 930–5.
2. The Royal Australian College of General Practitioners 2018, 'Diagnosis and management of hip and knee osteoarthritis algorithm'. In: *Guideline for the management of knee and hip osteoarthritis,* 2nd ed, RACGP, East Melbourne, Vic, p. 64.
3. McKenzie, S & Torkington, A 2010, 'Osteoarthritis. Management options in general practice', *Australian Family Physician,* vol. 39, no. 9, pp. 622–5.
4. Uthman, OA, van der Windt, DA, Jordan, JL, Dziedzic, KS, Healey, EL, Peat, GM et al. 2013, 'Exercise for lower limb osteoarthritis: systematic review incorporating trial sequential analysis and network meta-analysis', *British Medical Journal,* vol. 347, p. f5555.
5. Nuesch, E, Rutjes, AW, Husni, E, Welch, V & Juni, P 2009, 'Oral or transdermal opioids for osteoarthritis of the knee or hip', Cochrane Database of Systematic Reviews, CD003115.

Further reading

The Royal Australian College of General Practitioners 2018, *Guideline for the management of knee and hip osteoarthritis,* 2nd ed, RACGP, East Melbourne, Vic.

Case 54
Jeremy King

Instructions for the doctor

This is a short case.

Please take a history, conduct an appropriate examination and then outline your management plan to Jeremy.

Scenario

Jeremy King is a 25-year-old plumber who comes to see you for review following a car accident. He was driving to work when a truck went very slowly into the back of his car while he was stationary at traffic lights. He attended the hospital emergency department where he was examined. The doctor did not think X-rays were needed[1] and only did them following pressure from Jeremy. No fractures were identified.

Jeremy has returned for review a week after the accident. The brake and indicator light of Jeremy's work ute needed replacement but otherwise it was fine.

The following information is on his summary sheet:

Past medical history

Nil

Medication

Nil

Allergies

Nil known

Immunisations

Up-to-date

Social history

Self-employed plumber.

Instructions for the patient, Jeremy King

You are a 25-year-old self-employed plumber. Your business has been going badly and you have been getting increasingly tired and frustrated at work. You have wanted to take time off but cannot afford to.

Last week you were driving to work when a truck went very slowly into the back of your work ute while you were stationary at traffic lights. You attended the hospital emergency department where you were examined. The doctor said that you did not need X-rays but you insisted that they do some; no fractures were identified.

You have come to see your GP for review a week later.

The brake and indicator light of your work ute needed replacement but otherwise it was fine.

The truck driver's insurance company has already arranged for the repairs to your car, so you could get back to work next week. You have had one week off but want to take more time out. Your neck was a bit sore after the accident and you get mild pain at the end of the day. You have no other residual symptoms.

You want the GP to sign you off for more sick leave.

Clinical examination findings

Clinical examination is normal. There is a full range of pain-free movement.

The following information is on your medical record:

Past medical history
Nil
Medication
Nil
Allergies
Nil known
Immunisations
Up-to-date
Social history
Self-employed plumber.

Suggested approach to the case

Establish rapport
Open-ended questions to establish Jeremy's ideas and concerns about his injury, and expectations of this consultation.

Specific questions

Further history regarding neck pain
  —Interference with sleep, activities of daily living
  —Treatment so far
Enquire about other associated symptoms, such as headache, paraesthesiae, weakness
Explore potential impact of neck pain on work as a plumber
Request permission to examine neck.

Examination

Look—normal
Feel—no bony tenderness, no muscular spasm or increased tone
Move—full range of movement.

Management

Explain neck strains, reassure that symptoms will resolve, with no benefit from further time off
Suggest physiotherapy, simple analgesics; aim to maintain full range of movement
Empathise regarding business problems, screen for underlying mood disorder
A good doctor will also explore whether Jeremy smokes, drinks or uses drugs.

 CASE COMMENTARY

This case tests the GP's applied knowledge and skill and also their professional and ethical role. The car accident and resulting insurance claim has given Jeremy his first paid time off in years. He is still tired, and he thinks that more paid leave from the truck driver's insurance company would really help him.

A clinical assessment of the neck injury is required plus a decision about whether further sick leave is indicated. The minimal residual pain and absence of physical signs demonstrate that Jeremy is fit to return to work. The doctor must avoid collusion by endorsing further unjustified sick leave. Psychological, physiological and financial compensation factors all influence recovery from whiplash. The GP will need to make

Jeremy feel supported and understood with regard to his injury and his business pressures, but at the same time be clear that there is no justification for further sick leave.

The GP can offer follow-up about the accident, the business pressures and preventive health.

Reference

1. Ackland, H & Cameron, P 2012, 'Cervical spine. Assessment following trauma', *Australian Family Physician,* vol. 41 no. 4, pp. 196–201.

Further reading

Ferrari, R 2014, 'Predicting recovery from whiplash injury in the primary care setting', *Australian Family Physician,* vol. 43, no. 8, pp. 559–62.

Russell, G & Nicol, P 2009, '"I've broken my neck or something!" The general practice experience of whiplash', *Family Practice,* vol. 26, no. 2, pp. 115–20.

Teichtahl, A & McColl, G 2013, 'An approach to neck pain for the family physician', *Australian Family Physician,* vol. 42, no. 11, pp. 774–7.

Case 55
Geoff Sharp

Instructions for the doctor

This is a short case.

Please take a history from Geoff and conduct an appropriate focused examination. Outline to the facilitator your findings and suggestions for management.

Scenario

Geoff Sharp is a 54-year-old teacher. His wife has booked this appointment as she is fed up with listening to him complain about a pain in his right elbow. He says that he cannot make her cups of tea, as he can't pour the kettle.

The following information is on his medical record:

Past medical history
Nil significant
Medication
Nil
Allergies
Nil recorded
Immunisations
Up-to-date
Social history
Nil recorded.

Instructions for the patient, Geoff Sharp

You are a 54-year-old teacher. Normally you are fit and well and do not go to the doctor. For the last few weeks, you have noticed a pain in your right elbow. This makes it hard to carry books at school and you experience pain when trying to pour the kettle or open doors.

You have not sustained an injury to the elbow but do remember that the pain came on after you had spent the weekend gardening.

You have tried some paracetamol but it did not make much difference.

Clinical examination findings

You will demonstrate pain on pressure over the right lateral epicondyle and on active extension of the wrist. You have tennis elbow—extensor tendinopathy.

The following information is on your medical record:

Past medical history
Nil significant
Medication
Nil
Allergies
Nil recorded
Immunisations
Up-to-date
Social history
Nil recorded.

Suggested approach to the case

Establish rapport
Open questions to establish Geoff's ideas, concerns and expectations.

Specific questions

Duration of pain
Onset of pain
Precipitants of pain
General health
Treatment so far
Impact of problem on Geoff's life
Request permission to examine.

Examination

Ensure full view of both arms
Look
    —Exclude deformity or swelling
    —Muscle mass

Feel
>—Elicit tenderness
>—Exclude temperature increase in right arm

Move
>—Test range of movement of elbow joints—active, then passive
>—Flexion, extension and pronation/supination
>—Test movement against resistance

Pain is maximal on wrist extension against resistance.

Diagnosis

Tennis elbow—extensor tendinopathy.

Management

Education about the diagnosis
Rest
Range of treatment options starting with the least invasive[1, 2]
>—Wringing exercises[3, 4]
>—Topical non-steroidal anti-inflammatory drugs
>—Oral non-steroidal anti-inflammatory drugs—exclude
> contraindications prior to recommendation/prescription
>—Support bandage—epicondylitis brace
>—Referral for physiotherapy, ultrasonography treatment
>—Steroid/local anaesthetic injection[5]
>—Surgery—tendon transfer[2]

Occupational therapy review of work situation
Advice about the safety of driving
Arrange follow-up
If time allows, discuss preventive health measures such as smoking, blood
>pressure, exercise, diet, alcohol consumption, immunisation status.

CASE COMMENTARY

Geoff's symptoms should suggest the diagnosis to the doctor almost before the scenario begins. The doctor can then demonstrate their skills by excluding other serious pathology and clinch the diagnosis by identifying the epicondylar pain and reproduction of the pain on active resistance to wrist extension.

A good doctor will give a clear explanation of the problem in simple terms and then outline the options for treatment, carefully excluding any pre-existing contraindications. Tennis elbow typically presents after minor and often unrecognised trauma of the extensor muscles of the forearm.[1] It is a degenerative overuse–underuse tendinopathy of the common extensor origin of the lateral elbow.[2] Rehabilitation (exercise) based treatment is helpful,[3, 4] but to be effective patients must usually remove tendon overload.[2] Many cases of tennis elbow resolve spontaneously over 6–12 months. Steroid injection can give rapid pain relief in the short-term but is no longer recommended following evidence that it results in lower partial or full complete recovery, and greater recurrence after one year compared with a placebo injection.[5]

COMMON PITFALLS

There is time to complete the history, examination and management but only if the doctor focuses on the elbow. A poor doctor might be unnecessarily extensive with history-taking and examination, leaving no time for discussion regarding management. No investigations are needed for this diagnosis, nor is early referral to an orthopaedic surgeon.

References

1. The Royal Australian College of General Practitioners 2016, 'Exercise for tennis elbow'. In: *Handbook of Non-Drug Interventions (HANDI).* Available at: www.racgp.org.au/handi, accessed 1 December 2018.
2. Orchard, J & Kountouris, A 2011, 'The management of tennis elbow', *British Medical Journal,* vol. 342, p. d2687.
3. Murtagh, J, Rosenblatt, J, Coleman, J & Murtagh, C 2018, *Murtagh's General Practice,* 7th ed, McGraw-Hill Education, Sydney, pp. 726–8.
4. American Academy of Family Physicians 2007, 'Information from your family doctor. Exercises for tennis elbow', *American Family Physician,* vol. 76, no. 6, pp. 849–50.
5. Coombes, BK, Bisset, L, Brooks, P, Khan, A & Vicenzino, B 2013, 'Effect of corticosteroid injection, physiotherapy, or both on clinical outcomes in patients with unilateral lateral epicondylalgia: a randomized controlled trial', *Journal of the American Medical Association,* vol. 309, no. 5, pp. 461–9.

Case 56
Anna Wong

Instructions for the doctor

This is a short case.

Please take a focused history from Anna Wong, and then request appropriate examination and investigation findings from the facilitator. Based on the history, examination and investigation results, please outline your diagnostic impressions and initial management plan to Anna.

Scenario

Anna Wong is a 32-year-old mother of two. During the appointment for her four-month-old son's immunisation last week, she mentioned that she had been feeling tired and had aching joints. You recommended she try some simple analgesics and make an appointment to see you. She has come back today to discuss her symptoms.

The following information is on her summary sheet:

Past medical history
Nil significant
Medication
Nil
Allergies
Nil known
Immunisations
Up-to-date
Social history
Married, two children (four months and two years)
Hairdresser, currently on maternity leave
Non-smoker, non-drinker.

Instructions for the patient, Anna Wong

Six weeks ago, your left wrist became painful. Initially, you put it down to the way you were holding your baby to breastfeed. During the following fortnight your other wrist plus feet, ankles and hands started to hurt and have been steadily getting worse. You are also feeling really tired and run-down—a bit like the flu—although you suspect this is due to breastfeeding, lack of sleep and trying to look after your family. You have not noticed a fever.

Paracetamol does not provide much relief. You have avoided anti-inflammatories, as the pharmacist said they weren't safe to take when breastfeeding.

On specific questioning:

- You think your wrists and feet have been a bit swollen but you're not sure. The pain is worse on waking and you have stiffness for the first one to two hours of the day. You have lost three kg in two months without specifically trying, which you are very pleased about (getting rid of the 'baby bulge').
- You have not travelled anywhere recently and have no other contacts with similar symptoms.
- You have no personal or family history of auto-immune disease or allergies. Your only knowledge of arthritis is that it is a 'wear and tear disease that old people get'.

The following information is on your summary sheet:

Past medical history

Nil significant

Medication

Nil

Allergies

Nil known

Immunisations

Up-to-date

Social history

Married, two children (four months and two years)

Hairdresser, currently on maternity leave

Non-smoker, non-drinker.

Information for the facilitator

Clinical examination findings

Each aspect needs to be asked for specifically:

Looks tired but has normal colour

BP 125/75 mmHg
Pulse 82
Temperature 36.8°C
BMI 23.5

No thyroid enlargement
Cardiovascular, abdominal and respiratory examinations unremarkable
Musculoskeletal examination: no joint deformities; wrists, second and third
    MCP joints and second, third and fourth MTP joints slightly swollen
    and tender bilaterally, and painful on both active and passive movement;
    ankles painful but not swollen
No extra-articular signs.

Investigation findings

Each aspect needs to be asked for specifically:
FBC Hb 105, normocytic
ESR 38 (3–9 mm/hour)
CRP 22 (normal <5 mg/L)
Rheumatoid factor 28 (negative <30 IU/L)
Anticyclic citrullinated peptide (anti-CCP) antibody levels positive
Iron studies normal
Ross River virus serology negative
ANA low titre positive
TSH normal
No joint erosions on plain X-rays of hands and feet.

Suggested approach to the case

Develop rapport and show empathy regarding effects of symptoms on
    activities of daily living.

Specific questions for patients presenting with arthralgia

Onset—acute, subacute vs chronic
Temporal pattern
    —Migratory
    —Additive
    —Episodic/intermittent
Number of joints affected—1, 2–4, >5
Distribution of joint involvement
    —Proximal vs distal
    —Small vs large

—Symmetrical vs asymmetrical
—Spinal vs peripheral
Inflammatory vs non-inflammatory
Systemic symptoms
Extra-articular
—Ocular involvement
—Skin lesions
—Nail dystrophy
—Rheumatoid nodules.

Examination

Systematic approach
General examination plus specific examination of thyroid, skin (rash, bruises, nodules), nails and eyes
Joint examinations should include all affected joints, looking for swelling, deformity, tenderness and range of motion (active and passive).

Management

Recognise that clinical picture plus anti-CCP positive indicates diagnosis of rheumatoid arthritis
Arrange rheumatological referral
Relief of joint symptoms (seeking rheumatological opinion if needed)—e.g. paracetamol, NSAIDs/COX-2, prednisone
May consider starting DMARD (e.g. methotrexate), in conjunction with specialist advice if early appointment with rheumatologist is not possible
If medication is recommended, provide appropriate advice about breastfeeding
Patient information and education (e.g. referral to patient information and support service organisations, such as Arthritis Australia and the Australian Rheumatology Association)
Patient support regarding coping with diagnosis
Provide opportunity for questions
Arrange follow-up appointment.

 CASE COMMENTARY

This case assesses whether candidates:
- have an efficient and structured approach to conducting the history and examination on a patient presenting with polyarthralgia

- rationally and appropriately investigate suspected rheumatoid arthritis, and correctly interpret the test results
- provide appropriate patient education and support, after sensitively explaining the diagnosis
- refer this patient for specialist care in addition to considering immediate treatment.

The key features[1] that together raise suspicion of rheumatoid arthritis in Anna are:

- persistent joint pain and swelling (>6 weeks)
- joint pain and swelling affecting at least three joints (including at least one small joint)
- symmetrical involvement of MCP/MTP joints
- morning stiffness for more than 30 minutes.

Together with a positive anti-CCP and raised inflammatory markers, these allow a definitive diagnosis of rheumatoid arthritis (as per 2010 classification criteria[2]).

 COMMON PITFALLS

- Not diagnosing rheumatoid arthritis on basis of negative rheumatoid factor.
- Not treating joint symptoms while waiting for appointment with rheumatologist.

References

1. The Royal Australian College of General Practitioners 2014, 'Early diagnosis and management of rheumatoid arthritis'. Available at: www.racgp.org.au/guidelines/musculoskeletal-diseases, accessed 1 December 2018.
2. Wilsdon, T & Hill, C 2017, 'Managing the drug treatment of rheumatoid arthritis', *Australian Prescriber*, vol. 40, no. 2, pp. 51–8.

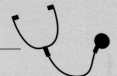

Section 16
Neurology

Case 57
Wilma Burns

Instructions for the doctor

This is a short case.

Please take a history, conduct a focused examination, outline the most likely diagnosis and negotiate a management plan with Wilma.

Scenario

Mrs Wilma Burns is 54 years old and has been a patient at the practice for several years. She is a keen gardener.

The following information is on her summary sheet:

Past medical history

Two children, normal pregnancies and delivery

Vaginal hysterectomy for prolapse aged 45

Mammogram normal this year

Medication

Nil

Allergies

Nil

Immunisations

Nil known

Social history

Non-smoker.

Instructions for the patient, Wilma Burns

You are a 54-year-old housewife and a keen gardener. For the last few weeks you have noticed pins and needles in your right hand on waking in the morning. This affects the pulps of the thumb, index, middle and half of the ring finger. Sometimes you get this after you have been gardening and in the last week the tingling sensation has woken you up at night. When you shake your right hand you can make some of the tingling go away and by doing this you can get back to sleep.

If the doctor asks, please say that you do not drink alcohol. You last had immunisations when you were at school.

Clinical examination findings

You have carpal tunnel syndrome. Please demonstrate an area of paraesthesia in the distribution of the right median nerve. Sensation is normal but power of thumb abduction is reduced. Tinel's sign* and Phalen's sign† are positive.

Neck and shoulder movements are normal.

The following information is on your medical record:

Past medical history
Two children, normal pregnancies and delivery
Vaginal hysterectomy for prolapse aged 45
Mammogram normal this year
Medication
Nil
Allergies
Nil
Immunisations
Nil known
Social history
Non-smoker.

Suggested approach to the case

Establish rapport
Open questions to explore patient's ideas, concerns and expectations.

Specific questions

Relevant to carpal tunnel syndrome
—Distribution of paraesthesiae

---

*Tinel's sign: tapping the flexor retinaculum on proximal part of palm reproduces median nerve paraesthesiae.

†Phalen's sign: flexion of both wrists for 30 seconds reproduces paraesthesiae in median nerve.

—Weakness of thumb movements
—Symptoms worse at night and early in the morning
Identify possible cause of carpal tunnel syndrome
   —Diabetes, obesity, rheumatoid arthritis, hypothyroidism,
     employment, hobbies
Exclude other causes
   —Neck or shoulder pathology, OA
   —Malignancy—Pancoast tumour, bone tumour
Request permission to examine.

Examination

Confirmation of area of paraesthesiae
Decreased sensation over the palm
Wasting of thenar eminence
Reduced power thumb abduction
Tinel's sign
Phalen's sign
Examination of the neck and shoulder.

Most likely diagnosis

Carpal tunnel syndrome.

Management

Discuss/explain diagnosis.

Investigations

TFTs
Glucose
Consider EMG depending on availability.

Treatment

Night splints
Consider corticosteroid injection
Refer for surgical decompression if conservative methods fail.

Opportunistic health promotion

Tetanus status—keen gardener
Alcohol intake.

CASE COMMENTARY

The history is suggestive of carpal tunnel syndrome. Most doctors suspect the diagnosis very quickly; the focus of the case becomes confirming this suspicion and excluding other causes.

The condition should be explained to Mrs Burns and then which investigations are needed and the treatment options. Some doctors will have easy access to nerve conduction studies but for doctors from rural areas, such investigations may be unavailable, and treatment will commence based on clinical grounds.

Tinel's sign and Phalen's sign are of doubtful value and so a doctor who does not perform these tests will not be penalised. The signs that correlate best with nerve conduction studies are the distribution of paraesthesiae and reduced strength of thumb abduction.[1]

Treatment of carpal tunnel syndrome usually starts with removing or modifying any underlying precipitants (such as use of vibration tools or keyboards, obesity or hypothyroidism), then trying night splints and/or local steroid injection before referring for surgery.[2,3]

References

1. D'Arcy, CA & McGee, S 2000, 'The rational clinical examination. Does this patient have carpal tunnel syndrome?' *Journal of the American Medical Association,* vol. 283, pp. 3110-7. Erratum appears in *Journal of the American Medical Association* 2000, vol. 284, no. 11, pp. 1384.
2. Wipperman, J & Goerl, K 2016, 'Carpal tunnel syndrome: diagnosis and management', *American Family Physician,* vol. 94, no. 12, pp. 993-9.
3. Simpson, MA & Day, B 2011, 'Painful numb hands', *Medical Journal of Australia,* vol. 195, pp. 388-91.

Case 58
Sybil Clarke

Instructions for the doctor

This is a long case.

Please take a history, examine this patient appropriately and discuss with her a management plan.

Scenario

A 65-year-old woman, Sybil Clarke, has booked a long appointment. She has noticed a tremor and her family have told her that they can no longer read her writing.

The following information is on her summary sheet:

Past medical history

Glaucoma, sees ophthalmologist regularly

Vaginal hysterectomy eight years ago for prolapse

First child, Terry, now aged 42

Second child, Malcolm, now aged 39

Medication

Timolol 0.25% 1 drop bd

Allergies

Nil

Immunisations

Up-to-date

Social history

Retired school secretary

Husband—retired credit union manager

Non-smoker

Alcohol intake—nil.

Instructions for the patient, Sybil Clarke

You are a 65-year-old retired school secretary. You have always been a very meticulous sort of person. Much to your embarrassment you now have a shake. You have made the appointment because your family said that they could not read your writing on the Christmas card that you sent them.

The shake has been getting worse gradually over the last couple of years, but it's now at a point that it is making it hard to complete day-to-day tasks such as doing up buttons. Your writing has deteriorated, becoming smaller and harder to read. You are finding it harder to move, and sometimes it can take a bit longer to get out of a chair. You are often fatigued. You had put this down to getting older but are starting to worry that you're getting older much quicker than your friends. You haven't had any falls. If asked, your voice has become softer and your family have complained they can't hear you when you're talking on the phone. You have had no issues with dribbling but do occasionally find it a little tricky to swallow foods like steak and bread. You are mostly continent of urine but have noticed some increased urgency over time. There have been no changes in your bowels.

You are mostly managing at home with cooking, cleaning, shopping and so forth, but are noticing that things take a bit more of a toll on you than in the past.

You have no mood symptoms or excessive anxiety, but you are worried about the cause of your tremor and deteriorating health.

Clinical examination findings

Please try to display a resting pill-rolling tremor, an expressionless face, persistent blinking on glabellar tap, cogwheel rigidity, a shuffling gait with a lack of arm swing, micrographia, poor balance and slow, stiff movements.

The following information is on your medical record:
Past medical history
Glaucoma, sees ophthalmologist regularly
Vaginal hysterectomy eight years ago for prolapse
First child, Terry, now aged 42
Second child, Malcolm, now aged 39
Medication
Timolol 0.25% 1 drop bd
Allergies
Nil
Immunisations
Up-to-date

Social history
Retired school secretary
Husband—retired credit union manager
Non-smoker
Alcohol intake—nil.

Suggested approach to the case

Establish rapport
Open-ended questions to explore Sybil's ideas, concerns and expectations.

Specific questions

Writing—what has changed?
Tremor—when does it occur?
Gait
Bradykinesia—slow movements, e.g. difficulty getting out of a chair, rolling over in bed
Falls
Dribbling/excess salivation
Dysphonia/dysphagia
Continence
Impact of symptoms on function and wellbeing
Mood symptoms—anxiety/depression
General health to exclude other causes—headaches, weight loss, fever, memory
Medication—exclude drug-induced Parkinsonism
Request permission to examine.

Examination

Pulse
BP
Neurological examination
  —Gait—shuffling
  —Balance—retropulsion test (the patient stands vertically and the doctor pulls them backwards to check for the speed of balance recovery. Parkinson disease patients are slower to recover)[1]
  —Tremor—at rest
Peripheral nervous system
  —Coordination—normal
  —Tone—cogwheel rigidity

–Power–slow movements but normal strength, writing shows micrographia
–Reflexes–normal
–Sensation–normal
Cranial nerve examination
–Normal except for expressionless face and glabellar tap–persistence of blinking reflex typical of Parkinson disease.

Most likely diagnosis

Parkinson disease.

Management

Explain condition
Demonstrate empathy and observe response to this diagnosis
Information–patient information leaflet/websites/support groups.

Investigations

TFTs[2]
UEC
LFTs.

Treatment

Drug therapy
    –Contraindication for anticholinergic drugs present
    –Aim to preserve quality of life[3]
    –Start with a low dose of levodopa/dopa-decarboxylase inhibitors (carbidopa or benserazide)[4]–for example, Sinemet
    –Dopamine agonist (e.g. pramipexole) or a monoamine oxidase type B inhibitor (e.g. selegiline) can be added later if needed
Consider neurology referral
Maintain function–healthy diet, regular exercise[4]
Consider occupational therapy/physiotherapy/exercise physiology/speech therapy referrals
Arrange follow-up.

 CASE COMMENTARY

Given the story of a new tremor plus difficulty writing, Parkinson disease is the most likely problem. Doctors who think of Parkinson can ask specific questions to confirm this and then demonstrate the cardinal signs of resting tremor, bradykinesia and rigidity on examination. Doctors who do not suspect Parkinson disease will need to take a more comprehensive history as well as doing the full neurological examination.

The doctor should consider other common causes of tremor, such as essential tremor, physiological tremor, hyperthyroidism, and potentially serious causes such as cerebellar disorders or a cerebral tumour. A good doctor will be able to demonstrate their clinical reasoning by asking relevant questions and conducting their examination appropriately so as to conclude that these disorders are less likely.

Mrs Clarke's history of glaucoma means that anticholinergic medication for the Parkinson disease is contraindicated.

Telling Mrs Clarke the likely diagnosis needs to be done sensitively. A good doctor may have been able to elicit her concerns at Parkinson being a possible cause. Such doctors will then be confirming her suspicions rather than breaking the news to her.

The doctor should consider the impact of the diagnosis on Mrs Clarke and provide appropriate support and follow up. Referral for assistance at home is not needed now but may be in the future. Likewise, Sybil's driving capacity will need to be assessed once her functioning on medication is known.

(The list of 'instructions for the patient' looks daunting, but it can be done. I found that playing Sybil was not only excellent revision for Parkinson but also gave me new insight into what it might feel like to have the 'shaking palsy'.)

References

1. Samii, A, Nutt, JG & Ransom, B 2004, 'Parkinson's disease', *Lancet,* vol. 363, pp. 1783–93.
2. Sirisena, D & Williams, DR 2009, 'My hands shake: classification and treatment of tremor', *Australian Family Physician,* vol. 9, pp. 678–83.
3. Hayes, MW, Fung, VS, Kimber, TE & O'Sullivan, JD 2010, 'Current concepts in the management of Parkinson disease', *Medical Journal of Australia,* vol. 192, pp. 144–9.
4. Gazewood, JD, Richards, DR & Clebak, K 2013, 'Parkinson disease: an update', *American Family Physician,* vol. 87, pp. 267–73.

Further reading

Sellbach, A & Silburn, P 2012, 'Management of Parkinson's disease', *Australian Prescriber,* vol. 35, pp. 183–8.

Case 59
Rosie Inkamala

Instructions for the doctor

This is a long case.

Please take a focused history from Rosie. Outline to Rosie your differential diagnosis and negotiate a management plan with her.

Scenario

Rosie Inkamala is a 36-year-old Indigenous woman. Rosie has come to see you because two days ago, on the weekend, she could not move her right side for about half an hour. She thought she was having a stroke and was relieved that her movement came back. She has come to see you for a check-up now that the clinic is open.

The following information is on her summary sheet:

Past medical history

Rheumatic fever aged 15

Atrial fibrillation (AF)

Alcoholic hepatitis

Hypercholesterolaemia

Medication

Atorvastatin 10 mg od

Aspirin 100 mg od

Digoxin 0.625 mg od

Ramipril 10 mg od

Etonogestrel intrauterine implant six months ago (Mirena)

Allergies

Nil known

Immunisations

Up-to-date

Cervical screening test
Normal this year
Social history
High alcohol use
Chews tobacco.

Instructions for the patient, Rosie Inkamala

You are a 36-year-old Indigenous woman. Two days ago, on the weekend, you could not move your right arm or leg for about half an hour. You thought that you were having a stroke and were relieved when the movement came back. Today you have decided to come to see the GP for a check-up, now that the clinic is open. You drink heavily whenever you can afford it, which works out at more than 10 standard drinks three to four days a week. When you drink you tend to forget your medications, which are in a Webster pack.

You live with extended family and your two children and feel safe at home.

You are very scared of having a stroke after seeing your aunt suffer from a big stroke last year; you are motivated to do what the doctor thinks you should do. If they suggest stopping drinking, tell them you will need help to stop.

You are fluent in four Aboriginal languages, but your English is limited.

Clinical examination findings

BP 124/82 mmHg
No evidence of cardiac failure
Rate-controlled atrial fibrillation (AF)
No residual neurological findings.

The following information is on your medical record:
Past medical history
Rheumatic fever aged 15
Atrial fibrillation (AF)
Alcoholic hepatitis
Hypercholesterolaemia
Medication
Atorvastatin 10 mg od
Aspirin 100 mg od
Digoxin 0.625 mg od
Ramipril 10 mg od
Etonogestrel intrauterine implant six months ago (Mirena)

Allergies
Nil known
Immunisations
Up-to-date
Cervical screening test
Normal this year
Social history
High alcohol use
Chews tobacco.

Suggested approach to the case

Request the assistance of an interpreter
Establish rapport
Open-ended questions to explore Rosie's ideas, concerns and expectations.

Specific questions

Details about loss of movement—duration, sites of loss of movement
Aura (suggests migraine)
Headache
Any associated loss, such as loss of vision, sensation, consciousness or
bladder control
Any residual problem
Previous episodes
Family history of stroke, heart disease
Systems review, e.g. exclude fever, weight change
Request permission to examine.

Examination

Temperature
Cardiovascular system
    —Pulse—rate, rhythm, volume
    —BP
    —Splinter haemorrhages
    —Apex beat
    —Heart sounds, added sounds
    —Carotid bruits
    —Evidence of CCF
        —JVP raised
        —Pulmonary oedema

  —Hepatomegaly
  —Pitting dependent oedema
Neurological system
  —Gait
  —Balance
  —Peripheral nervous system
    —Inspection—wasting, tremor, fasciculation
    —Tone
    —Sensation—light touch
    —Power
    —Reflexes
    —Coordination
  —Cranial nerve examination
  I   questions regarding change sense of smell
  II   acuity, fields, pupil reflexes, fundi
  III, IV, VI eye movements, exclude diplopia and nystagmus
  V   opening jaw and facial sensation
  VII   facial movements
  VIII   hearing, balance
  IX, X   swallowing
  XI   shrug shoulders
  XII   tongue movements.

Summary of findings

BP 124/82 mmHg
No evidence of cardiac failure, soft pansystolic murmur
Controlled AF
No residual neurological deficit
BMI 22 kg/m^2.

Most likely diagnosis

Transient ischaemic attack (TIA).

Differential diagnoses

Hemiplegic migraine
Postictal state
Intracranial bleed.

Management

Explain likely diagnosis

Educate about link with previous rheumatic fever—need to prevent future
stroke and need for control of cardiovascular risk factors

Encourage emergency call if symptoms recur—TIA = Take Immediate Action.

Investigations

FBC, ESR, UEC

BSL/HbA1c

Digoxin level

Fasting lipids

LFTs and coagulation studies (liver damage)

ECG

CT scan asap to exclude haemorrhagic event[1]

Carotid duplex ultrasound or CT angiogram

Echocardiogram.

Treatment

Continue current medications

Consider additional anticoagulation post CT scan result—low molecular
weight heparin plus warfarin is recommended; clopidogrel is an alternative. Doctors need to assess patient's safety regarding warfarin: the risks
can outweigh the benefits in patients who consume high volumes of
alcohol or cannot reliably attend for monitoring

Culturally appropriate, motivational interviewing regarding alcohol and
tobacco use. Offer support from drug and alcohol team regarding alcohol
cessation

Encourage regular exercise, eating healthy bush tucker

Arrange follow-up.

CASE COMMENTARY

The doctor should ask if an interpreter is available. In this scenario one
is not, so the doctor will need to communicate with Rosie in simple
English. The doctor should avoid using a loud voice or assuming that
an inability to understand English signifies intellectual disability. These
challenges can lead doctors to give up on communication and thus deny
patients essential information.

Rosie is at risk of a disabling stroke. A TIA is not a benign event but should be considered a warning for stroke. Sensitivity will be needed when encouraging Rosie to be investigated and to adopt a healthier lifestyle, and when helping her determine the relative risks and benefits of commencing warfarin. Rosie's atrial fibrillation is associated with mitral regurgitation following her rheumatic heart disease. Prescribing the newer oral anticoagulants for this situation would be off-label as these are only approved for non-valvular atrial fibrillation.

Rosie should be advised to seek assistance immediately if the paralysis returns. Urgent transfer to a hospital for thrombolytic therapy can then be arranged.[2-4]

References

1. Leung, ES, Hamilton-Bruce, MA & Koblar, SA 2010, 'Transient ischaemic attacks–assessment and management', *Australian Family Physician,* vol. 39, pp. 820-4.
2. Brieger, D 2014, 'Anticoagulation: a GP primer on the new oral anticoagulants', *Australian Family Physician,* vol. 43, pp. 254-9.
3. Wang, Y, Wang, Y, Zhao, X, Liu, L, Wang, D, Wang, C et al. 2013, 'Clopidogrel with aspirin in acute minor stroke or transient ischemic attack', *New England Journal of Medicine,* vol. 369, pp. 11-9.
4. Dhamija, RK & Donnan, GA 2007, 'Time is brain–acute stroke management', *Australian Family Physician,* vol. 36, pp. 892-5.

Case 60
Joe Summers

Instructions for the doctor

This is a short case.

Please read the following history and conduct a focused clinical examination. Tell the facilitator your findings and what initial investigations you would request.

Scenario

Joe Summers is a 67-year-old retired truck driver. He has been a patient at the practice for years but only attends to get his licence renewed. One year he went to a Pit Stop health promotion stand at the local show and he recorded a BMI of 39 kg/m^2 and a waist circumference of 115 cm.

Joe has noticed over the last few months that he cannot feel so well with his hands and feet. He assumed this was a normal part of ageing but he mentioned it when he went to buy some shoes and the shop assistant was concerned and told him that he had to come to see a doctor.

The following information is on his summary sheet:

Past medical history

Nil

Medication

Nil

Allergies

Nil

Immunisations

Nil known

Family history

Nil known

Social history

Retired truck driver.

Instructions for the patient, Joe Summers

You are a 67-year-old retired truck driver. You have been a patient at the practice for years but only attend to get your licence renewed. One year you went to a Pit Stop health promotion stand at the local show and you recorded a BMI of 39 kg/m^2 and a waist circumference of 115 cm. You already knew you were overweight and drank too much so did not see the point of going back to the GP to be told off again.

You have noticed over the last few months that you cannot feel so well with your hands and feet. You also get funny tingling feelings that are irritating. You assumed this was a normal part of ageing but you mentioned it when you went to buy some shoes. The shop assistant was concerned and told you to come to see a doctor for a check-up.

The following information is on your medical record:

Past medical history
Nil
Medication
Nil
Allergies
Nil
Immunisations
Nil known
Family history
Nil known
Social history
Retired truck driver.

Please mimic the absence of sensation to monofilament testing, and reduced vibration sense and joint position and pain sense of your feet to the level of your ankle, and hands to your wrist. Motor function, skin, pulses and reflexes are normal.

Instructions for the facilitator

The following equipment is needed: tendon hammer, sterile neurology pins, tuning fork and 10 g monofilament.

In the interests of time, examination of the hands is not required. When the doctor asks to examine the hands, please say that the signs are the equivalent to the signs in the feet. If the doctor does not examine the hands, do not volunteer this information.

Suggested approach to the case

Establish rapport
Summarise history
Request permission to examine.

Examination

Observe patient walking
Skin intact
No muscle wasting or fasciculation
Tone
Sensation
    —10 g monofilament testing
    —Pain sense with neuro-pin
    —Vibration sense
    —Joint position sense
Motor function
Coordination
Reflexes
Pulses
Random BSL or urinalysis.

Findings

Reduced sensation in both feet to ankle level and hands to wrists, i.e. glove
and stocking sensory neuropathy.

Initial investigations

Fasting blood glucose
FBC, ESR, B12, folate
Liver function tests, renal function, TSH
Fasting lipids and ratio
Further assessment
    —Drug and alcohol history.

 CASE COMMENTARY

Joe has developed a glove and stocking symmetrical sensory peripheral
neuropathy. There are multiple potential causes but the most common

are diabetes or alcohol.[1] A stepped approach to the investigations is appropriate, starting with routine blood tests. If these are normal, serum protein electrophoresis for a monoclonal gammopathy, and studies for HIV, sarcoidosis, heavy metal poisoning and vasculitis may be indicated.[2] The underlying cause of the neuropathy needs treatment, plus Joe needs advice on preventing damage to his hands and feet.

Foot ulcers are a significant burden for the individuals affected and for the health care system. Prevention is imperative. Testing for peripheral neuropathy is a key component of prevention.[3] Loss of ability to feel a standardised 10 g monofilament correlates with a risk of ulceration, making this test arguably more relevant in clinical practice than the more expensive nerve conduction test. Loss of vibration sense also correlates with the risk of ulceration but less so than the monofilament test.[4]

References

1. Azhary, H, Farooq, MU, Bhanushali, M, Majid, A & Kassab MY 2010, 'Peripheral neuropathy: differential diagnosis and management', *American Family Physician,* vol. 81, pp. 887–92.
2. Pascuzzi, RM 2009, 'Peripheral neuropathy', *Medical Clinics of North America,* vol. 93, pp. 317–42.
3. Ogrin, R & Sands, A 2006, 'Foot assessment in patients with diabetes', *Australian Family Physician,* vol. 35, pp. 419–21.
4. Singh, N, Armstrong, DG & Lipsky, BA 2005, 'Preventing foot ulcers in patients with diabetes', *Journal of the American Medical Association,* vol. 293, pp. 217–28.

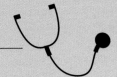

Section 17
Palliative care

Case 61
Liz Ross

Instructions for the doctor

This is a short case.

Please manage the patient's request as appropriate. Physical examination and investigations are not required.

Scenario

Liz Ross is 81 years old and a regular patient of yours. She has recently been diagnosed with metastatic ovarian cancer and her treatment is supportive rather than curative. She is currently feeling quite well physically and is pain free. Liz has come in to see you today because her daughter has told her to 'get her affairs in order'.

The following information is on her summary sheet:

Past medical history

Ovarian cancer

Mild hypertension

Medication

Paracetamol 1 g qid (antihypertensive stopped after cancer
   diagnosis)

Allergies

Nil

Immunisations

Influenza and pneumococcal vaccinations up-to-date

Social history

Widowed, four children; lives with her eldest daughter, Rosie

Non-smoker

Does not consume alcohol.

Instructions for the patient, Liz Ross

Your opening statement is 'As you know doctor my days are numbered, my daughter thinks I should get my affairs in order and talk to you about paperwork.'

You are an 81-year-old woman with recently diagnosed ovarian cancer. Your treatment will not cure your cancer but aims to keep you comfortable. At the moment you feel very well and live independently. You have limited health literacy and don't understand the legal or practical aspects of advance care planning. You don't need anything else today as you saw your specialist yesterday.

You have come to terms with your diagnosis and feel satisfied that you've lived a long and good life. You are not depressed and don't have any questions regarding your prognosis or treatment at this time.

You have heard there is a form that will stop hospital doctors 'giving you the paddles' if your heart stops. You think this is a reasonable idea, as you don't want to prolong your life if you are very ill with little chance of recovery.

Your understanding from what your daughter has told you, is that these forms will mean you don't have to make any future decisions, handing over the management of your health and financial affairs to your daughter. While this appeals in one sense, and you trust that your daughter will act in your best interests, you also feel like you would like to have a say in what happens while you still have your faculties and feel less comfortable with signing something that hands over decision-making at this point.

You have a simple will, leaving your estate to your children and your grandchildren and you are happy with that.

Initially answer questions about your understanding with a hesitant 'yes'; however, if asked to explain in your own words or for other appropriate assessments of understanding, you respond in a way that shows your understanding is very limited. If the matter is explained again in a clear and helpful way, your response indicates increased understanding of the issues.

Your reading level is mid-primary school and you don't use a computer.

Once the doctor explains the idea of an advance care plan or a living will, you want to pursue this. If the doctor indicates that they will give you the legal forms (Guardianship and Power of Attorney), you don't feel you need this right away. You would like another appointment to organise a living will and, if the doctor suggests it, you think it would be best if your daughter attends.

The following information is on your summary sheet:

Past medical history

Ovarian cancer

Mild hypertension
Medication
Paracetamol 1 g qid (antihypertensive stopped after cancer
    diagnosis)
Allergies
Nil
Immunisations
Influenza and pneumococcal vaccinations up-to-date
Social history
Widowed, four children; lives with her eldest daughter, Rosie
Non-smoker
Does not consume alcohol.

Suggested approach to the case

Establish rapport
Inquire into feelings regarding her recent diagnosis and prognosis
Assess level of understanding of advance care planning ('living will')
Provide information about advance care planning pitched at appropriate
    level and checking for understanding
Explore Liz's views towards advance care planning and her wishes for
    end-of-life care
Ask whether Liz has a legal will
Explain the difference in simple terms between an advance care plan,
    enduring guardianship and enduring power of attorney
Explain your ability to assist in advance care planning
Provide opportunity for questions in a supportive and non-confrontational
    way
Provide educational resources/hand-outs
Offer another appointment and suggest that her daughter (and/or another
    family member) attends with her.

 CASE COMMENTARY

The legislation for advance care planning and power of attorney documents vary between states and territories. Good candidates would be
expected to have a reasonable working knowledge of the legislative
requirements in their own jurisdiction. Key points include explaining the
concept of guardianship and that enduring power of attorney/enduring
guardianship (medical) and enduring power of attorney (financial) are

separate to advanced care planning. Many resources are now online, however, this will be of little help to Liz who does not use computers. Knowing reputable sites to access information relevant to your state and printing them for the patient would be the best approach.

 COMMON PITFALLS

Poor knowledge of advance care planning
Not recognising the patient's limited health literacy
Asking 'Do you understand?' and accepting a response of 'Yes' at face value.

Further reading

Advanced Care Planning Australia 2018, Factsheet for health professionals. What is advance care planning? Retrieved from: www.advancecareplanning. org.au/docs/default-source/acpa-resource-library/acpa-fact-sheets/acpa_ healthcare-professionals-factsheet-online_aug2018.pdf?sfvrsn=1, accessed 5 March 2019.

Bird, S 2014, 'Advance care planning', *Australian Family Physician,* vol. 43, no. 8, pp. 526–8.

Koay, K, Schofield, P & Jefford, M 2012, 'Importance of health literacy in oncology', *Asia Pacific Journal of Clinical Oncology,* vol. 8, no. 1, pp. 14–23.

Johnson, CE, McVey, P, Rhee, JJ et al. 2018, 'General practice palliative care: patient and carer expectations, advance care plans and place of death–a systematic review', *BMJ Supportive and Palliative Care,* Published Online First: 25 July 2018. doi: 10.1136/bmjspcare-2018-001549.

Case 62
Frank Stanley

Instructions for the doctor

This is a short viva.

Please discuss your management of this situation with a GP colleague.

Scenario

Frank is a 68-year-old retired postman who is dying from bowel cancer. He is now receiving palliative care and has a prognosis of weeks to months. He lives with his wife in a country town; their daughter lives nearby and helps a lot.

You visit Frank at home and glean the following:

- Frank is taking 20 mg oxycodone (Oxycontin) BD and 5 mg oxycodone (Endone) for breakthrough pain two to three hourly
- he sleeps badly as he is waking throughout the night to take breakthrough pain medication. It relieves the pain for about 90 minutes.

Please answer the examiner's questions about Frank.

Instructions for the facilitator

This is a viva. The doctor is expected to talk with you as a professional colleague.

Please ask the following questions:

1. How would you manage Frank's pain?
2. What are some of the symptoms you may need to consider in Frank's end-of-life care?

Prompts if needed:
> Do you think he is on the right pain medication?
> What do you think of the dose?
> Are there any non-opioid options to consider?
> Are there any non-pharmacological options?
3. Who else might be involved in Frank's care?

Suggested approach to the case

Overall aim is a 'good death' by managing Frank's pain and any other symptoms and taking a holistic approach to palliative care for him and his family.

1. Ask about the detail of his pain to determine best options for management:
   - consider if the pain is from the tumour, metastases, constipation or another new condition
   - Frank most likely needs a higher dose of slow-release pain medication
   - calculate his current total daily dose from the slow-release oxycodone and the total breakthrough doses of oxycodone
   - increase the slow-release oxycodone dose to the current total daily dose
   - provide breakthrough oxycodone at a sixth to a twelfth of the total dose
   - if a patient is on two different opioids, use an opioid conversion chart to calculate current total 24-hour dose of morphine, and then calculate the slow-release and breakthrough doses
   - ask Frank to document his breakthrough doses so that you can increase slow-release doses as needed in future
   - reassure that using opioids is appropriate
   - provide scripts for laxatives, as well as asking about constipation
   - add paracetamol regularly as this potentiates the action of opioids
   - consider the role of palliative radiotherapy, chemotherapy or nerve blocks, but these would require hospital care away from home
   - heat/cold packs, antispasmodics, nifedipine (for tenesmus) and corticosteroids could also be tried.

2. Palliative care patients can experience many complex symptoms and it is important to consider your patient and their family holistically.

   A helpful mnemonic is PAIN DOCTORSSS[1]

Pain
Anorexia
Insomnia
Nausea
Dyspnoea
Oedema
Constipation
Tiredness
Oral hygiene/mouth care
Restlessness
Spiritual
Social
p**S**ychological

Managing pain is a vital first step in relieving suffering; so too is open discussion about how Frank and his family are coping. What are their fears or concerns? Are there long-term worries or issues that could be addressed before he dies? Is his will up-to-date? Does he want to give his wife enduring power of attorney so that she can manage his financial affairs? Does he want to write an advanced health directive regarding his care? Are they receiving financial assistance through Centrelink? These topics can be addressed over time during visits to check on his pain and other physical symptoms.

3. Palliative care, given its many facets, is done best with a team. Others you may want to involve in end-of-life care include, but are not limited to:
   • spiritual care—pastor/priest/chaplain
   • palliative care teams, either locally or remotely. Most states have palliative care advice lines etc.
   • community care—visiting nurses, carers
   • home help, meals-on-wheels
   • respite for his family—hospital, local nursing home, local volunteers
   • psychologist/social worker.

 CASE COMMENTARY

This is a fairly straightforward case of end-of-life care. Frank appears to be on the right medication as it does work, but the need for regular breakthrough pain relief and waking from sleep suggests he is not on the right dose. You would not need to come up with actual doses in a viva, rather a structured approach to more effective pain management and care for Frank.

COMMON PITFALLS

Despite evidence that GP involvement in end-of-life care is beneficial, there are some GPs who opt out. Sometimes doctors are optimistic prognosticators and do not undertake end-of-life care planning early enough, resulting in late referrals to palliative care. It is important we have a solid understanding of end-of-life care in general practice and use help from palliative care teams and hotlines to continue providing excellent care.

Reference

1. Hart, A, Palliative care consultant, Western Australia (personal communication).

Further reading

Mitchell, G 2014, 'End-of-life care for patients with cancer', *Australian Family Physician,* vol. 43, no. 8, pp. 514–19.

Opioid Calculator–FPM ANZCA. App produced by the Faculty of Pain Medicine of the Australian and New Zealand College of Anaesthetists. Available for Apple and android.

www.palliaged.com.au. PalliAGED app available on android and Apple. Australian Government Department of Health palliative care resource.

Tait, P, Morris, B & To, T 2014, 'Core palliative medicines: meeting the needs of non-complex community patients', *Australian Family Physician,* vol. 43, no. 1–2, pp. 29–34.

Therapeutic Guidelines Ltd, Palliative Care Expert Group 2016, *Therapeutic Guidelines: Palliative Care. Version 4.* Therapeutic Guidelines Ltd, North Melbourne, Vic.

Case 63
Katrina Carroll

Instructions for the doctor

This is a short case.

Read the following scenario. Discuss the essential issues that arise with Katrina and suggest appropriate management. If you are considering anything that you do not wish to discuss with the patient at this stage, you should inform the observing examiner.

No physical examination is required and no further investigations are available.

Scenario

Katrina Carroll, a long-term patient of yours, is attending for an urgent appointment after scheduled routine follow-up with her breast surgeon. Your receptionist has obtained Dr Fisher's report from her recent review as follows:

Dear Doctor,

Re: Mrs Katrina Carroll, I saw Katrina for routine annual review following her T2 N1 M0 receptor negative left breast cancer four years ago. She has been well and had no specific complaints, but clinical examination revealed an enlarged, firm node in the left supraclavicular area. I organised an excision biopsy, which unfortunately returned results consistent with metastatic breast cancer. I organised staging scans which suggested she has metastasis in her T7 and L1 vertebrae, as well as two lesions in her liver.

We discussed her results today and I outlined that her condition is not operable. I have organised for her to see the oncologist next week.

Regards

The following information is on her summary sheet:

Past medical history

Mild episodic asthma

Left breast cancer—mastectomy, radiotherapy and chemotherapy
four years ago

Medication

Nil regular

Allergies

Nil known

Immunisations

Up-to-date

Social history

Non-smoker

Married to Paul

Six children

Works as a librarian.

Instructions for the patient, Katrina Carroll

You are Katrina Carroll, a 54-year-old woman who has been coming to this GP for several years. You are married to Paul (a high school English teacher) and you have six children. The youngest of your children is 17 and is the only one still at home. Your oldest two are married with children of their own.

You present to the doctor today following a visit to your surgeon, Dr Fisher, last week.

You came to this doctor with a breast lump four years ago and ended up having your left breast surgically removed because of breast cancer. Following this, you had radiotherapy to the left armpit and shoulder area and a course of chemotherapy. All this went pretty well and you've been healthy since then—back at work and feeling well.

About three weeks ago you went to see Dr Fisher for your annual check-up.

You weren't bothered by anything, but he found a lump around your left collarbone and cut it out a couple of days later. It came back as cancer in a lymph node and he then sent you for more tests—mostly scans. You saw him for the results of these last week, and he explained that your breast cancer has come back and has spread to your backbone in a couple of places, as well as your liver. He has explained that your situation is not one he can help with and has referred you to the oncology clinic. You're feeling abandoned by him and are glad to see your regular GP today.

You're scared but are prepared to concentrate on making the most of the time you have left. In contrast, your husband Paul is eager to pursue surgical or other cures and does not want to talk about death or dying. Paul has told you of an experimental light treatment in Mexico and is suggesting you sell the house to give it a go. You really don't think this is a good idea but are keen to know what the GP thinks.

You knew if it ever came back it would end your life and you are keen to know how long you've got. If your GP is reluctant to give any time frame, ask for their 'best guess' or a 'ballpark' idea. You're currently feeling well and if it is explored, you would like to spend the time you've got left with your children and grandchildren and you've always wanted to see Rome. You're not sure how long you would be prepared to keep having chemotherapy as it made you so very ill the first time around.

The following information is on your summary sheet:

Age
54
Past medical history
Mild episodic asthma
Left breast cancer—mastectomy, radiotherapy and chemotherapy four
     years ago
Medication
Nil regular
Allergies
Nil known
Immunisations
Up-to-date
Social history
Non-smoker
Married to Paul
Six children
Works as a librarian.

Suggested approach to the case

Establish rapport
Gently clarify Katrina's understanding of her condition and her prognosis
Recognise that Katrina and Paul are at different stages of acceptance.

Management

A good candidate should explore Katrina's concerns and recognise her husband's denial

Sensitively dismiss surgery as a curative option

Gently discourage the pursuit of an unorthodox cure at great expense to the family

Emphasise the GP's role in supporting Katrina and her family through the next stage of Katrina's care

Give compassionate but realistic information about Katrina's prognosis

Be prepared to sensitively encourage Katrina to face her mortality and maximise her time remaining

In response to the questions about prognosis you could introduce the concept of survival data and their value, given that each case is different

Katrina's five-year survival could be up 25% but it is dependent on receptors and her response to chemotherapy.

CASE COMMENTARY

Palliative care represents an unparalleled privilege for the GP. To care for your patient and their family through the last stage of life is both challenging and rewarding. Most are familiar with the stages of grief made popular by American psychiatrist Elisabeth Kübler-Ross. We now do not consider progress through these stages (in any order) as normative, but allow for a wide range of responses in our patients facing grief and loss. This case allows for practice in some important communication skills in a setting complicated by the husband's reluctance to accept his wife's prognosis.

While patients are free to elect to pursue alternative or unconventional treatment, there remains an important advocacy role for the GP in this setting. Encouraging the Carrolls to mortgage their house to expose Katrina to a non-evidence-based treatment is to betray that role. There are valuable skills to be practised in the discussion about her prognosis, with the extremes of being overly specific or overly evasive to be avoided.

COMMON PITFALLS

It is tempting to allow Katrina to join Paul in his optimism for a quick fix or miracle cure and, if you do, the case runs along a very positive line. Even Katrina can eventually be drawn into this. However, you have not been honest and she will be less prepared for what lies ahead as a result.

Sometimes we are quick to forcefully 'burst the bubble' of those we see in denial, forgetting that it can be a defence mechanism to allow continued functioning in the face of great loss. It's easy to side with Katrina as if she has the correct response and Paul must quickly 'catch up' with her. Helping Katrina to see that Paul's attitude is just as valid as hers is valuable.

When we raise referring our patients to various services—oncology, palliative care and so on—it can sound to the patient as though we are abandoning them and we have to work hard to emphasise our continued and central role in their care.

Michael Barbato's book, *Caring for the Palliative Care Patient,* deals with the role of denial and what to advise about alternative therapies.

Further reading

Barbato, M 2002, *Caring for the Palliative Care Patient,* McGraw-Hill, Sydney.

Kübler-Ross, E 1969, *On Death and Dying,* Routledge, London.

National Health and Medical Research Council 2011, 'An Ethical Framework for Integrating Palliative Care Principles into the Management of Advanced Chronic or Terminal Conditions'. Available at: www.nhmrc.gov.au/_files_ nhmrc/publications/attachments/rec31_ethical_framework_palliative_care_ terminal_110908.pdf, accessed 24 September 2014.

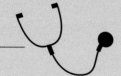

Section 18
Preventive health

Case 64
Bill Ferguson

Instructions for the doctor

This is a short case.

Please consult with Bill Ferguson, who wants help in giving up smoking.

Scenario

Bill Ferguson is a 60-year-old carpenter. He has smoked 30 cigarettes per day since leaving school at the age of 14. Yesterday he was diagnosed as having had a transient ischaemic attack. The doctor at the Emergency department told him that he had to stop smoking.

Bill has come to see you today to ask for advice about stopping smoking. He has previously resisted any discussion about giving up smoking whenever he attends for regular blood pressure and cholesterol checks.

The following information is on his medical record:
Past medical history
Hypertension five years
Hypercholesterolaemia three years
Medication
Perindopril 5 mg od
Atorvastatin 80 mg per day
Aspirin 100 mg per day
Allergies
Nil known
Immunisations
Up-to-date
Family history
Father died of a stroke, aged 64
Mother aged 93, moderate dementia living in a nursing home

Social history
Smokes 30 cigarettes per day
Alcohol intake—not known.

Instructions for the patient, Bill Ferguson

You are a 60-year-old carpenter. You have smoked 30 cigarettes per day since leaving school at the age of 14. Yesterday you had a funny turn. You suddenly could not use or feel your right arm and right leg. It only lasted about five minutes but it scared you and you went to the hospital. The letter from the hospital said it was a transient ischaemic attack or 'ministroke'. The doctor at the Emergency department told you that you had to stop smoking or you may have another attack or even a full stroke. Additionally, you could lose your driving licence.

You have come to your usual GP for advice on stopping smoking. You have previously resisted any discussion about giving up smoking when you come for regular blood pressure and cholesterol checks.

Lighting a cigarette has been the first activity of your day for over 40 years. You have tried to give up smoking before by going 'cold turkey' and only stopped for two weeks. You have never tried nicotine replacement therapy or tablets. Yesterday's funny turn has petrified you and you are now willing to do anything the doctor suggests.

The following information is on your medical record:
Past medical history
Hypertension five years
Hypercholesterolaemia three years
Medication
Perindopril 5 mg od
Atorvastatin 80 mg per day
Aspirin 100 mg per day
Allergies
Nil known
Immunisations
Up-to-date
Family history
Father died of a stroke, aged 64
Mother aged 93, moderate dementia living in a nursing home
Social history
Smokes 30 cigarettes per day
Alcohol intake—not known.

Suggested approach to the case

Introduction

Establish rapport and confirm reason for consult

Use the **5 A's** approach:[1]

1. Ask

How many cigarettes per day, for how long

2. Assess

Readiness to quit

Previous attempts/experience of quitting, longest period of abstinence

Assess nicotine dependence

—Minutes after waking to first cigarette

—Cravings or withdrawal symptoms in previous quit attempts

Personal preference of using nicotine replacement therapy (NRT) or medication, such as bupropion or varenicline

3. Advise

Specific advice on how to use NRT or medication

4. Assist

Talk through strategies when craves a smoke

—**4 D's**: **d**elay, **d**eep breathe, **d**rink, **d**istract

—Give information about Quitline

5. Arrange

Arrange follow-up

Relapse prevention advice.

CASE COMMENTARY

Assisting patients to stop smoking is a core skill for general practitioners, with clear evidence of health benefits. The research evidence is that Bill will have greater chance of success with quitting if he uses either NRT, bupropion (Zyban) or varenicline (Champix). He will also benefit from the support of those around him at work and at home, from agencies such as Quitline and from planned review with his GP.

All forms of NRT (gum, patch, spray or inhaler) are equally effective and have been shown to increase quit rates at 5 to 12 months approximately two-fold compared with a placebo. The choice of NRT product depends on personal preference and combining NRT with oral medication may improve success rates. Bill has smoked 30 cigarettes per day for many years and has his first cigarette within 30 minutes of waking up, so he has a high likelihood of nicotine dependence. Initially he should use the high-dose patch (21 mg/24 hr or 15 mg/16 hr patch) or gum (4 mg) and then follow the manufacturer's instructions on switching to the lower dose.[2]

Electronic cigarettes (e-cigarettes) are battery-powered devices that deliver nicotine in a vapour without tobacco or smoke. Some trials suggest that e-cigarettes could play a role in smoking cessation,[3] but long-term safety and efficacy data are needed. Acupuncture and hypnosis are not effective, but mindfulness is being explored to assist smoking cessation, especially in smokers with mental illness.

References

1. Zwar, N, Mendelsohn, C & Richmond, R 2014, 'Tobacco smoking: options for helping smokers to quit', *Australian Family Physician,* vol. 43, no. 6, pp. 348–54.
2. Mendelsohn, C 2013, 'Optimising nicotine replacement therapy in clinical practice', *Australian Family Physician,* vol. 42, no. 5, pp. 305–9.
3. McRobbie, H, Bullen, C, Hartmann-Boyce, J & Hajek, P 2014, 'Electronic cigarettes for smoking cessation and reduction', *Cochrane Database of Systematic Reviews,* vol. 12:CD010216.

Further reading

Australian Medical Association, Tobacco Smoking and E-cigarettes 2015. The AMA Position. Available at: https://ama.com.au/position-statement/tobacco-smoking-and-e-cigarettes-2015, accessed 1 December 2018.

The Royal Australian College of General Practitioners 2011, Supporting smoking cessation: a guide for health professionals, RACGP, Melbourne, Vic.

Case 65
Taylor Jordan

Instructions for the doctor

This is a short case.

Please take a history, assess this patient appropriately and discuss a management plan with her.

Scenario

Taylor Jordan is a 30-year-old woman not previously seen by you. She has made an appointment to ask you for advice on losing weight.

Three months ago, she attended the surgery and was examined and tested to exclude any organic cause for her obesity.

The following information is on her summary sheet:

Past medical history
Irritable bowel syndrome
Medication
Ethinyloestradiol 30 mcg, levonorgestrel 150 mcg (Microgynon 30 ED)
Allergies
Nil
Cervical smear
None recorded
Immunisations
Recall due for Hep A and for Hep B second injection
Social history
Single
Non-smoker
Alcohol intake not recorded.

Instructions for the patient, Taylor Jordan

You are 30 years old. You have always had a problem with your weight. You used to play hockey at state level but no longer exercise regularly. You work at a call centre about an hour's drive from home. Life is a constant series of diets but your height is 1.70 m, your weight is 90 kg and BMI is 30.2 kg/m^2 with an 80 cm waist. Three months ago, you attended the surgery and were examined and tested to exclude any organic cause for your obesity.

A friend at work lost weight through a very low-calorie diet but now she is putting the weight back on. You had thought of trying this diet but are now so uncertain about what to do that you have decided to see another GP for advice.

The following information is on your medical record:
Past medical history
Irritable bowel syndrome
Medication
Ethinyloestradiol 30 mcg, levonorgestrel 150 mcg (Microgynon 30 ED)
Allergies
Nil
Cervical smear
None recorded
Immunisations
Recall due for Hep A and Hep B second immunisation
Social history
Single
Non-smoker
Alcohol intake not recorded.

Suggested approach to the case

Establish rapport
Open questions to explore Taylor's ideas, concerns and expectations.

Specific questions

Review current weight, BMI, waist circumference and trend[1]
Review current diet and alcohol intake
Review current exercise level and attitude towards exercise
Exclude eating disorder
Brief review of Taylor's previous weight loss strategies.

Management[2]

Reassure that there is no need for further tests
Need for diet/activity balance and long-term sustainable change
Refer to reputable information sources regarding healthy eating, consider
dietitian referral
—Five serves of vegetable and two serves of fruit per day
—Drink 500 mL water half an hour before food[3]
Advise about use and interpretation of food labels, e.g. low in fat may
mean high in sugar
Increase activity—approximately an hour per day for weight loss
Set realistic goals—focus on health gains, not weight loss
Plan for regular follow-up and review
Plan for future consultations including hepatitis immunisations and cervical
screen.

 CASE COMMENTARY

This case tests the doctor's ability to engage with Taylor and encourage
her with the difficult task of lifestyle change. GPs need to skilfully support and motivate patients into action by exploring their readiness for
change and by being non-judgemental.[2] The formula for losing weight
is simple, but counteracting the multiple environmental, cultural, social
and personal factors[3] that have contributed to obesity in Australia is not.

Taylor's recent physical examination and tests mean that these do not
need to be repeated. The doctor should review Taylor's daily routine,
her diet and activity. Obesity results from a chronic imbalance between
energy intake from food and energy expenditure. Changes to her diet and
energy use (exercise) are needed. The doctor should encourage Taylor
to consider realistic changes that fit around her work. For example, is
there an option to park the car 15 minutes' walk away from work; can she
exercise during her lunch breaks; what exercise can she do at weekends?
Picking activities she enjoys will turn exercise from a chore to a hobby.
Can she gain needed support[4] by teaming up with a work colleague or
friend who also wishes to lose weight?

One pitfall is linking exercise with a reward of food and actually
putting on more weight. To burn off the kilojoules in one banana
(365 kJ), the average person would need to cycle for 11 minutes; to
burn off the kilojoules in one beer (585 kJ), they would need to walk
for 33 minutes—and one jam doughnut (1360 kJ) is equivalent to
55 minutes of dancing.

References

1. The Royal Australian College of General Practitioners 2018, *Guidelines for preventive activities in general practice,* 9th ed, updated, RACGP, East Melbourne, Vic, pp. 69–72.
2. Grima, M & Dixon, JB 2013, 'Obesity—recommendations for management in general practice and beyond', *Australian Family Physician,* vol. 42, pp. 532–41.
3. Handbook of Non-Drug Interventions (HANDI), Pre-meal water consumption for weight loss, Royal Australian College of General Practitioners.
4. Russell, HA, Rufus, C, Fogarty, CT, Fiscella, K & Carroll, J 2013, '"You need a support. When you don't have that . . . Chocolate looks real good". Barriers to and facilitators of behavioural changes among participants of a healthy living program', *Family Practice,* vol. 30, pp. 452–8.

Further Reading

The Royal Australian College of General Practitioners 2015, *Smoking, nutrition, alcohol, physical activity (SNAP): A population health guide to behavioural risk factors in general practice,* 2nd ed, RACGP, Melbourne, Vic.

Case 66
Ali Turnbull

Instructions for the doctor

This is a short case.

Please take a history and negotiate a management plan with Ali.

Scenario

Ali Turnbull is a 32-year-old artist who comes to see you requesting sleeping tablets. This is the first time that she has been to this surgery.

Prior to seeing you she completed the new patient questionnaire as below:

Past medical history

Recurrent tonsillitis

Medication

Nil

Allergies

Nil

Immunisations

Can't remember, will ask Mum

Cervical screen

Normal two years ago

Family history

Mum and Dad both fine, live interstate

Social history

Artist

Single

Smokes 15 cigarettes per day

No recreational drugs.

Instructions for the patient, Ali Turnbull

You are a 32-year-old artist who has come to the GP to request sleeping tablets. You used to combine your artwork with work as a Community Development Officer at the downtown youth centre. This year you sold enough paintings to be able to afford to paint full-time. You love the freedom and chance to express yourself and are happy to be earning enough money doing what you love to do.

Your timetable is flexible enough to fit around your inspiration to paint and you often end up painting all night if you are working well. You fit shopping, washing and cleaning in between painting sessions, sometimes taking your work outside for more inspiration. You drink about eight cups of coffee per day and do no regular exercise. You drink two to three beers a day. Your ideal evening is painting until late and then catching up with friends on social media from the comfort of your bed.

Your mood is stable and you have no weight loss or other symptoms suggestive of an organic illness.

The only frustration is that you cannot sleep and you have decided to see if the local GP can help. This is your first visit to this practice as you previously saw the GP near the youth centre.

Before seeing the GP you completed the new patient questionnaire as below:

Past medical history
Recurrent tonsillitis
Medication
Nil
Allergies
Nil
Cervical screen
Normal two years ago
Immunisations
Can't remember, will ask Mum
Family history
Mum and Dad both fine, live interstate
Social history
Artist
Single
Smoke 15 cigarettes per day
No recreational drugs.

Suggested approach to the case

Establish rapport
Open-ended questions to establish Ali's ideas, concerns and expectations.

Specific questions[1]

Sleep pattern and quality, bedtime regime
Lifestyle
   —Work
   —Family or community commitments
   —Alcohol and other drugs
   —Smoking
   —Exercise
General health
   —Brief systems review to exclude organic illness
Mental health
   —Mood, energy levels—exclude mania or depression
Strategies and treatments tried so far.

Diagnosis

Primary insomnia, secondary to lifestyle.

Management[1, 2]

Explain problem—need for significant lifestyle change to improve sleep quality in short-term and long-term health
No indication for medication
Appropriate sleep environment—quiet, dark, appropriate temperature, comfortable bedding
Regular routine—consistent daytime rising important
Develop regular night-time routine—keep bed for sleep, not the internet
Cut down caffeine
Stop smoking
Cut down alcohol consumption
Regular exercise (at least two hours ahead of bedtime)
If can't sleep, get up and try again
Bedtime restriction—limiting duration in bed to average calculated sleep time.

CASE COMMENTARY

Ali's success in her painting career has meant freedom from the restrictions imposed by paid external employment. Her love of her work means that it seems effortless to her to stay up for much of the night painting. However, this freedom comes at a price of poor sleep and a lifestyle that has the potential for harm in the long term. Ali needs specific advice on how to restore her circadian rhythms to promote good quality sleep and a non-judgemental space to discuss the implications of her smoking, alcohol consumption and lack of exercise.

The last thing that Ali needs is medication so that she can mask the problem of not sleeping and continue to push her body beyond the design specification!

COMMON PITFALLS

Poor sleep can be a sign of mental illness such as mania or depression, or might herald a new onset of an organic illness such as diabetes mellitus causing nocturia. While Ali's story seems immediately related to her lifestyle, it is vital to avoid 'premature closure' of the diagnosis and exclude the symptoms indicative of more sinister causes.

References

1. Cunnington, D, Junge, M, Fernando & A 2013, 'Insomnia: prevalence, consequences and effective treatment', *Medical Journal of Australia,* vol. 199, no. 8, pp. S36–40.
2. Therapeutics Guidelines Australia 2013, 'Patient information sheet: advice on good sleep practices'.

Further reading

Berk, M 2009, 'Sleep and depression—theory and practice', *Australian Family Physician,* vol. 38, no. 5, pp. 302–4.

Fernando 3rd, A, Arroll, B & Falloon, K 2013, 'A double-blind randomised controlled study of a brief intervention of bedtime restriction for adult patients with primary insomnia', *Journal of Primary Health Care,* vol. 5, no. 1, pp. 5–10.

Mansfield, D & McEvoy, R 2013, 'Sleep disorders: a practical guide for Australian health care practitioners', *Medical Journal of Australia,* vol. 199, issue 8 supplement, p. 8.

The Royal Australian College of General Practitioners, 'Brief behavioural therapy: insomnia in adults', *Handbook of Non-Drug Interventions (HANDI).*

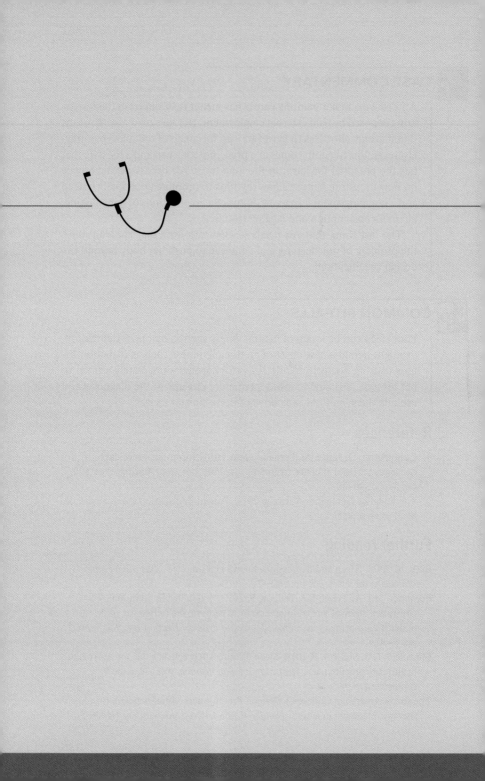

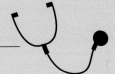

Section 19
Professional practice

Case 67
Vincent Butler

Instructions for the doctor

This is a short viva.

Please discuss your management of this situation with a GP colleague.

Scenario

You are on call and it is the end of the Saturday morning surgery. Your receptionist gives you a message from the laboratory to say that Mr Vincent Butler's INR level is 5.7.

You find the following information in Mr Butler's medical record:

Age

62

Past medical history

Mitral valve replacement six years ago

Hypertension

Medication

Warfarin 4 mg, alternate day 5 mg

Ramipril 10 mg per day

Atorvastatin 20 mg per day

Allergies

Nil recorded

Immunisations

Nil recorded

Social history

Retired chef.

Instructions for the facilitator

This is a viva.

The doctor is expected to talk with you as a professional colleague.
During the viva please ensure you ask the following questions:
1. What is your management of Mr Butler today?
2. What are the common causes of poor INR control?
3. What systems should there be in a practice to monitor the INR of patients on warfarin?
4. You decide to do a locum in a remote Aboriginal community. Would that make any difference to your management of patients on warfarin?

The following information is in Mr Butler's medical record:

Age
62
Past medical history
Mitral valve replacement six years ago
Hypertension
Medication
Warfarin 4 mg, alternate day 5 mg
Ramipril 10 mg per day
Atorvastatin 20 mg per day
Allergies
Nil recorded
Immunisations
Nil recorded
Social history
Retired chef.

Suggested approach to the case

1. **Management of the high result**
Clarify result with laboratory—preferably in writing/fax
Check that it is the correct result for the correct patient on the correct date
Search notes for:
- contact details—inform patient by phone if possible or via text message or through friends/family. If not by direct contact candidate must ensure that Mr Butler contacts you back to confirm receipt of the message and management plan. If not contactable may need to do home visit

- clinical information—reason for being on warfarin, target INR[1], any recent medication or dietary change likely to alter INR, pattern of INR control.[2]

Management plan[3]—to discuss with Mr Butler

- Plan for temporary cessation of warfarin, next test date and how to get results to find out next dose of warfarin
- Reiterate indications that would require hospital assessment: prolonged bleeding from a cut or unexpected bleeding
- Recommend quiet weekend, avoid contact sports
- Question to determine what affected control.

2. **Common causes of poor INR control**
   - Poorly calibrated machine/incorrect use of machine on point-of-care testing
   - Omissions or commissions taking warfarin, either deliberate or accidental
   - Medication interaction: patients should inform any prescriber that they are on warfarin, as NSAIDs and antibiotics (ciprofloxacin, metronidazole, doxycycline, erythromycin) are common causes of raised INR
   - Herbal products known to interact with warfarin include gingko, ginger, ginseng, garlic, St John's wort
   - Change to a different formulation—the formulations of warfarin are not interchangeable
   - Dietary change: increase in consumption of foods high in Vitamin K, such as green vegetables, can reduce INR; conversely a decrease in consumption can increase INR
   - Alcohol consumption.

3. **What systems should there be in a practice to monitor the INR of patients on warfarin?**

   Practices need systems that are not dependent on one person; they should be 'locum-proof' and 'holiday-proof'.

   The systems can be electronic or paper-based and should include the following:
   - a list of all patients on warfarin
   - for each patient on warfarin, their notes should say the indication, planned duration of treatment and target INR
   - each patient should be advised about the need for regular monitoring, to alert any prescriber that they are on warfarin, to maintain a stable diet, and of symptoms that would require urgent attention. A medical alert bracelet should be considered

- method of checking that each person being prescribed warfarin has regular INRs. The minimum recommended interval is monthly. Tests can be done at a laboratory or onsite using point-of-care testing equipment
- a result is received for each INR requested
- each INR result is checked on the day that the sample was taken
- patients get or receive their INR results on the day that the sample was taken. Each result to include the INR result, the current and recommended new dose and date of next test
- each result is signed, dated and filed
- if using point-of-care testing, calibrating and using instrument as per manufacturer's instructions
- system should include protocol for weekend and on-call handling of results.

4. **You decide to do a locum in a remote Aboriginal community. Would that make any difference to your management of patients on warfarin?**

Management may need to take into consideration the following:
- use of point-of-care testing very common
- if lab is used, potential delay in getting specimen to lab and getting results
- limited ability to contact patients by telephone. May need to liaise with clinic staff about how results are normally passed to patients, e.g. clinic bus or via Aboriginal liaison officer
- limited use of English. May need to use interpreters or in clinic use warfarin tablets to demonstrate how many of each colour to take
- intermittent access to food, including fruit and vegetables, may affect INR control
- lack of secure facilities to store warfarin
- patient may choose a nomadic lifestyle—need to assess risk/benefits of warfarin in this situation
- potential high use of alcohol—particularly in binges. What is the patient's individual risk/benefit equation?
- cultural factors—warfarin may need to be ceased ahead of some ceremonies/pay-back.

CASE COMMENTARY

This case requires the GP to talk with a professional colleague about a common clinical situation. The doctor will be assessed on their ability to listen and then talk concisely, clearly and appropriately answer the questions. Medical jargon can be used provided it is clear that both doctors use the same jargon or abbreviations to have the same meaning.

Warfarin is indicated for primary and secondary prevention of cardiovascular disease following evidence from randomised controlled trials of its benefits.[1] While there is evidence of benefit at the population level for those at high risk, it is up to the GP to assess the risks and benefits for an individual patient, taking into consideration that patient's psychological, social, cultural and biomedical factors and the clinic's ability to monitor the drug safely.[2, 3] The new anticoagulants that do not require INR monitoring are changing the treatment of non-valvular atrial fibrillation but are not licensed for use in patients like Mr Butler who have had valve replacements.[4]

COMMON PITFALLS

Medico-legal advice is that the prescription of warfarin requires patients 'who are well instructed, able to communicate clearly, cognitively intact, cooperative and compliant'.[5]

The duty of care that GPs have for following up and taking action on results depends on the clinical significance of the test results. Clinical significance is determined by the probability that the patient will be harmed if further medical advice is not obtained and the likely seriousness of the harm.[6] Warfarin and INR problems accounted for the largest proportion (18%) of medication errors in the Threats to Australian Patient Safety (TAPS) study.[7]

References

1. Whitlock, R, Sun, J, Fremes, S, Rubens, F & Teoh, K 2012, *Antithrombotic and thrombolytic therapy for valvular disease: Antithrombotic Therapy and Prevention of Thrombosis,* 9th ed, American College of Chest Physicians Evidence-Based Clinical Practice Guidelines, 141 (2 supplement) e:5765–e005.
2. Tideman, P, Tirimacco, R, St John, A & Roberts, G 2015, 'How to manage warfarin therapy', *Australian Prescriber,* vol. 38, no. 2, pp. 44–8.
3. Tran HA, Chunilal SD, Harper PL, Tran H, Wood EM & Gallus AS 2013, 'An update of consensus guidelines for warfarin reversal', *Medical Journal of Australia,* vol. 198, no. 4, pp. 198–9.
4. Brieger, D & Curnow, J 2014, 'Anticoagulation: a GP primer on the new oral anticoagulants', *Australian Family Physician,* vol. 43, no. 5, pp. 254–9.

5. Bird, S 2003, 'Medication errors: warfarin', *Australian Family Physician,* vol. 32, no. 12, pp. 1003–4.

6. The Royal Australian College of General Practitioners 2017, 'Follow-up systems', *Standards for general practices,* 5th ed, RACGP, East Melbourne, Vic.

7. Makeham, MAB, Saltman, DC & Kidd MR 2008, 'Lessons from the TAPS study. Warfarin: a major cause of threats to patient safety', *Australian Family Physician,* vol. 37, no. 10, pp. 817–18.

Case 68
Stephanie Clark

Instructions for the doctor

This is a short case.

You have arranged a meeting with your receptionist, Stephanie Clark, to manage the following situation.

Scenario

Stephanie Clark works as a receptionist at your single-doctor practice. Her 3-year-old child, Letitia, attends the local childcare centre. Last week another child, Daisy, attended the practice because of diarrhoea. Daisy's mum, Sally, was advised to keep Daisy at home until the results of the stool tests were available.

Sally brings Daisy to the practice today for a follow-up. Sally mentioned that she already knew that the stool test showed an infection that needed treatment, as Stephanie had told her when they met in the supermarket yesterday.

Breach of patient confidentiality is a reason for instant dismissal in all your staff contracts. Your practice manager is currently on leave and so you have to meet with Stephanie on your own.

Instructions for the receptionist, Stephanie Clark

You work as a receptionist at the local general practice. Your 3-year-old daughter, Letitia, attends the local childcare centre.

Children at the childcare centre have had a 'run' of diarrhoea. You have been hoping that Letitia would not catch the infection as you would have to take time-off work to care for her.

Letitia's best friend is Daisy. Last week Daisy attended the practice because of diarrhoea. Daisy's mum Sally was advised to keep Daisy at home until the results of the stool tests were available. When you chatted with Sally at the supermarket yesterday you told her the result showed Daisy needed treatment. Sally was happy to know this, as she could then reschedule her work.

You are a bit surprised that the GP has asked to see you this morning.

When the GP tells you about the breach of confidentiality and implications for your job, you react defensively. You consider that the rules are 'over-the-top' and stupid—Sally is your friend and you have a right to tell her what you know about her own child.

You show no appreciation of the seriousness of your error.

Suggested approach to the case

Arrange the meeting in a quiet, private office and ask Stephanie if she wishes to bring a support person

Explain the reason for meeting—Sally knew the results of Daisy's stool test prior to seeing the doctor

Sensitively ask for Stephanie's side of the story

Demonstrate active listening to Stephanie

Explore Stephanie's understanding and response to a reminder of the rules of patient confidentiality

Remind Stephanie that her employment can be terminated immediately if a breach of confidentiality occurs

State that Stephanie has breached confidentiality based on information from Sally and herself

Tell Stephanie that her employment is being ceased and that she will be paid outstanding leave entitlements. Ask her to leave the practice and remind her that her obligation to confidentiality continues after leaving the job

Document the meeting and its outcome in Stephanie's personnel folder.

CASE COMMENTARY

This case tests the doctor's knowledge of the legal and organisational domain of general practice and their skill in applying this knowledge in a difficult situation. All GPs need this core competence, even if many delegate such tasks to practice managers or choose to be an employee in a corporate entity.

Privacy of health information is a legislative requirement.[1] The Medical Board of Australia considers that 'Patients or clients have a right to expect that practitioners and their staff will hold information about them in confidence, unless information is required to be released by law or public interest considerations'.[2] Confidentiality is a particular issue for rural and remote practices where everybody knows everybody, but this does not mean that everybody has a right to know everybody's business.

Stephanie has committed a serious offence that threatens the reputation and potentially the future viability of the practice. The GP is fortunate that the patient has not lodged a formal complaint. Stephanie's response shows that she has little insight into the seriousness of her misconduct. Continuing her employment risks further breaches and so the GP must take the necessary step of terminating her employment immediately.

References

1. The Royal Australian College of General Practitioners National Expert Committee on Standards for General Practices. Standards for General Practices, 5th ed, RACGP, Launched 26 October 2017. Criterion C6.3: Confidentiality and privacy of health and other information. Available at: www.racgp.org.au/your-practice/standards/standards-for-general-practices-(5th-edition)/, accessed 3 September 2018.
2. Medical Board of Australia. Good medical practice: A code of conduct for doctors in Australia. 3.4 Confidentiality and privacy, www.medicalboard.gov.au/Codes-Guidelines-Policies/Code-of-conduct.aspx, accessed 3 September 2018.

Case 69
Debra and Declan Poole

Instructions for the doctor

This is a short case.

You are expected to discuss a clinical problem with the facilitator role playing your senior colleague.

Scenario

Last Friday you did your first evening on call for the practice. It was much busier than you had expected. As it was your wedding anniversary you were keen to get home as soon as possible.

You are a bit puzzled as to why the practice principal has asked to chat with you after this morning's surgery about a problem. Your memory is that you saw mostly kids with runny noses and one with an ear infection.

Instructions for the practice principal

Last weekend you were on call when you received a phone call from an angry and anxious mother, Debra Poole. Her son Declan, aged four, had a painful ear and they had come to see the new doctor at the practice. Debra said that the doctor seemed to be in a hurry and had a quick look in his ears but no further examination before prescribing amoxycillin.

Debra gave Declan the first dose of the medication but then looked more carefully at the packet and saw the drug was similar to penicillin. Two years previously Declan had had an allergic reaction to penicillin requiring him to stay overnight in hospital. Once she realised what had happened she went straight to the emergency department. As a precaution he was admitted to hospital for observation. Fortunately, Declan did not react to the single dose of amoxycillin but Debra lost a day's pay because she monitored him the following day.

When you talked with Debra on the weekend you promised that you would discuss this with your colleague on Monday.

Suggested approach to the case

Doctor to listen carefully to the practice principal's concerns
Doctor demonstrates understanding of different issues involved
  −Problem of a cursory clinical examination and risk of missing other more serious pathology
  −Impact of hurrying the consultation
  −Inappropriate prescribing of amoxycillin despite allergy−an avoidable and potentially fatal mistake
  −Financial impact of mistake on patient's family
  −Impact of the error on the practice reputation/business
Doctor acknowledges mistakes and outlines plans for action
  −Apologise to the family for the mistake
  −Apologise to the practice principal for impact on practice/reputation
  −Conduct more appropriate full physical examinations in the future
  −Check with patients about allergies and use information in the records
  −Check if Declan's file includes his penicillin allergy and update it if required
  −Undertaking prescribing modules from RACGP or NPS MedicineWise
  −Seek assistance with consultation techniques such as asking senior doctor to sit in or observe videotaped consultations
  −Ask practice principal if there is anything else that should be done
  −Inform their medical defence organisation.

CASE COMMENTARY

This case tests a doctor's ability to talk to a colleague, to recognise a mistake and to learn from it. The Medical Board of Australia's code of conduct states that 'When adverse events occur, you have a responsibility to be open and honest in your communication with your patient, to review what has occurred and to report appropriately'.[1] In this instance, formal reporting seems unnecessary as no severe reaction occurred, but the doctor should apologise to the family and the practice principal for the error. Next, there should be reflection on the precipitants of the problem. In this case, it was the tension between a work and a home commitment—a common scenario for GPs. This does not mean that GPs should not have a home life but that, in most instances, it should take second place when on call. A useful acronym is HALT: a GP should take extra care when Hungry, Angry, Late or Tired.

The doctor should outline to the practice principal what they intend to do differently in the future to prevent another similar event. Regular reviews of critical incidents and complaints are recommended, so that individuals and practices can learn from errors and modify processes to reduce risks.[2] A counterbalance to negative feedback can be 'compliments received', so that good practice is also acknowledged and reinforced.

Computerised alerts embedded in electronic health records have the potential to reduce prescribing errors by warning prescribers of possible risks such as allergies, but many studies report that doctors override computerised alerts up to 95% of the time.[3-5] 'Alert fatigue' resulting from excessive numbers of alerts has been identified as the primary reason for this but there is evidence that the timing of the alerts (often in the final stages of prescribing) also contributes to an alert being regarded as intrusive and unwelcome, and subsequently being ignored.[6]

 ## COMMON PITFALLS

The doctor in this scenario must avoid defending their actions and blaming the mother for not mentioning the penicillin allergy. Checking an allergy history is good practice whenever a medication is being prescribed. Absence of a documented allergy is not evidence of an absence of allergy. Such errors in the process of care are more common than errors due to lack of knowledge or skills.[7]

References

1. Medical Board of Australia. Good medical practice: A code of conduct for doctors in Australia. 3.10 Adverse events, www.medicalboard.gov.au/Codes-Guidelines-Policies/Code-of-conduct.aspx, accessed 3 September 2018.
2. Steer, N 2010, 'Managing clinical risks—tips from the toolkit 9', *Australian Family Physician,* vol. 39, no. 10, pp. 791–2.
3. Weingart, SN, Toth, M, Sands, DZ, Aronson, MD, Davis, RB & Phillips, RS 2003, 'Physicians' decisions to override computerised drug alerts in primary care', *Archives of Internal Medicine,* vol. 163, pp. 2625–31.

4. van der Sijs, H, Aarts, J, Vulto, A & Berg, M 2006, 'Overriding of drug safety alerts in computerized physician order entry', *Journal of the American Medical Informatics Association,* vol. 13, no. 2, pp. 138–47.
5. Sweidan, M, Reeve, JF, Brien, JE, Jayasuriya, P, Martin, JH & Vernon, GM 2009, 'Quality of drug interaction alerts in prescribing and dispensing software', *Medical Journal of Australia,* vol. 190, pp. 251–4.
6. Hayward, J, Thomson, F, Milne, H, et al. 2013, 'Too much, too late: mixed methods multi-channel video recording study of computerized decision support systems and GP prescribing', *Journal of the American Medical Informics Association,* vol. 20, pp. e76–e84.
7. Makeham, M, Stromer, S, Bridges-Webb, C, Mira, M, Saltman, D, Cooper, C, et al. 2008, 'Patient safety events reported in general practice: a taxonomy', *Quality & Safety in Health Care,* vol. 17, no. 1, pp. 53–7.

Further reading

Australian Commission on Safety and Quality in Health Care 2013, Implementing the Australian Open Disclosure Framework in small practices. ACSQHC, Sydney.

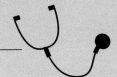

Section 20
Respiratory medicine

Case 70
Andrew Bond

Instructions for the doctor

This is a long case.

Please take a history and conduct an appropriate clinical examination. Outline to Andrew your differential diagnosis and plans for initial management.

Scenario

Mr Andrew Bond is a 65-year-old man who has not been to the surgery for a while. He is usually well. You spent time with him a year ago when he was giving up smoking. You are not sure why he has booked this appointment with you today.

The following information is on his summary sheet:

Past medical history

Vasectomy aged 42

Medication

Nil

Allergies

Nil

Immunisations

Up-to-date

Social history

Retired bus driver

Gave up cigarette smoking last year—was 20 per day for 40 years.

Instructions for the patient, Andrew Bond

You are a 65-year-old retired bus driver who gave up cigarette smoking last year. The final spur to giving up was when your older brother was diagnosed with lung cancer. Like you, he had smoked since leaving school. You had a bit of a cough for the weeks after you gave up but then you were fine and felt better than you had for years.

You have developed a new cough in the last three to four weeks. It is worst first thing in the morning. You have coughed up some blood but mostly it is a dry cough. You have lost weight and your appetite is not so good. You get puffed more easily than you used to but you are still managing to do the wood-turning you enjoy.

At the back of your mind is the thought that this might be cancer. You are not going to tell the GP that this is your concern but will talk about it if the GP mentions it.

Clinical examination findings

Height 1.7 m
Weight 67 kg (weight five years ago 73 kg)
BMI 22.1 kg/m^2
No abnormal clinical findings.

The following information is on your medical record:
Past medical history
Vasectomy aged 42
Medication
Nil
Allergies
Nil
Immunisations
Up-to-date
Social history
Retired bus driver
Gave up cigarette smoking last year—was 20 per day for 40 years.

Suggested approach to the case

Establish rapport
Open-ended questions to establish Andrew's ideas, concerns and expectations.

Specific questions

Cough
Haemoptysis

Sputum
Pain
Shortness of breath
Fever
Family history
Social history
    —Confirm smoking history
    —Occupational history—exposure to asbestos
    —Travel
Systems review—to include weight loss/appetite/energy/sleep
Request permission to examine.

Examination

General signs
    —Weight loss
    —Cyanosis
    —Clubbing
Respiratory system
    —Respiratory rate
    —Use of accessory muscles
    —Trachea
    —Chest expansion
    —Percussion
    —Auscultation
    —Lymph node enlargement
Abdominal examination looking for evidence of metastatic spread to the
    liver.

Differential diagnosis

Lung cancer—doctor must mention this as a possibility
Acute respiratory tract infection
Chronic obstructive pulmonary disease
Tuberculosis (less likely without risk factors).

Initial investigations

FBC
ESR or CRP
UEC

LFTs
Chest X-ray
Consider spirometry
Sputum for cytology and MCS.

Management

While not an initial investigation, Mr Bond has risk factors for lung cancer
and will require a chest CT and specialist referral irrespective of initial
results
Assure Mr Bond of ongoing support
Non-urgently need to find out about alcohol consumption and check of
immunisation status
No proven benefit for cough medicine
Arrange follow-up.

 CASE COMMENTARY

Mr Bond's story of past long-term smoking, loss of weight and appetite,
and a new cough and haemoptysis indicates lung cancer until proved
otherwise. Haemoptysis is the only symptom that in isolation consistently
predicts lung cancer.[1] As there is high clinical suspicion of lung cancer, a
CT chest and urgent referral to a specialist linked with a lung cancer multidisciplinary team is indicated even if the initial chest X-ray is negative.[2, 3]

It is essential that the doctor includes lung cancer in the differential
diagnosis. In clinical practice the timing of when to share the potential
diagnosis of cancer is determined by many factors. These include the
GP's prior relationship to the patient and the patient's level of interest
in finding out the diagnosis. Patients have the right to information and
evidence suggests that patients are keen to find out more than doctors
are willing to tell them. True patient-centred medicine gives the right
level of information, in understandable terms, at the right pace and at
the right time, as determined by the patient.

Poor doctors will either tell Mr Bond a definite diagnosis of cancer
with blunt disregard for his feelings or be too embarrassed or anxious
to mention the word cancer. Try to avoid these extremes. Mr Bond is
already concerned regarding cancer. A good doctor will explore these
pre-existing concerns and sensitively talk about the differential diagnosis
in the light of this and the clinical situation. Empathy with Mr Bond's
reactions will also be demonstrated.

References

1. Shim, J, Brindle, L, Simon, M & George, S 2014, 'A systematic review of symptomatic diagnosis of lung cancer', *Family Practice,* vol. 31, no. 2, pp. 137–48.
2. Earwood, JS, Dwight, D & Thompson, TD 2015, 'Hemoptysis: evaluation and management', *American Family Physician,* vol. 91, no. 4, pp. 243–9.
3. Cancer Australia. Investigating symptoms of lung cancer: a guide for GPs, 2012. Available at: www.canceraustralia.gov.au/publications-and-resources/cancer-australia-publications/investigating-symptoms-lung-cancer-guide-gps, accessed on 23 June 2018.

Case 71
Kerrie Griffiths

Instructions for the doctor

This is a short case.

Please take a history from Kerrie and conduct an appropriate focused clinical examination. Outline your differential diagnosis to the facilitator.

Scenario

Kerrie Griffiths is a 32-year-old woman whose first child was born by caesarean section a week ago. Baby Eloise is doing fine and Kerrie was discharged home yesterday.

This morning Kerrie has noticed a sharp pain on the left side of the chest. The pain is worse on breathing in. You are called to see Kerrie at home.

The following information is on her medical record:

Past medical history

Asthma

Medication

Fluticasone 250 mcg 1 puff bd

Salbutamol inhaler prn

Allergies

Nil

Immunisations

Up-to-date, rubella booster pre-pregnancy

Family history

Nil significant

Social history

Non-smoker.

Instructions for the patient, Kerrie Griffiths

You are 32 years old and your first child was born by caesarean section a week ago. Baby Eloise is doing fine and you were discharged home yesterday. This morning you have noticed a sharp pain on the left side of your chest. This is worse on breathing in and you feel short of breath. You have asked the doctor to see you at home.

This is a new pain. It is preventing you from breathing comfortably. You have had a cough this morning and have coughed up a bit of blood. You do not have a temperature and do not have any pain or symptoms suggestive of a deep vein thrombosis in your legs. You are breastfeeding without difficulty.

The following information is on your medical record:

Past medical history
Asthma

Medication
Fluticasone 250 mcg 1 puff bd
Salbutamol inhaler prn

Allergies
Nil

Immunisations
Up-to-date, rubella booster pre-pregnancy

Family history
Nil significant

Social history
Non-smoker.

Clinical examination findings

When the doctor examines you, please tell them the following:
- Temperature 37.2°C
- Pulse 106 regular
- BP 112/78 mmHg
- Respiratory rate 20 per minute.

You will experience pain in your left lower lobe on inspiration and be reluctant to take deep breaths

The chest is clear

Legs are normal (the most likely diagnosis is that you have a pulmonary embolus).

Suggested approach to the case

Establish rapport
Ask after the baby, feeding, sleep etc.
Open questions to explore Kerrie's ideas, concerns and expectations.

Specific questions

Details about the pain
Check for haemoptysis, dizziness, syncope, shortness of breath
Enquire about asthma control
Exclude infection as likely cause—ask about fever, systemic upset
Leg pain or swelling
Past history of thromboembolism or known thrombophilia disorders
Exclude mastitis/feeding problem
Reason for caesarean section—epidural or general anaesthetic?
Social history—does she smoke?
Family history of thromboembolism or thrombophilia disorders
Request permission to examine.

Examination

Temperature
Pulse
BP
Respiratory rate
Chest
   —Use of accessory muscles
   —Palpation—chest expansion
   —Percussion
   —Auscultation
Heart sounds
Legs—for signs of a DVT.

Differential diagnosis

Must mention pulmonary embolus
Basal atelectasis
Pneumonia
Other options including musculoskeletal chest wall pain—less likely.

CASE COMMENTARY

This case provides doctors an opportunity to practise, time and demonstrate their skills in taking a history and conducting an examination of both the cardiovascular and respiratory systems. The doctor must sensitively ask permission to examine the breasts, as mastitis is one of the potential diagnoses. The need for a chaperone should be discussed even though arranging this can be difficult on a home visit. The facilitator will explain that examination of the breasts is normal and that this is not required in this case.

The combination of new pleuritic chest pain, shortness of breath, a cough, haemoptysis and recent delivery requires the doctor to consider pulmonary embolus as a potential cause.[1] Pulmonary embolus is more common (relative risk over four) during pregnancy and is 15 times more common in the postpartum period,[2] hence this serious condition requires careful consideration during these times.

Although this case does not ask the doctor for management, it is worth noting that pulmonary embolism cannot be excluded from just a history and examination. Kerrie requires transfer to hospital for further tests. Risk stratification tools such as the Wells score and PERC rule[3] are less useful in the pregnancy and postpartum setting. Likewise, D-Dimer testing is inappropriate postpartum and post-surgery, and indeed her high risk of pulmonary embolism means that a negative D-Dimer test would NOT rule out this diagnosis.[4]

References

1. Chapman, NH, Brighton, T, Harris, MF, Caplan, GA, Braithwaite, J & Chong, BH 2009, 'Venous thromboembolism—management in general practice', *Australian Family Physician,* vol. 38, pp. 36–40.
2. Tapson, VF 2008, 'Acute pulmonary embolism', *New England Journal of Medicine,* vol. 358, pp. 1037–52.
3. Doherty, S 2017, 'Pulmonary embolism: an update', *Australian Family Physician,* vol. 46, pp. 816–20.
4. Agnelli, G & Becattini, C 2010, 'Acute pulmonary embolism', *New England Journal of Medicine,* vol. 363, pp. 266–74.

Case 72
Paul Jackson

Instructions for the doctor

This is a short case.

Please read the following history. The results of the examination will be available from the facilitator. Using this history and the examination findings, outline your diagnosis and management plan to Paul.

Scenario

Paul Jackson is a 20-year-old man who is about to start a painting and decorating apprenticeship. Paul had asthma as a child but has been well since. Four weeks ago, he had a viral upper respiratory tract infection. Since then he has had a cough, which is keeping him awake at night. He has to stop playing soccer after only 10 minutes due to shortness of breath and wheeze. He is noticing some wheeze occasionally during the day, maybe two to three times per week.

The following information is on his summary sheet:

Past medical history
Childhood asthma
Medication
Nil
Allergies
Nil
Immunisations
Up-to-date
Family history
Maternal osteoporosis
Social history
Lives with de facto partner
Non-smoker.

Instructions for the patient, Paul Jackson

You are 20 years old and will soon start a painting and decorating apprenticeship.

As a child you had asthma. Four weeks ago, you had a cold and since then you have had a cough. The cough is dry and worse at night; your girlfriend is getting really irritated by it. You are worried because you are short of breath and wheezy after exercise. You can manage only around 10 minutes of playing soccer before coming off. You have occasionally (two to three times per week) felt a little wheezy at other times during the day. It feels as though your asthma has come back.

The following information is on your medical record:

Past medical history
Childhood asthma

Medication
Nil

Allergies
Nil

Immunisations
Up-to-date

Family history
Maternal osteoporosis

Social history
Lives with de-facto partner
Non-smoker.

Instructions for the facilitator

Please give the doctor the following information when requested specifically:
- Height 1.85 m
- Pulse 92
- Blood pressure 106/70 mmHg
- No cyanosis
- Talking in sentences
- Respiratory
  —Respiratory rate 14/min
  —No use of accessory muscles
  —Chest expansion normal
  —Percussion note normal
  —Widespread wheeze on auscultation
  —Oxygen saturation 99% in room air.

Peak expiratory flow rate actual   350 L/min
Peak expiratory flow rate predicted   580 L/min
Peak expiratory flow rate after salbutamol   450 L/min

Please hand these results to the doctor if spirometry is requested:

Actual:	FEV1 3.5 L	FVC 5.78 L	Ratio FEV1/FVC 60.5%
Predicted:	FEV1 5.05 L	FVC 6.09 L	Ratio FEV1/FVC 82.9%
After salbutamol:	FEV1 4.3 L	FVC 5.82 L	Ratio FEV1/FVC 73.9%

Suggested approach to the case

Establish rapport
Brief summary of history—for example, 'So I have read that you used to have asthma. You had a cold recently and you are now wheezy and out of breath. I'm going to find out the results of the physical examination and then we can chat about what to do.'
Request permission to examine.

Ask for the examination findings

General appearance and colour
Heart rate and blood pressure
Oxygen saturation
Ability to talk in sentences
Respiratory examination
    —Respiratory rate
    —Use of accessory muscles
    —Chest expansion
    —Percussion
    —Auscultation
    —Oxygen saturation 99% in room air
    —Peak expiratory flow rate
    —Spirometry.

Diagnosis

Poorly controlled asthma.

Management

Explain likely recurrence of asthma
Asthma can recur in adulthood
Reassure Paul that asthma can be treated

Poorly controlled asthma—start both preventer (low-dose inhaled corticosteroid) and reliever (e.g. salbutamol)

Discuss rationale and mechanisms of action of both medications

Demonstrate/explain the use of inhalers and spacer

On suggestion of starting inhaled steroids, watch for emotional reaction and respond appropriately

Enquire sensitively about the reasons for the concern about steroids, for example, Paul's mother developed osteoporosis

Outline risks and benefits of inhaled steroids, in particular addressing any concerns raised by Paul

Plan follow-up and development of an asthma action plan

Assure Paul that asthma should not stop him starting his apprenticeship but to observe any impact from paint fumes

Advise on when to return for follow-up, and to contact urgently if condition worsens

Discuss asthma first aid and emergencies

Other health promotion—use of alcohol and other drugs

Advice regarding influenza vaccination.

 ## CASE COMMENTARY

The key issue in this case is to explain to Paul that it is most likely his asthma has returned.

According to the National Asthma Council's *Australian Asthma Handbook,* Paul has poorly controlled asthma, requiring management with preventer therapy. Most patients can be well-managed on a low-dose inhaled corticosteroid, e.g. 100–200 mcg fluticasone propionate or beclomethasone dipropionate or 250–400 mcg budesonide.[1, 2]

Optimal management will involve an inhaled beta-agonist administered through a spacer, commencement of inhaled steroids as above and early review to ensure best lung function is achieved, preferably assessed by spirometry.[1, 2] Subsequent visits can be used to maintain best lung function, minimise the dose of medication while encouraging adherence[3] and give Paul an asthma action plan.[1, 2] Paul can be encouraged by pointing out that avoiding cigarette smoke and maintaining his fitness by returning to soccer training should help to control his asthma.[4] Paul can commence his apprenticeship but will need to observe any impact of paint fumes on his breathing.

References

1. National Asthma Council 2017, *Australian Asthma Handbook,* Version 1.3. National Asthma Council Australia, Melbourne. Available at: www. asthmahandbook.org.au, accessed 5 July 2018.
2. Hancock, K 2014, 'Long-term management of asthma: the new Australian guidelines', *Medicine Today,* vol. 15, no.11, Suppl, pp. 6–19.
3. Martinez, FD & Vercelli, D 2013, 'Asthma', *Lancet,* vol. 382, pp. 1360–72.
4. Carson, KV, Chandratilleke, MG, Picot, J, Brinn, MP, Esterman, AJ & Smith, BJ 2013, 'Physical training for asthma', Cochrane Database of Systematic Reviews 9:CD001116.

Case 73
Nicholas Morris

Instructions for the doctor

This is a long case.

Please take a history and conduct an appropriate clinical examination. Discuss with the patient the most likely diagnosis, your differential diagnoses and negotiate a plan for management.

Scenario

Nicholas Morris is 63 years old and has booked in to see you this morning. The last entry in the notes was five years ago when he attended after a dog bite.

The following information is on his summary sheet:
Past medical history
Dog bite
Medication
Nil
Allergies
Nil
Immunisations
Nil recorded
Social history
Maths teacher
Single
Smokes 30 cigarettes per day.

Instructions for the patient, Nicholas Morris

You are a 63-year-old maths teacher and a lifelong smoker. You enjoy smoking and get quite offended when people suggest that you should give up. Even the pupils at school keep telling you to stop when they see you smoking around town at the weekends. You only go to the doctor when you really have to.

In the last few months you have become increasingly short of breath. You take your dog for walks in the morning and this is getting more difficult. You have begun to arrive earlier to school so that you can get a parking space near the staffroom.

When asked by the GP you will reveal that you have had a productive cough in the mornings for the last few years. You have never coughed up blood. Colds 'always go to your chest' and when this happens you get a wheeze.

You have been saving up to visit your relatives overseas and are due to fly soon. You have made the appointment to discuss your breathlessness with the GP and want to know if there is any medication that will fix the problem.

Clinical examination findings

Height 1.72 m
Weight 75 kg
BMI 25.3 kg/m^2
Tobacco stains on the fingers
No respiratory distress, respiratory rate 16 breaths per minute
Chest shape and expansion normal
Percussion normal
Auscultation reveals scattered wheezes
PEFR 320 L/min, predicted 620 L/min
ECG shows normal sinus rhythm.

The following information is on your medical record:
Past medical history
Dog bite
Medication
Nil
Allergies
Nil
Immunisations
Nil recorded
Social history
Maths teacher
Single
Smokes 30 cigarettes per day.

Information for the facilitator

If requested, please hand these spirometry results to the doctor:

Actual: FEV1 2.0L FVC 3.3L Ratio FEV1/FVC 60.6%
Predicted: FEV1 3.2L FVC 4.3L Ratio FEV1/FVC 75.1%
After salbutamol: FEV1 2.1 FVC3.3L Ratio FEV1/FVC 63.6%

Suggested approach to the case

Establish rapport

Open-ended questions to establish Nicholas' ideas, concerns and expectations.

Specific questions

Shortness of breath, including exercise tolerance
Cough
Sputum
Haemoptysis
Wheeze
Fever
Chest pain
Orthopnoea/paroxysmal nocturnal dyspnoea
Ankle swelling
Impact of symptoms on lifestyle and ability to work
Smoking history
Alcohol history
Family history
Systems review—include energy levels, sleep, weight loss or change in appetite
Request permission to examine.

Examination

General signs
    —Weight and BMI
    —Cyanosis
    —Clubbing
    —Tobacco stains on the fingers
Respiratory system
    —Respiratory rate
    —Use of accessory muscles
    —Trachea
    —Nodes
    —Chest shape

—Chest expansion
—Percussion
—Auscultation
Cardiovascular system
    —Pulse
    —Blood pressure
    —Heart sounds
    —Signs of heart failure.

Most likely diagnosis

Chronic obstructive pulmonary disease

Differential diagnoses

Carcinoma of the bronchus
Tuberculosis
Infection
Heart failure.

Investigations

FBC
ESR or CRP
UEC
LFTs
Fasting lipids
Fasting BSL
Chest X-ray.

Management

Using the **COPD-X** management plan:
Confirm diagnosis and assess severity
    Explain most likely diagnosis chronic obstructive pulmonary disease
    Inform that this illness is related to smoking
    Assess ability to travel overseas.
Optimise function
    Inhaled bronchodilators
    Pulmonary rehabilitation.
Prevent deterioration
    Use motivational interviewing techniques to discuss smoking
    Outline options for assistance in giving up smoking

Immunisations—influenza, pneumococcal vaccines as per *Australian Immunisation Handbook.*

Develop support network and self-management plan

GP and primary care team follow-up

Develop written action plan to aid in recognition and response to exacerbations.

Manage eXacerbations (cover in subsequent consultations)

Increased bronchodilators

Systemic steroids

Early treatment with antibiotics if signs of infection.

Other issues

Check alcohol consumption

Offer follow-up to address other preventative health issues.

 CASE COMMENTARY

This case tests the doctor's ability to identify chronic obstructive pulmonary disease (COPD) as the most likely diagnosis and to engage with Mr Morris about the importance of giving up smoking. The COPD-X framework provides a useful mnemonic for the key information that should be covered in the next few consultations with Mr Morris. Further detail may be relevant to some patients and is available in the full guideline.

 COMMON PITFALLS

A poor doctor might display a judgemental attitude to the smoking and ignore the issue of the forthcoming holiday. A good doctor will use motivational interviewing to assess Mr Morris's readiness to change and give practical advice about smoking cessation tailored to his readiness to quit (see Case 64).

A good doctor will acknowledge the importance of the holiday and assess Mr Morris's fitness to fly. If Mr Morris can climb a flight of 15 stairs and walk 50 metres without symptoms, he should not experience problems during the flight (see Case 79). He is unlikely to get travel insurance to cover his respiratory condition, so buying a flexible ticket so that he can travel when medically stable is recommended.

Further reading

Lim, ML, Brazzale, DJ & McDonald, CF 2012, '"Is it okay for me to. . .?" Assessment of recreational activity risk in patients with chronic lung conditions', *Australian Family Physician,* vol. 41, no. 1, pp. 852-4.

Seccombe, L & Peters, M 2010, 'Patients with lung disease. Fit to fly?', *Australian Family Physician,* vol. 39, no 3, pp. 112-5.

Walters, J 2010, 'COPD–diagnosis, management and the role of the GP', *Australian Family Physician,* vol. 39, no. 3, pp. 100-3.

Yang, IA, Brown, JL, P George, J, Jenkins, S, McDonald, CF, McDonald, V, et al. 2017, 'COPD-X Concise Guide for Primary Care'. Available at: www.lungfoundation.com.au, accessed 20 November 2018.

Case 74
Jonty McLeod

Instructions for the doctor

This is a short case.

Please take a history from Jonty and his father, Matt. The results of a focused physical examination will be available on specific request from the facilitator. Outline the most likely diagnosis to Jonty and Matt and discuss your suggested management plan with them.

Scenario

Jonty McLeod is 12 years old. Following his parents' divorce, he spends half his time with his mum, Elspeth, and half with his dad, Matt. Jonty has mild persistent asthma, which is well controlled with inhaled corticosteroids.

The following information is on Jonty's medical record:

Past medical history
Asthma
Medication
Fluticasone 100 mcg bd
Salbutamol 200 mcg prn via spacer
Allergies
Nil known
Immunisations
Up-to-date
Family history
Mother has severe eczema
Social history
Attends high school.

Instructions for Jonty and Matt

Jonty

You are 12 years old. You are quite settled in the routine of spending half your time with your father, Matt, and half with your Mum, Elspeth. You enjoy being in your Mum's city flat, which has a nearby cinema and ice-cream shop. Time with your Dad is also enjoyable but more chaotic, as his house is packed with half-finished custom-made furniture, plus his ever-loyal, kelpie-cross Homer.

You have had asthma since you were a baby and it is well controlled. For the last few months you have noticed it has been worse when you are at Dad's and you also seem to sneeze a lot. Your nose is often itchy, runny and blocked, so that you can find it difficult to sleep.

You are in grade seven at a school half-way between Mum and Dad's and are generally a happy kid. There are no problems at either home or at school, other than finding blowing your nose all the time annoying and embarrassing!

Matt

You are a self-employed carpenter. Your marriage to Elspeth fell apart because she wanted to live in the city, whereas you wanted a more relaxed country lifestyle. You have both been much happier since the divorce and Jonty seems to thrive on the variety of having two very different homes.

In recent months you have been nagging Jonty to blow his nose and often hear him sneezing and awake during the night. When you finally caught up with Elspeth after one of her overseas trips, you were surprised to find out that Jonty sleeps through when he is at her house and seems well most of the time.

You have now come to see your own doctor to plan what to do.

Note: If you are unable to persuade someone to play Jonty's role, please change the scenario so that the consultation takes place with Matt on his own.

The following information is on Jonty's medical record:

Past medical history
Asthma

Medication
Fluticasone 100 mcg bd
Salbutamol 200 mcg prn via spacer

Allergies
Nil known

Immunisations
Up-to-date
Family history
Mother has severe eczema
Social history
Attends high school.

Information for the facilitator

Please give the candidate the results of examination findings on specific request.

Examination

Apyrexial, pulse 84, respiratory rate 14/minute
Ears normal
Throat normal
Nose—blocked, with serous discharge
Chest—no respiratory distress, clear on auscultation
Height 1.55 m (over 50th percentile)
Weight 51 kg
BMI 21 kg/m^2
Predicted PEFR rate 323 L/min
Actual PEFR 255 L/min = 79% of predicted.

Suggested approach to the case

Establish rapport with both Jonty and Matt
Open questions to explore their ideas, concerns and expectations
Closed questions
  —Nasal symptoms: itch, sneeze, nature of discharge, blockage or
    bleeding, facial pain
  —Asthma: wheeze, cough, shortness of breath, exercise tolerance,
    need for salbutamol
  —Eyes: itch, discharge, swelling, erythema
  —Brief systems review: sleep, energy levels, appetite, growth
  —Timing of current symptoms
  —Exclude acute illness: no fever, no sore throat, no headache, no ear
    pain
  —Treatment tried so far.

Examination

Temperature, pulse, respiratory rate
Ears, nose, throat
Chest: movement, breath sounds, percussion note, PEFR
Growth.

Management

Most likely diagnosis of allergic rhinitis
Explain condition and its link with asthma.

Investigations

Observation of environmental precipitants
Consider skin-prick test or serum-specific IgE.

Treatment options

Non-pharmacological
    –Identify and avoid allergens
Pharmacological
    –Antihistamines
    –Intranasal corticosteroids
    –Saline nasal spray may help with congestion
Arrange follow-up and consider referral for immunotherapy.

 CASE COMMENTARY

Allergic rhinitis is a common problem that is often underdiagnosed and undertreated. Improving Jonty's symptoms is likely to improve his asthma as well as his sleep and thus his quality of life. The most common environmental allergens to consider are house dust mites, grasses, pollen, animal dander and mould. The potential causes in this case include sawdust from Matt's carpentry and dander from Homer, the kelpie-cross. The GP will need to give this information sensitively: if there is ongoing tension between the two parents about living styles, the fact that Jonty gets unwell each time he visits his Dad has the potential to upset the dynamics and arrangements.

Depending on your location, it is worth considering the potential for thunderstorm asthma in anyone with allergic rhinitis, and particularly those with concomitant asthma (as poorly controlled asthma is associated with worse outcomes). Risk is greatest in those with seasonal (springtime) allergic rhinitis, as they can be assumed to be sensitised to ryegrass pollens. Jonty does not give a history of seasonal rhinitis and hence ryegrass is less likely a trigger in this case. Risk of thunderstorm asthma is greatest in south-eastern Australia, hence the importance of considering this varies by location.

The increased number of children who have two homes under shared parenting arrangements makes this an area where GPs need to avoid escalating any difficult situations. If a child has more than one GP, a shared electronic health record can facilitate communication and avoid duplication of tests, or Matt's GP could give the other GP a hard copy of the record. As Jonty enters his teenage years, this may become further complicated by his right to confidentiality and this should be discussed when using an electronic health record.

Further reading

Australasian Society of Clinical Immunology and Allergy 2017, 'Allergic rhinitis clinical update'. Available at: www.allergy.org.au/hp/papers/allergic-rhinitis-clinical-update, accessed 23 November 2018.

National Asthma Council 2014, 'Australian Asthma Handbook, version 1.0', National Asthma Council, Melbourne. Available at: www.asthmahandbook.org.au, accessed 23 November 2018.

National Asthma Council 2017, 'Epidemic thunderstorm asthma', National Asthma Council, Melbourne. Available at: www.assets.nationalasthma.org.au/resources/Thunderstorm-Full-WEB-JRD.pdf, accessed 23 November 2018.

Rueter, K & Prescott, S 2014, 'Hot topics in paediatric immunology: IgE-mediated food allergy and allergic rhinitis', *Australian Family Physician,* vol. 43, no. 10, pp. 680–5.

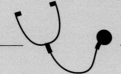

Section 21
Sexual health

Case 75
Ben Ramsay

Instructions for the doctor

This is a short case.

Please conduct this consultation as you would in your clinical practice. There is no need to conduct an examination.

Scenario

Ben Ramsay is a 33-year-old engineer who recently ended a long-term relationship with his partner Tim. He has presented to you today to discuss taking PrEP to lower his risk of HIV. Please discuss his suitability for PrEP and answer his questions.

The following information is on his summary sheet:

Past medical history

Rectal gonorrhoea 2000

Medication

Nil recorded

Allergies

Nil known

Immunisations

Nil known

Social history

Homosexual

Smokes five to ten cigarettes per day.

Instructions for the patient, Ben Ramsay

You are a 33-year-old engineer who recently ended a long-term relationship with your partner Tim. You think of yourself as pretty sensible and your friends know you as 'Mr Safe Sex' from all the reminders you've given over the years, but have found being back on the single scene difficult. You had unprotected receptive anal intercourse once after using methamphetamine at a music festival and a condom broke last month. You had a negative STI check six months ago. Despite going out more and burning the candle at both ends you've not had any infections recently. You're happy to have whatever tests the doctor suggests today.

Some of your friends have started taking PrEP and after these two episodes you think this might be a good idea. You've heard the rates of new HIV cases are starting to go down with PrEP on the PBS and have some questions for the doctor:

- Would I be eligible for PrEP?
- Are there any tests I need to have before I start?
- What's the best way to take it? Some friends just take it if they know they are going to have a big weekend of drugs and sex.
- What side effects can you expect?
- How often will you need to see a doctor and get tests while taking PrEP?

The following information is on your summary sheet:
Past medical history
Rectal gonorrhoea 2000
Medication
Nil recorded
Allergies
Nil known
Immunisations
Nil known
Social history
Homosexual
Smokes five to ten cigarettes per day.

Instruction for the facilitator

Please provide a hard and/or electronic copy of the *Australian Medicines Handbook* or *Therapeutic Guidelines*.

Suggested approach to the case

Establish rapport
Demonstrate a non-judgemental empathic response to his request for PrEP
Listen carefully to his ideas and concerns
Exclude symptoms suggestive of recent STI
Assess his current risk of HIV and other STIs
Check details of PrEP using drug resource available and discuss with Ben
Reinforce value of using condoms.

The steps to prescribing PrEP are as follows:

1. Determine eligibility—medium to high risk eligible
   Those at high risk of acquiring HIV include men who have sex with men who have a concurrent STI-rectal gonorrhoea, chlamydia; those who have had condomless anal intercourse with a HIV positive partner or partner of unknown status in the previous six months, methamphetamine use.
2. Confirm HIV status—the patient must be confirmed HIV negative prior to commencing PrEP
   PrEP should be commenced within seven days of a negative HIV test being performed. This is because PrEP is inadequate in the treatment of undiagnosed acute or chronic HIV.
3. STI and hepatitis testing
   Screen for hepatitis B, hepatitis C, kidney function and STIs. Treat STIs as required, and consult an expert in the case of a positive hepatitis B or C test, or impaired kidney function. (PrEP can negatively impact kidney function.) Review and update immunisations for HPV, hepatitis A and B and meningococcus. Measure bone density if there are risk factors for low bone density, and actively monitor.
4. Prescribe PrEP
   Daily, continuing, oral dose PrEP. Patients need to take a daily dose of PrEP for seven days before high levels of protection are achieved for both vaginal and rectal exposure to HIV.
   There is an 'on demand' regime of PrEP whereby the patient takes it only at high-risk times. This is not as effective and should be discussed with an experienced prescriber.
5. Review the patient every three months
   Review sexual practices and adherence to PrEP to reassess continuation of PrEP. Test kidney function and test for HIV and STIs. This is an ideal chance to attend to preventative health and primary health care needs of the patient.

CASE COMMENTARY

Ben has recognised his risks and is taking steps to proactively reduce them. Asking for PrEP may be difficult and so the doctor must not judge him.

This is a new area of medicine and you may not know the details of PrEP prescribing but this will not prevent you taking an appropriate history and forming a management plan with Ben. When new medicines become available doctors need to be able to use appropriate resources in the consultation to guide patient care. Being able to check drug details while showing empathy and maintaining patient contact are important skills.

Australian data from 2015 show that men who have sex with men accounted for 73% of new HIV diagnoses. The Aboriginal and Torres Strait Islander population is over represented in new cases of HIV and yet is not getting access to PrEP at the same level as their non-Indigenous counterparts.

GPs can prescribe PrEP (Truvada) as HIV pre-exposure prophylaxis to eligible patients. People without Medicare cards can access PrEP under the TGA personal importation scheme. PrEP is effective at preventing new HIV infections in those who take it correctly. San Francisco has seen a 50% drop in new HIV infections since PrEP was approved by the US Food and Drug Administration in 2012.

There are concerns that PrEP may change sexual practices and lead to more STIs. Regular follow-up to prescribe PrEP is an opportunity to discuss overall health, including preventing other STIs and use of drugs, for example, methamphetamines in Ben's case.

COMMON PITFALLS

In cases discussing new developments in medicine, if you are not across the developments, you may freeze momentarily. Remember to return to first principles and you will realise there is a lot you will be able to do, while sourcing the up-to-date information.

Further reading

Cornelisse, V 2018, *PrEP on the PBS: An opportunity in HIV prevention.* Retrieved from: www.nps.org.au/news/prep-on-the-pbs-an-opportunity-in-hiv-prevention, accessed 25 February 2019.

Decision making in PrEP Australasian Society for HIV, Viral Hepatitis and Sexual Health Medicine 2018. Retrieved from: www.Ashm.Org.Au/Products/Product/3000100092, accessed 25 February 2019.

Ward, J, Hawke, K & Guy, RJ 2018, 'Priorities for preventing a concentrated HIV epidemic among Aboriginal and Torres Strait Islander Australians', *Medical Journal of Australia,* vol. 209, no. 1, pp. 5–6.

Wright, E, Grulich, A, Roy, K, Boyd, M, Cornelisse, V, Russell, D, Zablotska, I 2017, 'Australasian Society for HIV, Viral Hepatitis and Sexual Health Medicine HIV pre-exposure prophylaxis: clinical guidelines', *Journal of Virus Eradication,* vol. 3, no. 3, pp. 168–84.

Case 76
Vinay Singh

Instructions for the doctor

This is a long case.

This consultation may be conducted as if it is more than one session.

Please take a history from Vinay. Examination findings are available from the facilitator. When you are ready, outline your diagnostic impressions and initial management to Vinay. Investigation results will then be available from the facilitator. Discuss these results with Vinay, together with any further management, if required.

Scenario

Vinay Singh is a 35-year-old management consultant whom you've seen a few times for minor ailments. His wife and children are regular patients of yours. His wife rang the surgery this morning to say Vinay is sick with the flu and has a strange non-itchy rash on his palms and soles. Upon arrival Vinay is put in a spare consulting room for quarantine purposes. His wife and children are in the waiting room.

The following information is on his summary sheet:

Past medical history
Nil significant
Medication
Nil
Allergies
Nil
Immunisations
None recorded
Social history
Married, two children (aged four and six), management consultant.

Instructions for the patient, Vinay Singh

A week ago you started feeling unwell—joint pains, fatigue, malaise—as though you were getting the flu. You weren't particularly worried until a rash developed on your palms and soles. It is not itchy or painful. You looked on the internet and self-diagnosed hand, foot and mouth disease but the rash does not look like the picture on the internet and has now started spreading to your chest. Having returned from a business trip to the northern United States a month ago, you were also wondering about Lyme disease.

On specific questioning

You travel overseas about five times per year, for one to two weeks, to either the United States or South-East Asia for work. Your family does not accompany you on these trips. Not uncommonly on these overseas trips you'll have sex with male and/or female sex workers (vaginal, oral and anal—receptive and penetrative). You use condoms 'most' of the time. You have never had a sexually transmitted infection (STI) screening or any previous STI (to your knowledge).

You see these trips as well-deserved opportunities to let your hair down and have some fun. You compartmentalise your life: you see yourself as a 'different person' when working overseas and believe that your trips away enhance your ability to be a good husband and father, as they allow you to 'blow off steam'. You categorically see yourself as a heterosexual loving father and husband. You deny any mood problems or guilty feelings—while life has its ups and downs, you see yourself as a relatively happy and confident person.

You were born in India and have lived in Australia since the age of 10. You are not religious and don't have any particularly strong cultural or extended family ties. You have not been back to India for more than 10 years.

You did not visit any wooded/rural areas during your recent trip to the United States and have no particular reason for thinking you have Lyme disease except that you have heard that it is 'common over there'.

You do not smoke and rarely drink alcohol, as it tends to give you a headache and to make you feel sleepy. If asked about other drugs, you pause, look uncomfortable and say 'not really'. If asked to expand in a sensitive and non-judgemental way, you admit to using methamphetamine ('meth'/'ice') as a party drug when overseas for work. You also use it to help you to keep awake and alert when jetlagged (e.g. before a big meeting). You have used it in tablet form but prefer 'snorting' it (intranasally). You've never used IV drugs. You used marijuana a few times in college but not since then. You do not consider yourself an addict and you're not interested in giving it up. You've never used drugs in front of your wife or kids (they are unaware of your drug use). You purchase drugs from local dealers (usually in nightclubs). You never carry drugs while travelling and you've never been in trouble with the law. You have had some dental decay requiring crowns and veneers to be fitted, but otherwise no adverse effects from the meth use.

About three months ago (two to three weeks after returning from a trip to Thailand), you noticed a painless ulcer around your anus. It healed in about three weeks. You have been otherwise well until last week. You have noticed some new, painful lumps around your anus.

Suggested prompt: 'Is there any chance this could be something I got overseas?'

When the diagnosis is given

You are devastated by the syphilis diagnosis and initially disbelieving: 'Could there be some mistake?'

You thought syphilis was an old disease that had been eradicated, like polio. You thought you may have been vaccinated against it in the past. You know nothing else about it, other than it can 'send you crazy'.

You are initially resistant to the idea of informing your wife, but you agree that if the reasons (including the health risks to your wife) are explained sensitively and with empathy you will sit down and talk with her this evening. You would prefer to talk to her alone initially, rather than her finding out another way. If suggested, you are willing to return for a follow-up visit with your wife and to follow an appropriate management plan.

Suggested prompts:
- 'What should I tell my wife?'
- 'Do I need tests to see if it's cured?'
- 'You did say that this consultation was confidential, didn't you?'

The following information is on your summary sheet:
Past medical history
Nil significant
Medication
Nil
Allergies
Nil
Immunisations
None recorded
Social history
Married, two children (aged four and six), management consultant.

Information for the facilitator

Clinical examination findings

Each finding needs to be asked for specifically.
General appearance—looks mildly unwell
Temperature 37.8°C
BP 120/75 mmHg
Pulse 80 and regular
Pale red, discrete, round, symmetrically bilateral macules on palms, soles and trunk; lesions measure 5–10 mm in diameter
No oral lesions
No alopecia
Anogenital area—reddish-brown tender papular lesions coalescing into plaques in places
Generalised non-tender lymphadenopathy (cervical, axillary and inguinal)
Rest of examination is unremarkable.

Investigation results

FBE within normal limits
Urea and electrolytes within normal limits
LFTs within normal limits
First pass urine PCR—negative for *Chlamydia* and gonorrhoea
Oral and anal swabs PCR—negative for *Chlamydia* and gonorrhoea
Swabs of lesions on palms/soles PCR—negative for enteroviruses
Anogenital lesions, wet mount preparation of expressed exudate—dark field microscopy reveals syphilitic spirochaetes
Syphilis serology—positive ELISA, followed by positive results on confirmatory testing
Hepatitis A, B and C serology negative, non-immune
HIV Ab negative
Lyme disease serology—result pending (three-to-four week turnaround)
Chest X-ray normal.

Suggested approach to the case

Establish rapport
Empathic, open and non-judgemental approach
Thorough history of presenting complaint, past history, social history and systems review.

Specific questions

Sexual history should include partners (number and gender), sexual practices, protection from STIs, previous STIs

Drug history should include drug type/s, frequency of use, route of administration and readiness to modify behaviour

Relationship with wife/family, beliefs and self/cultural identity, mood.

Examination

Ask the facilitator for specific examination findings as per above list

Must ask for description of skin lesions

Must ask for examination of anogenital area.

Investigations

As per above list

Key investigations include

   —First pass urine PCR

   —Oral and anal swabs: PCR and wet mount preparation

   —Syphilis/Hepatitis B/HIV serology.

Management

Sensitively break news of secondary syphilis infection

Patient education about syphilis, including explaining cause, transmission, stages (primary, secondary and tertiary) and correcting any misconceptions

Treat infection

   —Benzathine penicillin G 1.8 g IM single dose OR

   —Procaine penicillin G 1.0 g IM daily for 10 days OR

   —Doxycycline 100 mg twice daily for 14 days (if allergic to penicillin)

Vaccinate against hepatitis A and B

Talk to sexual health unit/clinic

Tracing of all sexual partners, if possible

Wife needs to be informed and tested (encourage Vinay to inform her, but offer assistance: yourself and/or contact tracing service)

Refrain from sexual activity until seven days after treatment of both partners is complete

Safe sex messages

Follow-up—regular STI screening

Follow-up—clinical and lab testing (syphilis serology) at 3, 6 and 12 months Harm reduction regarding methamphetamine use. Aim to move from precontemplation to contemplation.

 CASE COMMENTARY

This case assesses a candidate's ability to suspect, identify and manage sexually transmitted infections and 'party drug' use. A detailed and sensitively taken sexual and drug-taking history is crucial. The approach should be open and non-judgemental, and questions should be normalised/depersonalised whenever possible, for example: 'There are some personal questions I ask all patients with symptoms like these to help lead us to a diagnosis. Some of them might be quite confronting but I would appreciate any information you're willing to share with me.'

Sensitively and successfully negotiating the issues of confidentiality with the patient (balancing doctor–patient confidentiality with the need for contact tracing to reduce harm to others) is another key feature of this case.

People taking 'party drugs' at social functions may not be ready to change their behaviour. The best outcome in such cases is likely to be achieved by using a non-judgemental approach and focusing on informing patients on how to reduce harm and risk when using substances. During this consultation, Vinay realises that, while he compartmentalises his life, infections and illness transcend the compartments he has established. Not only is his health threatened, but so is his marriage and his wife's health; skill is needed to help him to use this realisation to motivate change.

 COMMON PITFALLS

Many patients prefer to see their GP for sexually acquired infections rather than to attend sexual health clinics. However, sexual health is an aspect of clinical practice where a GP's background and personal values can significantly affect their professional effectiveness. It is easy to jump to erroneous conclusions regarding sexuality, belief systems and/or cultural identity based on a patient's marital status, socioeconomic status and racial background. GPs who are uncomfortable asking about sexual or drug practices risk missing important clues in the history. Practising asking open and specific questions and learning to respond to the answers is time well spent.

Further reading

Australasian Sexual Health Alliance 2018, 'Australasian STI management guidelines for use in primary care; Syphilis'. Retrieved from http://www.sti. guidelines.org.au/sexually-transmissible-infections/syphilis.

Cornelisse, V, Fairley, CK & Roth, NJ 2016, 'Optimising healthcare for men who have sex with men: A role for general practitioners', *Australian Family Physician,* vol. 45, no. 4, pp. 182–5.

Frei, M 2010, 'Party drugs: use and harm reduction', *Australian Family Physician,* vol. 39, no. 8, pp. 548–52.

Hopwood, M, Cama, E & Treloar, C 2016, Methamphetamine use among men who have sex with men in Australia: A literature review. Sydney: Centre for Social Research in Health, UNSW Australia. http://doi.org/10.4225/53/58d4 418d0a14b.

Ong, JJ & Towns, JM 2017, 'Occult syphilitic chancres in the rectum and oropharynx', *Australian Family Physician,* vol. 46, no. 9, pp. 673–5.

Case 77
Samantha Heyward

Instructions for the doctor

This is a short case.

Please take a history from your regular patient, Samantha Heyward. The facilitator will give you the results of any relevant physical examination on request. Then outline a management plan with Samantha.

Scenario

Samantha Heyward is 21 years old and her family have been your patients for many years. She has mostly enjoyed good health and has been on the oral contraceptive pill for about five years, initially for irregular periods and then for contraception.

She has also had some depression, which got quite severe during her final year of school and she has been on sertraline since then. She has tried a couple of times to stop taking it, but within a month or so her mood drops and she recommences. Sam has a close relationship with her parents and has two older brothers who are both married with children but live nearby. You see Sam every several months and at her last appointment she was doing well. She told you she had a new boyfriend, Glen, and was enjoying her work as a clerk in the courthouse.

The following information is on her summary sheet:

Age

21

Past medical history

Depression

Medication

Sertraline 100 mg od

Ethinylestradiol 30 mcg/levonorgestrel 150 mcg (Microgynon 30)
one daily

Allergies
Nil known
Immunisations
Up-to-date
Social history
Non-smoker
Non-drinker.

Instructions for the patient, Samantha Heyward

Your name is Samantha (Sam) Heyward and you are a 21-year-old long-term patient of this doctor. You've had some trouble with depression in the past but have generally been healthy. You have come to the doctor because you are confused. You are having problems with your partner, Glen, and are not sure which one of you is normal and who is 'to blame'. Your opening line can be something like, 'Glen and I are having problems and I don't know if there's something wrong with me or him'.

Let the candidate ask questions to draw the story out. You are initially somewhat embarrassed and reticent but respond to the doctor's approach. If the doctor seems embarrassed, you can become more shy and awkward. Alternatively, if the questions are being asked skilfully in a relaxed manner, you can also relax and open up more.

You've been living with Glen for about nine months now and have been together for a little over a year. He seems really nice but you're having problems in the 'bedroom department' and this is starting to affect your relationship. He wants to have sex a couple of times a day and perpetually seems excited and ready. At first you didn't mind because you thought it would settle down with time, but it hasn't.

As far as you are concerned, sex is enjoyable and you feel you have a healthy interest and libido, but most days you'd rather read a book or watch TV than have intercourse again. You've had some talks with Glen about the problem and as a compromise you have sex once a day. Neither of you are very happy about this. Glen says you have something wrong with your libido, and you've had a brief look at some women's magazines (like *Cleo* and *Cosmo*), which do seem to suggest you might have a problem. Women that you read about in those magazines (and see on TV and in movies) all seem to have incredible libidos, and this seems a long way from your own experience. You talked with your Mum about it and she seemed embarrassed, saying dismissively, 'Don't worry about those magazines—all the women in our family have very low libidos'. You're wondering if it is as simple as that.

If asked:

You had three partners before Glen, each of them monogamous at the time and each lasting three to six months. Your first partner was when you were 17 (he was 18).

You've never been sexually abused or pressured into having sex. You've never been tested for STIs. You don't feel scared of Glen or pressured, you just feel you would like to satisfy his desires.

You used condoms in your previous relationships but after a few months you and Glen decided it would be OK not to use them because you were on the pill.

You have no concerns about Glen's faithfulness, but do worry that if you had sex less often he might start looking elsewhere.

You do get aroused when having sex but have never climaxed. This doesn't really bother you—sex is enjoyable and you're not bothered about a lack of orgasm.

Sometimes lubrication seems to be an issue but you think this is probably normal and is just because he is always ready to go and you don't have time to 'warm-up'.

If asked more detail about your sexual practices, you can be a bit reluctant and ask if that is really necessary but if the doctor pushes for details you can say that it is vaginal and oral sex.

You've never been pregnant and are not keen to be pregnant at the moment. You have good cycle control on your contraceptive pill and if it is suggested you stop it you are quite anxious about pregnancy and irregular periods. You suspect Glen would not be keen to have to go back to using condoms.

If ceasing your antidepressant is raised, you are very reluctant because you have tried to get off it a few times and each time your mood plummets and your anxiety skyrockets.

You've been on both the oral contraceptive pill and the antidepressant since before you were sexually active and hadn't considered that either could be affecting your interest or performance negatively.

Your mood is good, your appetite, energy and sleep are fine and you are enjoying your work at the courthouse.

The following information is on your summary sheet:

Age
21
Past medical history
Depression

Medication
Sertraline 100 mg od
Ethinylestradiol 30 mcg/levonorgestrel 150 mcg (Microgynon 30)
  one daily
Allergies
Nil known
Immunisations
Up-to-date
Social history
Non-smoker
Non-drinker.

Information for the facilitator

Clinical examination findings

General appearance: Young adult female in no distress
BMI 21 kg/m^2
BSL 5 (random) mmol/L
Urinalysis normal
All physical examination findings are normal.

Suggested approach to the case

Establish rapport
Open questions to elicit Sam's concerns.

Specific questions

Explore libido mismatch
Explore the relationship
Exclude abuse
Explore arousal, orgasm and dyspareunia
Explore general health and medications.

Examination

General appearance
BMI
BSL
Urinalysis.

Management

Explanation of libido mismatch
Reassurance
Explanation that anorgasmia likely to be related to SSRI use
Resources and simple suggestions regarding libido mismatch
Offer to see Sam and her partner together
Follow-up.

 CASE COMMENTARY

Sex is an important part of human experience, but often patients (like Sam in this case) can find themselves having problems and feeling that they have no one to help them. A GP does not have to be a trained sex therapist, but the basic tools of taking a sexual history, giving appropriate reassurance, offering simple, common sense advice and exploring this vital but sensitive area should be in the GP's armament. Female sexual issues include painful intercourse, lack of libido (up to four in ten women) and anorgasmia (up to one in three women). Sam should be reassured that there is nothing 'wrong' with her but that as a couple she and her partner are experiencing libido mismatch. Libido mismatch (also referred to as desire discrepancy) is the most common reason for a person to seek out a sex counsellor. Both her SSRI and the OCP can dampen libido, but a careful history should reveal that Sam's libido is healthy and she should be reassured about this. Libido is typically classified as high or low, but it is actually much 'more complex than how often a person desires sex. It has elements including what triggers arousal and what dampens it, the importance of sex compared to other parts of a relationship, the meaning of sex for each individual, what is pleasurable during sexual activity'. When a couple has mismatched libidos, a 'pursuer–distancer' cycle can develop that will threaten the relationship if it continues.

Australia's Bettina Arndt is a prolific author and researcher on attitudes towards sex and sexuality. She has followed a large number of Australian couples and encouraged them to document their thoughts and experiences regarding the sexual aspect of their relationship. She provides in-depth understanding into the interpersonal dynamics of desire discrepancy, as well as some excellent practical advice for couples trying to manage it. Having identified the issue, the GP can give patients education and resources about the condition, as well as some management principles, and should offer to counsel the couple together in order to facilitate communication.

As an added issue, Sam describes primary anorgasmia, an adverse effect of the SSRI. It should be noted that this is not why she has presented and is not a problem for her. She is anxious about ceasing her sertraline but a watchful trial of a lower dose might be discussed.

 ## COMMON PITFALLS

GPs can be uncomfortable taking a sexual history and may skip important issues as a result. This will lead to an inadequate understanding of the situation, which in turn will mean less helpful management suggestions. Diagnostic algorithms exist for primary anorgasmia, and it is easy to progress through these and forget that this is not a problem for Sam. Her instructions are to respond to the doctor's manner: relaxing and being more forthcoming if the doctor seems relaxed and skilful in their questioning and vice versa if they are not. This is realistic, but one of the disadvantages of exam anxiety is that it's hard to appear relaxed. Practice can definitely help here.

Further reading

Arndt, B 2009, *The Sex Diaries,* Melbourne University Press, Melbourne.

Goodwach, R 2017, 'Let's talk about sex', *Australian Family Physician,* vol. 46, no. 1–2, pp. 14–18

Phillips, N 2000, 'Female sexual dysfunction: evaluation and treatment', *American Family Physician,* no. 62, no. 1, pp. 127–36.

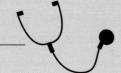

Section 22
Travel health

Case 78
Tanya Hardy

Instructions for the doctor

This is a long case.

Please take a history from Tanya Hardy, who is a 23-year-old patient of your practice. Conduct any relevant physical examination and discuss an appropriate management plan with Tanya.

Scenario

Tanya is a nursing student who has generally been very healthy but has presented in the past for immunisations, an episode of bronchitis and once for emergency contraception.

The following information is on her summary sheet:

Past medical history
Lower respiratory tract infection
Cervical screen
Normal this year
Medication
Ethinyloestradiol 30 mcg/levonorgestrel 150 mcg (Microgynon 30)
Allergies
Nil known
Social history
Nursing student
Single
Smokes 10–15 cigarettes per day
Immunisations
Up-to-date.

Instructions for the patient, Tanya Hardy

You are coming to the doctor today because you and a friend are planning a backpacking holiday after you both graduate. In two months you will go to Thailand, Laos, Vietnam and then party in the Thai islands before going to Malaysia and finishing in Singapore.

You have read about a backpacker track where you can get food and accommodation for a couple of dollars a day and alcohol is 'super-cheap'. If asked, you are hoping to do some jungle trekking, see wild monkeys, ride an elephant, learn to ride a scooter, try scuba diving and do lots of partying.

You have never travelled overseas before and aren't big on planning. Nothing is booked apart from your flights. You're very excited about the trip but haven't thought much about any health issues. You are receptive to issues the doctor raises and listen attentively to their advice, asking the sort of practical questions you think the real Tanya would ask.

Your health is good, and your only regular medication is your contraceptive pill. Your family are all healthy but live interstate.

If asked, you are not currently sexually active, having broken up with your boyfriend six months ago. You've heard men in Asia are very friendly and fun-loving so you're looking forward to making new friends on your trip. You have used marijuana in the past and ecstasy on occasion when you've gone dancing. You've heard about the magic mushroom shakes you can get in Asia and can't wait to try them.

You had various immunisations three years ago when you started nursing. You're not exactly sure which ones, but you think they included hepatitis B, pertussis and measles/mumps/rubella. You currently smoke about 10 to 15 cigarettes a day and have done so since you started nursing. You plan to give up one day, but certainly not on your big holiday. You don't drink alcohol every day but about once a week you go out with your friends and drink up to 10 to 12 drinks. This doesn't really bother you, apart from the hangovers, which you plan to sleep through on your holiday. If explored, a couple of times in the past you have had too much to drink and ended up sleeping with guys you don't know very well. About half of the times this has happened you have not remembered to use condoms. You are forthcoming about all this if asked, but will clam up if you feel the doctor is lecturing you.

The following information is on your summary sheet:
Past medical history
Lower respiratory tract infection
Cervical screen
Normal this year

399

Medication
Ethinyloestradiol 30 mcg/levonorgestrel 150 mcg (Microgynon 30)
Allergies
Nil known
Social history
Nursing student
Single
Smokes 10–15 cigarettes per day
Immunisations
Up-to-date.

Information for the facilitator

Clinical examination findings

General appearance: healthy-looking female
BMI 21 kg/m^2
BP 121/78 mmHg
Physical examination is normal.

Suggested approach to the case

Establish rapport
Open questions to elicit the nature of her trip.

Specific questions[1]

Previous travel history
Specific travel questions
    —Intended activities
    —Precise itinerary
    —Style and mode of travel
    —Type of accommodation
    —Time of year
    —Length of stay
    —Any travel/health insurance
Drug (including recreational drugs) and alcohol history
Smoking history
Previous vaccinations
General health and systems review
Request permission to examine.

Examination

General appearance
BMI
Vital signs.

Management

Food and water advice—should be practical and specific
Accidents and safety—alcohol and road safety, wearing helmets, hiking/
  jungle safety
Safe sex/contraception
Malaria/dengue prevention, zika advice
Rabies prevention
Drug awareness
Travel insurance
Simple medical/first aid kit
Vaccinations[2]
  —Typhoid
  —Hepatitis A +/− Salmonella
  —Japanese encephalitis
  —Cholera
  —+/− Rabies
Advise her to seek medical attention if she becomes unwell within the first
  few weeks of her return to Australia
Provide written information as well.

CASE COMMENTARY

People are travelling more and, while travel offers wonderful new experiences, it comes with health risks, which GPs should be equipped to
manage. The main challenge in this case will be managing your time as
you work your way through a long agenda of relevant issues for Tanya,
a healthy but naïve traveller. It is good to begin with open questions
exploring the nature of the intended trip, followed by a checklist of
specific questions to further define the key issues.

The backpacker circuit through South-East Asia is well worn and often
appeals to the people seeking cheap food, accommodation, alcohol and
adventures. The associated health problems include infections transmitted through contaminated food and water and insect bites, as well as

sexually transmitted infections and motor vehicle accidents, either as driver or pedestrian.

Food and water hygiene advice should be delivered in an efficient and practical way, indicative of lots of previous experience. Supplement the health advice with written material to improve recall and compliance. In exams, reference can be made to these as if they have been provided.

The risk of cholera infection is low, but cholera vaccination does afford some partial short-term protection against travellers' diarrhoea caused by enterotoxigenic *Escherichia coli* (ETEC) because cholera and ETEC share the same toxin. The combined Hepatitis A/Salmonella Typhi vaccination has similar benefits.

Tanya's attitude to alcohol and other drugs should raise alarms and be addressed sensitively but clearly.

Rabies prevention includes discussion about the risk of the disease from bites or scratches from infected animals such as dogs, monkeys, bats and rodents. Tanya's itinerary is reasonably high risk and she is spending considerable time in rabies-endemic areas, some of which are isolated regions where access to appropriate medical care, such as effective and timely post-exposure prophylaxis is limited, so vaccination is recommended.

Tanya risks catching malaria on her trip, and a discussion about prevention should include the pros, cons and costs of chemoprophylaxis alternatives (probably doxycycline or mefloquine), as well as mosquito bite prevention measures.

 COMMON PITFALLS

Often travel advice focuses on recommended vaccinations but it includes much more. A common error is to ask only about the itinerary, but a few additional questions allow us to accurately assess risk. We also shouldn't miss the opportunity of preventive health care by exploring Tanya's attitude to her smoking, episodic binge drinking and risky sexual practice. To be thorough, post-travel illness presentation and management should be addressed as well.

References

1. Chen, LH, Hochberg, NS & Magill, AJ 2015, 'The pre-travel consultation', Centers for Disease Control and Prevention, Atlanta, GA.

2. Henderson, J, Harrison, C, Bayram, C & Britt, H 2015, 'Travel advice and vaccination', *Australian Family Physician,* vol. 44, no. 1-2, pp. 14-15.

Further reading

Batchelor, T & Gherardin, T 2007, 'Prevention of malaria in travellers', *Australian Family Physician,* vol. 36, no. 5, pp. 316-20.

Centers for Disease Control and Prevention 2017, *CDC Yellow Book 2018: Health Information for International Travel,* Oxford University Press, New York.

Leder, K 2015 'Advising travellers about management of travellers' diarrhea', *Australian Family Physician.* Vol. 44, no. 9, pp. 34-37.

Neilson, A & Mayer, C 2010, 'Cholera—recommendations for prevention in travellers', *Australian Family Physician,* vol. 39, no. 4, pp. 222-5.

Neilson, A & Mayer, C 2010, 'Hepatitis A: prevention in travellers', *Australian Family Physician,* vol. 39, no. 12, pp. 942-8.

Neilson, A & Mayer, C 2010, 'Rabies: prevention in travellers', *Australian Family Physician,* vol. 39, no. 9, pp. 641-5.

Case 79
Betty Ward

Instructions for the doctor

This is a short case.

Please take a focused history from Betty and manage the issues that arise.

Scenario

During her routine check-up last week, 68-year-old Betty Ward mentioned that she had just booked to go on an overseas holiday. Today she has returned with her planned itinerary.

Last week you noted:

Feeling well, no new issues

BP 110/70

Pulse 95 bpm irregularly irregular

CVS—heart sounds dual, nil added, JVP three cm above sternum, no swelling of ankles

Respiratory—respiratory rate: 26 breaths/min, sats 94% on room air, no dyspnoea at rest, decreased breath sounds globally on auscultation (long-standing)

Spirometry—FEV1 54% predicted, no significant reversibility (FEV1 58% six months earlier)[1]

FBE, LFTs and electrolytes all in normal range

INR 2.7.

The following information is on her summary sheet:

Past medical history

Atrial fibrillation (non-valvular)

COPD

Hypertension

Medication
Warfarin (dose variable, currently 3 mg OD)
Perindopril 4 mg
Salbutamol 100 mcg 2 puffs prn
Fluticasone propionate/salmeterol xinafoate 250/50 mcg 1 puff bd
Tiotropium bromide 18 mcg one daily
Allergies
Nil
Immunisations
ADT, influenza and pneumococcal immunisations up-to-date
Social history
Retired school teacher, lives alone
Widowed 18 months ago, no children
Ex-smoker (40 pack/year history; quit three years ago)
No alcohol.

Instructions for the patient, Betty Ward

Last week you booked a last-minute non-refundable special deal to go on a three-week trip to Europe (Germany, France, Switzerland, Italy), leaving in four weeks' time. You don't have a travel companion but will be joining a tour group of older travellers the day after you land in Europe. It has been a lifetime dream to 'see Europe' but your husband didn't like to travel, and you've never been overseas before.

On specific questioning:

Your travel agent reassured you that the pace of the tour will be 'sedate' and that they 'will take good care of you'. You have not yet investigated travel insurance options. You live independently but can walk only 30 to 40 metres without 'stopping to catch a breath'. You have been on warfarin for four years and have monthly INR tests. Your INR results have been stable and you have not required any dose adjustment for more than six months.

You are happy to see a respiratory physician if this is recommended, as long as it can be done before your trip.

The following information is on your summary sheet:
Past medical history
Atrial fibrillation (non-valvular)
COPD
Hypertension

Medication
Warfarin (dose variable, currently 3 mg OD)
Perindopril 4 mg
Salbutamol 100 mcg 2 puffs prn
Fluticasone propionate/salmeterol xinafoate 250/50 mcg 1 puff bd
Tiotropium bromide 18 mcg one daily
Allergies
Nil
Immunisations
ADT, influenza and pneumococcal immunisations up-to-date
Social history
Retired school teacher, lives alone
Widowed 18 months ago, no children
Ex-smoker (40 pack/year history; quit three years ago)
No alcohol.

Suggested approach to the case

Develop rapport.

Specific questions[2]

Previous travel experience
Itinerary (places/activities/length of stay)
Method of travel (flights/rail/bus/vehicle; independent/tour)
Travel companion? Support available?
Travel insurance? Health insurance?
Current exercise tolerance
Immunisation status.

Management[3]

Medical and medication summary
Letter from GP stating medication is for personal use
Carry list of emergency contacts
Consider medical alert bracelet
Find travel companion, if possible
Advice about importance of travel insurance (warn her that she may have
    difficulty finding insurance to cover pre-existing conditions)
Advice about carrying medication (e.g. in original packaging, spare supplies
    split between cabin and checked luggage)

Discuss mobility needs with tour group company and airline

Send for specialist assessment/get specialist advice about need for inflight supplemental oxygen (Clearance to Fly certificate)[4]

Test INR just before departure or consider switching to new orally active anticoagulants[5, 6]

Warn about INR variations due to unfamiliar diet etc. and possible need for testing while overseas (provide letter)

Advice about travel medical kit

General safety precautions (e.g. motor vehicle, theft)

Discuss impact of jet lag (tends to be more severe in older travellers; consider scheduling 'recovery' days/stopover if possible).

Register with SmartTraveller website.[3]

 CASE COMMENTARY

With cheaper flights and increased numbers of older Australians wanting to travel, GPs are commonly in the position of needing to give travel advice to those with chronic medical conditions. It is important for GPs to have a good working knowledge of the special health issues that can arise during travel and how best to manage these.[2]

This case is aimed at determining the candidate's ability to take a focused pre-travel history, identify risk factors in this patient (age, travelling alone, COPD and warfarin therapy) and provide both general and specific travel advice.

For those with chronic lung disease, the effects of decreased partial pressure of oxygen in an aircraft cabin and, if applicable, destination altitude (especially if travelling to Nepal, Peru, Tibet or Bolivia) need to be considered.[1] Aircraft cabins are generally pressurised at 1524–2438 m, which results in a concomitant fall in oxygen saturation of around 5%. This is generally well tolerated in those with mild respiratory disease but for those with dyspnoea or angina at rest, with hypoxaemia (resting saturation <95%) and/or those who cannot walk 50 m or 15 steps without breathlessness, such a drop in oxygen saturation may significantly compromise their function.[4] In these patients, inflight supplemental oxygen should be considered, preferably following assessment by a respiratory physician. High-altitude simulation tests (HASTs) can be performed in respiratory laboratories to determine the need for oxygen during flight. It is important to discuss the need for comprehensive travel insurance in detail with patients, highlighting the possible costs if medical care and/or medical repatriation is necessary while overseas.

References

1. Yang, IA, Brown, JL, George, J, Jenkins, S, McDonald, CF, McDonald, V, Smith, B et al. 2018, The COPD-X Plan: Australian and New Zealand Guidelines for the management of Chronic Obstructive Pulmonary Disease Version 2.56.
2. Chen LH, Hochberg NS & Magill AJ 2015, 'The pre-travel consultation', Centers for Disease Control and Prevention, Atlanta, GA.
3. Australian Government, Smart Traveller. Available at: www.smartraveller .gov.au/.
4. Lung Foundation Australia 2016, Fitness to Fly Factsheet.
5. Brieger, D & Curnow, J 2014, 'Anticoagulation: a GP primer on the new oral anticoagulants', *Australian Family Physician,* vol. 43, no. 5, pp. 254-9.
6. NPS MedicineWise, NOAC indications and PBS listings. Available at: www. nps.-org.au/noac-indications-and-pbs-listings, accessed 1 December 2018.

Further reading

Lim, M, Brazzale, D & McDonald, C 2012, '"Is it okay for me to. . .?" Assessment of recreational activity risk in patients with chronic lung conditions', *Australian Family Physician,* vol. 41, no. 11, pp. 852-4.
Henderson, J, Harrison, C, Bayram, C & Britt, H 2015, 'Travel advice and vaccination', *Australian Family Physician,* vol. 44, no. 1-2, pp. 14-15.

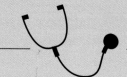

Section 23
Women's health

Case 80
Jenny Butterfield

Instructions for the doctor

This is a short case.

Please discuss with Jenny what you think may be causing the problem and how you plan to manage this situation.

Scenario

Jenny Butterfield is a 35-year-old woman who has heavy periods. Her periods are regular but last up to 10 days. For the first three to four days she is leaking despite wearing both tampons and sanitary pads. She has to change protection every half an hour and takes time off work during her period because of this. The periods are not painful. She has no other gynaecological symptoms and she does not pass clots. She is separated from her husband.

The following information is on her medical record:

Past medical history
Two normal vaginal deliveries
Medication
Nil known
Allergies
Nil
Immunisations
Up-to-date
Pap smear
Normal this year
Family history
Mother died of pancreatic cancer, aged 53
Social history
Separated

Two children
Non-smoker
Clinical examination findings
Normal abdominal and pelvic examination.

Instructions for the patient, Jenny Butterfield

You are 35 years old and work as a receptionist. It is not easy to leave the reception desk to go to the toilet. Your last three periods have come on time but have been very heavy. The periods last up to 10 days. For the first three to four days you leak despite wearing both tampons and sanitary pads. You have to change protection every half an hour and because of this take time-off work during your periods. The periods are not painful. You have no other gynaecological symptoms and do not pass clots.

You are separated from your husband. You will soon run out of sick leave and this worries you as you are bringing up two teenage children on your own.

If specifically asked
—You sometimes have a heavy dragging sensation in your lower
  abdomen
—You have felt much more tired than normal. The other day you'd
  forgotten to put out the bins and made a mad dash in your pyjamas,
  your heart was pounding out of its chest, you were short of breath
  and nearly fainted. You assumed you've just become really unfit.
  You are reluctant to attend your normal gym classes because of the
  flooding
—Your weight is stable and you don't particularly feel the heat or the
  cold
—Your bowel habit has not changed.
Please make sure you ask the doctor to outline your options for treatment.

The following information is on your medical record:
Past medical history
Two normal vaginal deliveries
Medication
Nil known
Allergies
Nil
Immunisations
Up-to-date
Pap smear
Normal this year

Family history
Mother died of pancreatic cancer, aged 53
Social history
Separated
Two children
Non-smoker
Clinical examination findings
Normal abdominal and pelvic examination.

Suggested approach to the case

Establish rapport
Open questions to explore Jenny's ideas, concerns and expectations
Explain menorrhagia—probably idiopathic
Reassure Jenny that symptoms can be improved.

Investigations

FBC and iron studies
Consider clotting factors and thyroid function tests.

Treatment options

Levonorgestrel releasing intrauterine device (Mirena)
NSAIDs—check no contraindication
Antifibrinolytic such as tranexamic acid
Oral contraceptive pill—if no other risk factors
Ultrasound scan and endometrial sampling not needed initially
Consider referral for danazol, endometrial resection or ablation or
    hysterectomy if medical treatment is not effective
Offer to discuss with employer if Jenny wishes
Arrange follow-up.

 CASE COMMENTARY

This case tests the doctor's ability to manage a common clinical problem, to recognise the impact of this problem on the patient's life and to negotiate management with the patient.

The regularity of the periods, and the absence of pain or any abnormalities on clinical examination make it most likely that this menorrhagia is idiopathic. A full blood count and iron studies should be done to exclude anaemia. Further tests such as an ultrasound scan and endometrial sampling are indicated if initial medical therapy is ineffective.

There is a range of effective options for menorrhagia with the levonorgestrel releasing intrauterine system (Mirena) now recommended as first-line therapy in primary care. The doctor should outline the options, avoiding medical jargon, and listen to Jenny's preferences.

Further reading

Australian Commission on Safety and Quality in Health Care 2017, Heavy Menstrual Bleeding Clinical Care Standard, Sydney, ACSQHC.

Bano, R, Datta, S & Mahmood, TA 2016, 'Heavy menstrual bleeding', *Obstetrics, Gynaecology and Reproductive Medicine*, vol. 26, no. 6, pp. 167–74.

Gupta, J, Kai, J, Middleton, L, Pattison, H, Gray R & Daniels, J et al. 2013, 'Levonorgestrel intrauterine system versus medical therapy for menorrhagia', vol. 368, pp. 128–37.

Lethaby, A, Duckitt, K & Farquhar, C 2013, 'Non-steroidal anti-inflammatory drugs for heavy menstrual bleeding', Cochrane Database of Systematic Reviews 1:CD000400.

Lethaby, A, Penninx, J, Hickey, M, Garry, R & Marjoribanks, J 2013, 'Endometrial resection and ablation techniques for heavy menstrual bleeding', Cochrane Database of Systematic Reviews 8:CD001501.

Middleton, LJ, Champaneria, R, Daniels, JP, Bhattacharya, S, Cooper, KG, Hilken, NH et al. 2010, 'Hysterectomy, endometrial destruction, and levonorgestrel releasing intrauterine system (Mirena) for heavy menstrual bleeding: systematic review and meta-analysis of data from individual patients', *British Medical Journal*, vol. 341, p. c3929.

Case 81
Vikki Nicolaides

Instructions for the doctor

This is a short case.
Please conduct this consultation as you would in clinical practice.

Scenario

Vikki Nicolaides is a 34-year-old accountant. She and Nico, her boyfriend, have been together for four years and they are considering starting a family. She has made this appointment to find out about when to stop the pill.

The following information is on her summary sheet:

Past medical history
Glandular fever
Mild anxiety—postgraduate exams 2005

Medication
Ethinyloestradiol 30 mcg/levonorgestrel 150 mcg (Microgynon 30)

Allergies
Nil

Immunisations
Nil recorded

Cervical screening
2018 normal

Social history
Parents migrated from Cyprus in 1960s
Non-smoker
Binge drinking at university.

Instructions for the patient, Vikki Nicolaides

You are 34 years old and work long hours as an accountant. Over the past year you have been discussing with your boyfriend the possibility of starting a family. You want to find out from the GP when to stop taking the pill and would be happy to have any other advice that you are offered.

You have regular periods on the pill and your BMI is 24 kg/m^2.

Your Mum and sister have diabetes. They were both diagnosed in their 30s. Your maternal grandmother is now on dialysis due to her kidney trouble and also was diagnosed young with diabetes. But they're all heavyset and you think you got your Dad's genes. You're hoping this won't be an issue for you.

The following information is on your medical record:

Past medical history
Glandular fever
Mild anxiety—postgraduate exams 2005

Medication
Ethinyloestradiol 30 mcg/levonorgestrel 150 mcg (Microgynon 30)

Allergies
Nil

Immunisations
Up-to-date

Cervical screening
2018 normal

Social history
Parents migrated from Cyprus in 1960s
Non-smoker
Binge drinking at university.

Suggested approach to the case

Establish rapport
Open questions to explore Vikki's ideas, concerns and expectations regarding this consultation
General health
 —Diet, check BMI, BP
 —Smoking
 —Caffeine and alcohol intake—note past history
 —Exercise
Briefly review past medical history—include drug use (prescribed, over the counter and illicit), exclude diabetes, epilepsy, depression
Cervical screening test.

Specific advice

Tailor advice to the answers given to the questions above, plus:
Diet and toxin avoidance
   —Folic acid (500 mcg od) and iodine supplements (150 mcg od)
   —Avoid eating liver
   —Eat fish twice a week
   —Hygiene—fresh food, care with cat litter
   —Avoid environmental toxins
Physical activity
   —Aim for 30 minutes/day of physical activity to optimise fitness
Smoking and alcohol
   —Enquire about substance use and advise regarding dangers of
      smoking, alcohol or other drugs during conception or pregnancy
Optimising fertility
   —When to stop contraceptive pill—explore understanding of fertile time
   —Decreased fertility after age 35—information needs to be given sensitively
Immunisations and blood tests
   —Check rubella immunity and herpes zoster immunity
   —Consider HIV test, hep B/C test, RPR, TFTs, vitamin D
   —Consider need for dTpa booster
Chromosomal, genetic abnormalities
   —Need to check if any family history of thalassaemia or other
      inherited disorders, and offer screening prenatal carrier screening.
      The table below from RANZCOG Prenatal screening and diagnosis
      of chromosomal and genetic conditions in the foetus in pregnancy
      gives you an idea of which conditions to consider based on ethnicity.
   —Availability of foetal anomaly screening tests non-invasive prenatal
      testing (NIPT), first trimester screening

	Cystic fibrosis	Haemoglobinopathies/ thalassaemia	Common Ashkenazi mutations	Spinal muscular atrophy	Fragile X syndrome[1]
European	X			X	X
Ashkenazi Jewish	X		X	X	X
Asian		X		X	X
African		X		X	X
Mediterranean		X		X	X

[1]Only women need be offered FXS screening. FXS screening is particularly important if there is a family history of intellectual disability.

—Consider health insurance cover
—Early OGTT given family history of diabetes
—Future travel advise against travel to Zika areas pre-conception and during pregnancy.

CASE COMMENTARY

Vikki attends this consultation just wanting to know about when to stop the pill. A good doctor will offer her preconception counselling and look for any modifiable risk factors to optimise her health prior to falling pregnant. Fertility issues related to her age also need to be identified.

Vikki's personal background that her parents migrated from Cyprus should alert doctors to ask about a family history of thalassaemia. Screening can be offered by a full blood count and red cell indices. A doctor would not necessarily remember the detail of the screening test but should know that it is available. If thalassaemia is confirmed Vikki's partner would require testing.

A leaflet summarising prenatal advice can supplement the information given during the consultation. The doctor needs to offer the advice such that Vikki wants to comply with it but is not so scared that she ignores it.

Pre-conception care can prevent a lifetime of problems for another human being, such as Foetal Alcohol Syndrome or congenital rubella, and is worth incorporating into routine care when discussing contraception.

Further reading

Dorney, E & Black, K 2018, 'Preconception care', *Australian Journal of General Practice,* vol. 47, no. 7, pp. 424–9.

Royal Australian and New Zealand College of Obstetrics and Gynaecology 2019, Prenatal screening for Fetal Genetic or Structural Conditions. Accessed at: www.ranzcog.edu.au/RANZCOG_SITE/media/RANZCOG-MEDIA/Women%27s%20Health/Statement%20and%20guidelines/Clinical-Obstetrics/Prenatal-Screening-for-Fetal-Genetic-or-Structural-Conditions-(C-Obs-35)-Review-March-2016.pdf?ext=.pdf, accessed 8 June 2019.

Tan, YL & Kidson-Gerber, G 2016, 'Antenatal haemaglobinopathy screening in Australia', *Medical Journal of Australia,* vol. 204, no. 6, pp. 226–30.

Case 82
Shantelle Kickett

Instructions for the doctor

This is a short case.

Please read the following scenario, and then take a focused history from Shantelle. Ask the facilitator for the results of a relevant physical examination and surgery tests. Outline the most likely diagnosis and discuss further testing required, your initial management, and recommendations with Shantelle.

Scenario

Shantelle Kickett is a 31-year-old Noongar woman from Western Australia. She has moved in with her long-term partner and is planning a family soon. She is concerned about her fertility as she only gets five periods a year. A colleague ordered tests and Shantelle has come to you for the results today.

Pelvic USS

The uterus and both ovaries were clearly identified. No abnormality demonstrated. No hydronephrosis.

FSH 6 (5–20) mIU/mL
LH 18 (5–20) mIU/mL
FSH/LH ratio 1:3 (elevated)
FAI 12 (normal 7–10)
SHBG 20 (18–114) nmol/L

The following is on her summary sheet:

Past medical history

Acne

Medications

On Ethinyloestradiol 35 mcg/cyproterone 2 mg (Diane 35) until 12 months ago

Tretinoin cream 0.05% (Retin-A) nocte

Immunisations

Childhood immunisations as per schedule.

Cervical screening

Last pap negative September 2017

Family history

Mother and maternal grandparents–type 2 diabetes

Sister–gestational diabetes mellitus

Father–high cholesterol

Social history

Lives with de facto partner David (34)

Works as a school teacher

Non-smoker

Alcohol three to fourth drinks one day a week

Not taking any recreational drugs or OTC medications.

Instructions for the patient, Shantelle Kickett

You and David have started to think about the long-term and planning kids. You stopped the contraceptive pill 12 months ago as you had irregular periods in your twenties and wanted to check your natural cycle before trying to fall pregnant. You have never been pregnant and use condoms for contraception.

Your period tracker shows you have had five periods in the last year. You are worried because the app suggests you are not ovulating and you need to see a doctor.

Your periods started at age 13 and were irregular until you started ethinyloestradiol 35 mcg/cyproterone 2 mg (Diane) for moderately severe acne when you were 20. You have always struggled with your weight. Your family are all big people. You thought that stopping the pill might help with this but you haven't lost any weight despite your efforts to do so.

You have a good knowledge of nutrition and eat healthy meals most of the time but admit there is room for improvement.

You are physically active and play tennis twice a week and walk around a lot at school.

Your mood is good. You are not lethargic or tired and get a good amount of sleep, six to eight hours a night, feeling refreshed when you wake. You do not snore. You have a good libido and no problems in your sex life.

You had some mild acne while on ethinyloestradiol 35 mcg/cyproterone 2 mg (Diane) but it has worsened since stopping. You are using benzyl peroxide and vitamin A–derived cream and you feel you are well informed and managing it adequately (you do not wish to discuss this further today).

You used to have dark hairs on your upper lip and chin but laser treatment has 'cured' you of this. You have new dark hairs appearing around your nipples and belly button which you've been plucking out.

The following is on your summary sheet:

Past medical history

Acne

Medications

On Ethinyloestradiol 35 mcg/cyproterone 2 mg (Diane 35) until 12 months ago

Tretinoin cream 0.05% (Retin-A) nocte

Immunisations

Childhood immunisations as per schedule

Cervical screening

Last pap negative September 2017

Family history

Mother and maternal grandparents—type 2 diabetes

Sister—gestational diabetes mellitus

Father—high cholesterol

Social history

Lives with de facto partner David (34)

Works as a school teacher

Non-smoker

Alcohol three to four drinks one day a week

Not taking any recreational drugs or OTC medications.

Information for the facilitator

Clinical examination findings

Each aspect needs to be asked for specifically:

BP 120/70 mm Hg

Pulse 75 bpm
Height 175 cm
Weight 87 kg
BMI 28 kg/m^2
Waist circumference 87 cm
Striae (old) on abdomen, upper thighs, breasts and upper arms
Central obesity.

Suggested approach to the case

Establish rapport
Elicit her concerns
Consider her need for an interpreter—none in this case
Take history
—Menstrual and reproductive history
—Current contraception; planning to become pregnant?
—History of acne and hirsutism, treatments tried
—How her symptoms are affecting/have affected her life
—Mental health screen for anxiety and depression
—Family history (polycystic ovarian syndrome (PCOS), diabetes,
cardiovascular disease)
—SNAP (Smoking, Nutrition, Alcohol, Physical activity)
—Social history
An excellent candidate may do the following:
- screen for obstructive sleep apnoea—snoring, daytime somnolence
- screen for eating disorder—prevalence in PCOS 21% with less than
half clinically significant eating disorders picked up (Jean Hailes)
- screen for psychosexual dysfunction.

Examination

Height/weight/BMI
Signs of hyperandrogenism (acne, hirstusim, central obesity, striae)
BSL
Urinary bHCG.

Diagnosis

Polycystic ovarian syndrome (PCOS) with oligomenorrhoea—possibly
anovulatory cycles.

Management

Metabolic screen—oral glucose tolerance test (OGTT) gold standard—HbA1c appropriate if OGTT difficult/not practical. No place for fasting insulin

Cardiovascular risk screen—lipids

Advise lifestyle and benefit of 5% weight loss—likely to help with menstrual irregularity and decrease cardiovascular risk

Vigorous exercise five times a week for 30 minutes (enough to break a sweat or not be able to sustain normal conversation due to being out of breath)

Commence metformin and consider referral for clomiphene

Advise need to cease topical retinoid prior to stopping contraception

An excellent candidate will consider preconception counselling and commencement of folic acid and iodine supplement (see Case 81 Vikki Nicolaides).

 CASE COMMENTARY

This case tests candidates' ability to diagnose polycystic ovarian syndrome. A good candidate will screen for its metabolic, cardiovascular and psychosocial effects.

The Rotterdam diagnostic criteria require two of the following three features:

1. Hyperandrogenism (biochemical or clinical)
2. Irregular anovulatory menstrual cycles
3. Polycystic ovaries on ultrasound.

Polycystic ovarian syndrome is the most common endocrine disorder in women of reproductive age (12-18% and up to 21% in Aboriginal and Torres Strait Islander women). Studies estimate up to 70% of women remain undiagnosed. It is a complex and heterogeneous condition with significant reproductive, metabolic and psychological sequalae. Depression has a prevalence of 28-64% and anxiety a prevalence of 34-57%.

 COMMON PITFALLS

Doctors need to ask about hirsutism because women often self-treat to hide their abnormal hair growth. A normal ultrasound result does not exclude PCOS and patients must be off the contraceptive pill for three months before biochemistry testing for PCOS.

Further reading

Ellis, E, Gibson-Helm, M & Boyle, JA 2018, 'Polycystic ovary syndrome in Central Australia: Diagnosis and screening of cardiometabolic risk and emotional wellbeing', *Australian Journal of General Practice,* vol. 47, no. 4, pp. 227–32.

International evidence-based guideline for the assessment and management of polycystic ovary syndrome 2018, copyright Monash University, Melbourne, Vic. Retrieved from: https://jeanhailes.org.au/contents/documents/ Resources/Tools/PCOS_evidence-based_guideline_for_assessment_and_ management_pcos.pdf, accessed 26 February 2019.

Jean Hailes PCOS Australian Alliance 2016 Indigenous health, 'Polycystic Ovary Syndrome'. Retrieved from: https://jeanhailes.org.au/health-a-z/indigenous-health/polycystic-ovary-syndrome-pcos, accessed 26 February 2019.

Norman, RJ & Teede, HJ 2018, 'A new evidence-based guideline for assessment and management of polycystic ovary syndrome', *Medical Journal of Australia,* vol. 209, no. 7, pp. 299–300.

Therapeutic Guidelines Ltd 2015, 'Polycystic Ovary Syndrome'. In: *eTG complete* (Internet). October, Therapeutic Guidelines Ltd, Melbourne, Vic.

Case 83
Zahra Mohammed Ibrahim

Instructions for the doctor

This is a long case.

Please take a history, ask for examination findings and discuss your management plan with the patient.

Scenario

Zahra Mohammed Ibrahim is a 36-year-old Somali refugee who arrived in Australia 18 months ago. She presents with a two-month history of missed periods and is asking for a pregnancy test. Your practice nurse has completed a urine pregnancy test that is positive.

The following information is on her summary sheet:

Past medical history

G9P6M2

Miscarriage (nine months ago)

Hepatitis B (HBeAg negative)

Latent TB (completed nine months isoniazid therapy under guidance of TB clinic)

Medication

Nil prescribed

Allergies

Nil known

Immunisations

Completed standard refugee catch-up schedule

Family history

Unknown

Social History

Alcohol—nil

Smoking—nil

Lives with husband and six children (ages 2–12)
Cervical screening
None recorded.

Instructions for the patient, Zahra Mohammed Ibrahim

You have presented today because you think you are pregnant. Your last period was about eight weeks ago (you are uncertain of the exact dates). You speak Somali and have very little English, although attend English classes three days per week when the children aren't at home sick. Please accept an interpreter if offered, and if not, give single-word answers or feign confusion.

You are happy about the pregnancy but a little worried because of your miscarriage last year. You have had one other miscarriage 10 years ago when you were living in a refugee camp. You did not seek any preconception counselling and are not taking any medications or vitamin tablets. Large families are normal in your culture. You are mildly concerned about where you are going to fit another child in your three-bedroom housing commission home.

You have been pregnant many times before but have not delivered in Australia. Your previous deliveries have been at home or in a refugee camp without medical assistance. You have delivered naturally without complications in the past. You have little knowledge regarding what to expect in an Australian system.

You've never heard about Down syndrome screening but would never terminate a pregnancy. You would accept any child that you were given.

You are feeling well other than occasional mild nausea.

You have hepatitis B and have only a superficial understanding of this, knowing that it could affect your liver (which you understand is something inside your belly but don't really know much more than this). You have had blood tests and an ultrasound 12 months ago and were told everything was okay; you have not been back to see your doctor since then.

Your two older children were also diagnosed with hepatitis B on arrival in Australia. Your husband was told he was immune to hepatitis B, and your younger children were vaccinated on arrival in Australia. You are aware that you passed on hepatitis B to your older children and are worried that this may happen again in this pregnancy.

You do not know what a pap smear/cervical screening test is and have never had one.

If asked, you have a history of female cutting/female genital mutilation (FGM) as a young girl. Your initial delivery was difficult and prolonged due to this but after this you have not had any obstetric problems related to FGM.

Your husband is supportive and is also studying English. There is no history of domestic violence. You receive Centrelink benefits but are hopeful that your husband will be able to soon find a job.

Prompts:
'Who will deliver my baby?'
'Will my baby get hepatitis B?'

The following information is on your summary sheet:

Past medical history
G9P6M2
Miscarriage (nine months ago)
Hepatitis B (HBeAg negative)
Latent TB (completed nine months isoniazid therapy under guidance of TB clinic)

Medication
Nil prescribed

Allergies
Nil known

Immunisations
Completed standard refugee catch-up schedule

Family history
Unknown

Social history
Alcohol—nil
Smoking—nil
Lives with husband and six children (ages 2–12)

Cervical screening
None recorded.

Information for the facilitator

Clinical examination findings

Well-looking 36-year-old female with dark skin wearing traditional Somali clothing including hijab
Height 167 cm
Weight 89 kg
BMI 36 kg/m^2

BP 125/76 mmHg
Pulse 78/min regular
Cardiovascular/respiratory/thyroid examinations normal
Abdomen—no peripheral signs of cirrhosis, abdomen soft non-tender, no
    masses including no fundus felt
Cervical screening/genital examination—to be deferred to later consult
Urine pregnancy test is positive
Urine dipstick negative
Finger-prick blood sugar level 6.1 mmol/L (non-fasting)
Edinburgh postnatal depression score 0.

Suggested approach to the case

Establish rapport
Level of English and need for interpreter should be established early
Open-ended questions to explore Zahra's ideas, concerns and expectations
A good candidate will explore Zahra's pre-existing knowledge/health literacy
    rather than assuming a level of knowledge or lack of knowledge.

Specific questions

Determine whether pregnancy is planned and wanted
Date of last menstrual period
Ask about previous pregnancies and complications
Ensure Zahra is well
Clarify past medical history, current medications, allergies, family history
Smoking/alcohol
Ask regarding previous cervical screening and FGM
Explore social history and support network, and mental wellbeing.

Examination

General appearance
Blood pressure and heart rate
Height, weight and BMI
Cardiovascular/respiratory/thyroid examination
Abdominal examination—palpate for fundus and liver examination
Urine dipstick
Finger-prick BSL
Edinburgh postnatal depression scale.

Management

Explain briefly about models of antenatal care in Australia (noting that Zahra is inappropriate for shared care due to obesity and hepatitis B)

Discuss need for folate and iodine. As Zahra's BMI is >35, she will require a 5 mg dose of folate

Advise regarding smoking and alcohol recommendations

Discuss healthy diet in pregnancy and avoiding high-risk foods

Mention cervical screening, this may require an additional specific appointment to further discuss and explain

Consider influenza vaccination

Dating scan is appropriate as Zahra does not know exact dates

Routine antenatal blood tests including FBC, blood group and antibodies, hep C, syphilis, HIV serology, rubella serology, urine MCS

Hepatitis B:

- request LFTs and hepatitis B quantitative DNA level given known hepatitis B
- good candidates will recognise she is also overdue screening for hepatocellular carcinoma
- candidate should reassure Zahra that her hepatitis B will be monitored and treated if necessary, and that baby will have immediate vaccination and hepatitis B immunoglobulin and that it is highly unlikely that she will transmit hepatitis B to this baby.

Zahra is at risk of vitamin D deficiency and should have this checked

She has risk factors for gestational diabetes, including obesity and ethnicity and should have an early oral glucose tolerance test or HbA1c depending on local hospital recommendations

Urine protein: creatinine ratio is appropriate given high BMI

Consider checking TSH and varicella serology

First trimester screening can be mentioned but full discussion may be deferred to a later consult

Likewise, non-invasive prenatal testing can be mentioned, although it is unlikely Zahra will have the funds to access this

Candidates should recognise that Zahra has a high-risk pregnancy and should be referred early for antenatal care and management of her hepatitis B.

 CASE COMMENTARY

Candidates require a good knowledge of routine antenatal care, plus some knowledge and understanding of the challenges involved in refugee

health care. About a third of women who give birth in Australia were not born in Australia and this can provide challenges with regards to differing cultural expectations or views surrounding the birthing experience. In particular, women with migrant or refugee backgrounds may present later for antenatal care and may have other more complex medical and psychosocial problems.[1]

A phone interpreter should be offered early in the consult. Phone interpreters are available free of charge to healthcare providers via the National Translating and Interpreting Service (www.tisnational.gov.au). Some tips for working with interpreters include:

- speak to the patient not the interpreter
- use eye contact and speak in the first person
- allow time for the interpreter to interpret what you say
- ensure that both you and the patient are in proximity to the speaker phone, and that you are speaking clearly for the interpreter to hear you.[2]

Candidates should be mindful that interpreters are not medically trained and may have low health literacy themselves. Care needs to be taken when using interpreters to avoid the use of complex language or jargon that is hard to translate. Small amounts of information at a time should be given to ensure things are not forgotten or missed. It can be tempting to use family members or children as translators, but this should be avoided when possible.[3]

Health information handouts can be given in English or Somali, but it is worth keeping in mind that many refugees (women in particular) may not have attended school and will not understand written information in either language.

Female genital mutilation is extremely common in Somalia and should be considered as it can complicate deliveries and result in difficult and/or traumatic examinations.[4]

Chronic hepatitis B is also common throughout Africa, usually through vertical transmission. More than 90% of infants infected at birth will go on to have chronic hepatitis B and its associated health outcomes. In contrast 95% of infected older children and adults will clear the infection without developing chronic disease. Fortunately, in Australia, perinatal transmission can be easily prevented through strategies including antiviral medication in the 3rd trimester for women with high viral loads, hepatitis B immunoglobulin and immediate vaccination for infants at birth, followed by a full hepatitis B vaccination course. Infants born to mothers with hepatitis B should have hepatitis B serology at 9–12 months of age.[5]

References

1. Department of Health 2018, Clinical Practice Guidelines: Pregnancy Care. Australian Government Department of Health, Canberra.
2. Phillips, C 2010, 'Using interpreters—a guide for GPs', *Australian Family Physician,* vol. 39, pp. 188–95.
3. Bird, S 2010, 'Failure to use an interpreter', *Australian Family Physician,* vol. 39, pp. 241–2.
4. Royal Australian and New Zealand College of Obstetricians and Gynaecologists 1994, revised November 2017. Female Genital Mutilation. Available at: www.ranzcog.edu.au/RANZCOG_SITE/media/RANZCOG-MEDIA/Women%27s%20Health/Statement%20and%20guidelines/Clinical%20-%20Gynaecology/Female-Genital-Mutilation-(C-Gyn-1)-Nov17.pdf?ext=.pdf, accessed 1 July 2018.
5. Mathews, G, Robotin, M & Allard, N (eds) 2014, 'B Positive—all you wanted to know about hepatitis B: a guide for primary care providers', Australasian Society for HIV, Viral Hepatitis and Sexual Health Medicine, Darlinghurst. Available at: www.hepatitisb.org.au, accessed 1 July 2018.

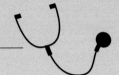

Section 24
Vivas

Case 84
Lori Dalton

Instructions for the doctor

This is a short case.

Mrs Lori Dalton is a 67-year-old retired journalist. She is a keen bush-walker but is frustrated because of pain in her osteoarthritic knees, for which she takes oral ibuprofen 200 mg three times daily as needed. She has brought in the following abstract from an article in *Australian Family Physician* on rosehip powder. She will ask you questions about this.

> **Rosehip powder for arthritis and inflammatory bowel disease**
>
> **Background:** Rosehips—which contain a particular type of galactolipid—have a specific anti-inflammatory action. A standardised rosehip powder has been developed to maximise the retention of phytochemicals. This powder has demonstrated antioxidant and anti-inflammatory activity as well as clinical benefits in conditions such as osteoarthritis, rheumatoid arthritis and inflammatory bowel disease.
>
> **Objective:** To examine the evidence suggesting that standardised rosehip powder may be a viable replacement or supplement for conventional therapies used in inflammatory diseases such as arthritis.
>
> **Discussion:** A meta-analysis of three randomised controlled trials involving 287 patients with a median treatment period of three months reported that treatment with standardised rosehip powder consistently reduced pain scores and that patients allocated to rosehip powder were twice as likely to respond to rosehip compared to placebo. In contrast to non-steroidal anti-inflammatory drugs and aspirin, rosehip has anti-inflammatory actions that do not have ulcerogenic effects and do not inhibit platelets nor influence the coagulation cascade or fibrinolysis.[1]

Instructions for the patient, Lori Dalton

You are a 67-year-old retired journalist. You are a keen bushwalker but get frustrated because of the pain in your osteoarthritic knees. You have seen an advert for rosehip powder at your local health food shop and want to know whether to use this during your planned trekking holiday in Nepal. The advert quoted an article in the *Australian Family Physician*,[1] so you have brought in the abstract to ask your GP about it.

You will ask the GP the following questions:

1. What do you think about this article, doctor? Do you think that the information is reliable? (Supplementary question: Why do you think that?)
2. The article talks about randomised controlled trials. Please would you explain what these are. And I've heard of some trials being 'double blind'. What does this mean?
3. Do you think the rosehip powder is worth trying?
4. Will the rosehip powder be safe for me to take while also taking ibuprofen?
5. Should I take it with me when I go on my trekking holiday to Nepal?

Suggested answers

1. What do you think about this article, doctor? Do you think that the information is reliable? (Supplementary question: Why do you think that?)

This article is about using rosehip powder to help with inflammatory conditions such as arthritis.

Factors to consider[2, 3]

- *Journal:* the *Australian Family Physician* is a peer-reviewed, professional journal, indexed by Medline. Reputable journals with high impact factors are regarded as reliable, but they still require systematic scrutiny.
- *Article:* sponsored or not? Are there conflicts of interest?
- *Level of evidence:* meta-analysis, but not clear in abstract who conducted this, or what methods were used. There is no indication on the inclusion or exclusion criteria.
- *Gold standard* is methodology used by the Cochrane collaboration.[4] Consider and explain what the levels of evidence are and how these support recommendations.
- *Trials:* were all trials of rosehip powder included or only those published?

- *Statistical and clinical significance:* in this paper, response is described as 'twice as likely'; it is not clear if this is the absolute or relative risk of benefit. There is no indication of the sample sizes or statistical power.
- *Author(s):* publication history, qualifications, academic affiliations, financial ties to research topic or conflicts of interest.

2. The article talks about randomised-controlled trials. Please would you explain what these are. And I've heard of some trials being 'double blind'. What does this mean?
   - Randomised controlled trials test whether treatments work.[2]
   - A group of people, all with the same clinical problem, are randomly allocated to have different treatments. The effect of a new treatment is compared to an inert, look-alike pill (the placebo) or another treatment.
   - Ideally trials are 'double blinded' so that neither the patient nor the person who assesses the effects of the treatments know which treatment the patient is on. This reduces the potential for bias among the groups.
   - Calculations are done before the trial to work out how many participants are needed (the power of the trial) to be sure any result is both clinically and statistically significant.

3. Do you think the rosehip powder is worth trying?
   From the information in this article it may be worth trying, but it is not something that I have previously studied or recommended. The Therapeutic Goods Administration (TGA)—the Australian government organisation that checks whether medicines work and are safe—lists products that are approved for use; we can examine the TGA and other sources of information. Within the article the number of people who have tried it seems very low compared to the number who have used other anti-inflammatories and painkillers. Also, the article mentions people who have taken it for a short time only and so its long-term safety is uncertain from this information.

   It is not clear what type of arthritis the participants in this study had, whether they were men or women and what age they were. This makes it more difficult to know if the results apply to you.

4. Will the rosehip powder be safe to take while also taking ibuprofen?
   I'm sorry, Mrs Dalton, but I cannot answer that question from this article. The participants were on either the rosehip powder or a dummy placebo pill. There is no information on the safety of mixing the rosehip powder with other medications.

5. Should I take it with me when I go on my trekking holiday to Nepal?
A general rule is to not start taking a medication for the first time while overseas. If you do want to take it with you, I would suggest a trial of several weeks before you go, so that if you have a bad response to it you will know while you are still in Australia and will have time to recover before you actually go away. It is also worth checking to see if rosehip powder can legally be taken into Nepal.

There's another option. Your dose of ibuprofen is quite low. Providing you are not getting any side effects from it, you could increase the dose, add regular paracetamol, and try walking poles and leg strengthening exercises.

 CASE COMMENTARY

This case tests the doctor's ability to appraise an abstract and then apply the information to the care of individual patients. General practitioners are not usually expected to conduct research but all should be able to read research information and apply it to their practice. One trap to avoid is for GPs to concur with the belief that 'natural' automatically equates to it being harmless.[5] The origin of a product is much less important than its proven efficacy and short and long-term safety.

References

1. Cohen, M 2012, 'Rosehip—an evidence-based herbal medicine for inflammation and arthritis', *Australian Family Physician,* vol. 41, no. 7, pp. 495–8.
2. Greenhalgh, T 2014, *How to read a paper: the basics of evidence-based medicine,* 5th ed, British Medical Journal Books.
3. Margolis, S 2018, 'Evidence-based medicine', *Australian Journal of General Practice,* vol 4, no. 6.
4. Spurling G, Mitchell B & van Driel M 2018, 'Unlocking the value of Cochrane reviews for general practitioners', *Australian Journal of General Practice,* vol. 47, no. 6, pp. 333–6.
5. Smith, A 2002, 'It's natural so it must be safe', *Australian Prescriber,* vol. 25, pp. 50–1.

Further reading

1. van Driel, M & Spurling, G 2017, 'Guidelines and systematic reviews: Sizing up guidelines in general practice', *Australian Family Physician,* vol. 46, no. 6, pp. 438–40
2. The Royal Australian College of General Practitioners 2018, *Guideline for the management of knee and hip osteoarthritis,* 2nd ed, RACGP, East Melbourne, Vic.

Case 85
Kaitlin Johansen

Instructions for the doctor

This is a short viva station.

Please discuss your management of this situation with a GP colleague.

Scenario

You are working an evening clinic in general practice and a patient of your practice, Kaitlin Johansen, comes in unexpectedly, tearful, reporting she has been raped at a party. Your last patient cancelled, so you can see Kaitlin now.

The following information is on her summary sheet:

Age

19

Past medical history

Asthma

Medications

Fluticasone 250 mcg/salmeterol 25 mcg (Seretide) 1 puff bd

Salbutamol inhaler 100 mcg 1–2 puffs prn

Social

Studying beauty therapy

Allergies

Nil known

Immunisations

Up-to-date

Cervical screening

None.

Instructions for the facilitator

This is a viva station.

Please ask the candidate the following questions about the case:

1. What are your immediate medical (including psychological) concerns for Kaitlin?
2. She tells you that she does not want to involve the police. How would you respond?
3. You arrange for the Sexual Assault Referral Centre to perform a forensic examination in two hours. She needs to go to the toilet. Is there anything you need to advise her?
4. Tell me the important things to consider about your notes regarding this consult?
5. What follow-up will you arrange for Kaitlin?

Suggested approach to the case

1. Medical priorities

   Physical injuries: assess Kaitlin with an initial primary survey and then more detailed secondary survey for specific injuries.

   STI screening and *bloodborne viruses*: possible prophylactic treatment for chlamydia, gonorrhoea, HIV and syphilis, and hepatitis B immunisation depending on her predicted risk.

   Pregnancy prevention: offer emergency contraception.

   Mental health: assess Kaitlin's current mental state, and her ongoing safety and support. She may wish to call a support person and may need help to find a safe place to go following examination.

   Most areas have a Sexual Assault Resource Centre (SARC) and/or telephone hotline which provide expert support. General practitioners often follow up patients who have experienced trauma.
2. When alleged assault is disclosed it is important to offer police involvement. As an adult, this is Kaitlin's choice. If she would like to report the offence you can call the police immediately. However, if she doesn't wish to involve them, then forensic specimens can still be collected in case she changes her mind. Forensic specimens have to be collected promptly.
3. Contact the local SARC services and establish the most appropriate place for a timely forensic examination. If there will be some waiting time and Kaitlin is wanting to go to the toilet you might be asked to collect initial forensic samples, such as gauze swab of perineum

and anal region, first pass urine and mouth washings, depending on details of the assault. SARC staff will help you decide necessary initial specimens.

4. Your notes may be used in legal proceedings so they must be written objectively and without judgement. Contemporaneous notes are imperative. It is recommended to write her history verbatim and distinguish this clearly from your clinical observations and management.

5. Follow-up may include a multidisciplinary team. Follow up two to three days post-incident to reassess injuries and wellbeing. After two weeks repeat a pregnancy test and follow up STI checks, assess her coping, healing and mental state. After three months repeat STI/bloodborne virus tests. Do a mental health assessment, offer ongoing counselling if necessary and SARC/legal follow-up as desired.

 ## CASE COMMENTARY

In 2011 there were 17 238 reports of sexual assault in Australia. This is likely to be lower than the true prevalence as the majority of victims do not report incidents to the police. The Australian Bureau of Statistics Personal Safety survey in 2016 showed that 18% of women and 4.7% of men had experienced at least one episode of sexual violence since the age of 15.

The risk factors for sexual assault include:
- young age
- Aboriginal or Torres Strait Islander people
- female
- substance users
- those suffering mental health issues and/or disability
- previous history of sexual assault
- homelessness
- poverty
- sex workers.

Disclosures of assault may happen immediately or years after. Other presentations to a GP following assault may be for emergency contraception or STI check and a thorough history and good rapport will be essential to exploring the presentation.

COMMON PITFALLS

It is common to feel unqualified in a presentation such as this, however, despite specialist services being available, immediate care often needs to be given by the first treating practitioner. A general practitioner is often a key part of the ongoing care of someone post-sexual assault. A history of assault is often implicated in other presentations such as chronic pelvic pain. Considering this, it is important to understand the basics in responding to an alleged assault.

Suggested resources

Daisy App helps people connect to local resources. Available at: https://www.1800respect.org.au/daisy/

RACGP White Book. Available at: https://www.racgp.org.au/clinical-resources/clinical-guidelines/key-racgp-guidelines/view-all-racgp-guidelines/white-book/interpersonal-abuse

For local resources in your state check this website: https://au.reachout.com/articles/sexual-assault-support

Further reading

The Royal Australian College of General Practitioners 2014, *Abuse and violence: Working with our patients in general practice,* 4th ed, RACGP, Melbourne, Vic.

Guidelines for medico-legal care for victims of sexual violence © World Health Organization 2003 Retrieved from: http://apps.who.int/iris/bitstream/handle/10665/42788/924154628X.pdf;jsessionid=83BD690CD8FE199FB8EB39ABA1385216?sequence=1, accessed 26 February 2019.

Tarczon, C & Quadara, A 2012, 'The nature and extent of sexual assault and abuse in Australia', Australia Centre for the Study of Sexual assault, Melbourne. Retrieved from: https://aifs.gov.au/sites/default/files/publication-documents/rs5.pdf, accessed 26 February 2019.

Australian Bureau of Statistics' 2016 Personal Safety Survey. Available at: https://www.abs.gov.au/ausstats/abs@.nsf/Lookup/4906.0main+features12016, accessed 9 March 2019.

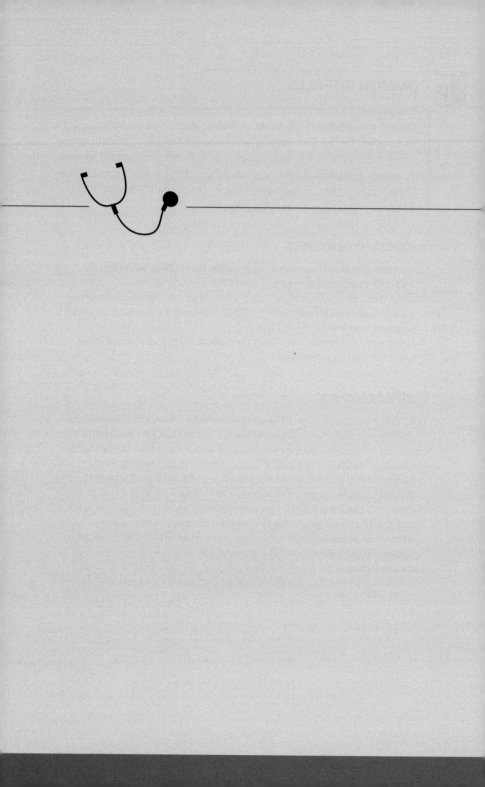

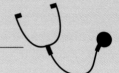

Section 25
Vulnerable populations

Case 86
Jill Krecher

Instructions for the doctor

This is a long case.

Please take a history from Jill and ask for the physical examination findings from the facilitator. Talk to Jill about your initial diagnosis or concerns and discuss an initial plan of management with her.

Scenario

Jill Krecher is a 29-year-old woman who has been to the surgery four times for minor ailments in the last few months. The receptionist told you she sounded teary on the phone when she booked for an appointment today.

The following information is on her summary sheet:

Past medical history

Anxiety—treated 2013-14

Menorrhagia—inactive

Medication

Mirena inserted September 2017

Allergies

Nil known

Immunisations

As per schedule

Social history

Teacher at local primary school

Lives with fiancé Paul, who is an accountant

Non-smoker

Social drinker with friends on the weekend

No recreational drugs

Family history

Dad—hypertension

Mum—osteoarthritis knees.

Instructions for the patient, Jill Krecher

You have asked to see the doctor urgently as you can't teach today due to your bruises. You have a black eye, which you can't cover with make-up and bruises on your arms. Your partner Paul has become increasingly violent. You haven't been able to tell anyone and have hidden the bruises. This weekend he has been very violent. He's never hit you in the face before.

You have had some time off work recently as his behaviour has been upsetting you so much, but you've told the doctors it's either gastro or a viral illness.

Today you think the doctor will probably notice the bruises and if they ask you will tell them what's going on. You feel so much shame about being in this situation you can't bring it up unprompted.

Initially, tell the doctor you've had trouble sleeping and don't think you can teach today.

If you trust them and they ask questions about your situation you will tell them you had an argument with your partner and 'things have been a bit rough lately'. If they ask about violence or if you feel safe you will confide in them.

You've been with Paul for two years. The first year he was like a dream come true and he swept you off your feet. All your friends and family loved him too. But he then became jealous and slowly you've stopped seeing friends and family.

He first hit you six months ago after a male colleague chatted to you at a local café. He thought you were cheating. His violence is getting more frequent and last night he strangled you until you almost passed out.

Your friends seem worried about you, but they have stopped ringing as often as you have been withdrawn.

There are no children involved.

You would like to consider leaving but have no idea where to start and you are scared about what Paul will do if you leave.

The following is on your summary sheet:
Past medical history
Anxiety—treated 2013–14
Menorrhagia—inactive
Medication
Mirena inserted September 2017
Allergies
Nil known
Immunisations
As per schedule

Social history
School teacher at local primary school
Lives with fiancé Paul who is an accountant
Non-smoker
Social drinker with friends on the weekend
No recreational drugs
Family history
Dad hypertension
Mum osteoarthritis knees.

Information for the facilitator

Each aspect is to be asked for specifically.
General appearance: pale, teary woman; obvious bruising to right eye and
   some conjunctival injection
BP 110/70 mmHg
Pulse 76 bpm
Height 165 cm
Weight 60 kg
BMI 22.1 kg/m^2
Waist circumference 76 cm
Urine NAD
If skin exposed, slight bruising to neck
Different-aged bruises to both arms
All other systems NAD.

Suggested approach to the case

Establish rapport
Empathic, open and non-judgemental approach
Start with open questions: 'How are things at home?'
Specific questions: 'Are you ever afraid of your partner?'
In response to this patients' specific injuries you might say something
   along the lines of:
   'When I see injuries like this, I wonder if someone could have hurt you?'
   'You seem very anxious and nervous. Is everything alright at home?'

Validate

Use statements such as:
   'You deserve to feel safe'

'You do not deserve to be treated this way'
'I am here to help you'
'I am concerned about your safety'
Avoid statements such as:
    'Why don't you leave?'
    'Why did he hit you?'
    'You should leave'
Traumatised patients often need time. You may not have much time in an
    initial consultation, but early follow-up and enlisting the help of a team
    help the patient to get the time they may need.

Assess safety

Does the patient feel safe?
Are there any red flags?
Is the violence escalating?
In this case the patient has experienced non-lethal strangulation. Studies
    show this increases the risk of attempted and completed homicide four
    to six fold in the future. This behaviour needs to be recognised as a
    significant risk.

Assist in safety planning

The elements of safety planning include a list of emergency numbers, access
to money, important documents such as passport, birth certificate, driver's
licence, Medicare card, clothing and keys.
    Establish where she would go if she had to leave
    How would she get there?
    What would she take with her?
    Who are the people she could contact for support?
    Does she need referral to domestic violence services to assist with
    planning?
    Document any plans made, for future reference
    Organise early follow-up.

 CASE COMMENTARY

GPs often comment that they do not see many victims of domestic
violence; however, it is estimated that on average GPs see five women
a week who are affected. 17% of all women and 5.3% of all men aged >
18 years have experienced violence from a partner.

Evidence shows that four to ten pregnant women out of every 100 experience intimate partner violence. Aboriginal and Torres Strait Islander people are over-represented in domestic and family violence statistics.

Domestic violence has a devastating effect on individuals and communities. Victims of domestic violence often suffer adverse outcomes, including depression and anxiety, post-traumatic stress disorder, physical injury and disability. Injuries can be severe and sometimes fatal, which is why increasing resources are available to deal with this important health issue.

The World Health Organization recommends that GPs ask women about intimate partner abuse as a part of assessing the conditions that may be caused or complicated by intimate partner abuse. These include mental health symptoms, alcohol and other substance use, chronic pain or chronic digestive or reproductive symptoms.

GPs can offer frontline support to the victims of domestic violence, including asking about violence, listening, validating the patient's experience and providing non-judgemental practical support. Directing patients to resources and support helps to enhance their safety.

When children are involved and at risk, GPs need to practise according to the mandatory reporting requirements in their jurisdiction.

A multidisciplinary approach is important; social workers, nurses, counsellors and psychologists can all provide assistance. Dedicated domestic violence services within the police department may also be able to assist, particularly in a case where patients would like to press charges or seek protective measures such as restraining orders.

 COMMON PITFALLS

Most women don't mind being asked about family violence by their GP but a minority are actually asked. Given the high prevalence of family violence, we need to remember to ask about the safety of our patients.

Suggested resources

Daisy App helps people connect to local resources. Available at: https://www.1800respect.org.au/daisy/

RACGP White Book, Chapter 2 Intimate partner violence. Available at: https://www.racgp.org.au/clinical-resources/clinical-guidelines/key-racgp-guidelines/view-all-racgp-guidelines/white-book/interpersonal-abuse

Further reading

Australian Domestic and Family Violence Death Review Network (2018) Data Report. Retrieved from: www.coroners.justice.nsw. gov.au/Documents/ADFVDRN_Data_Report_2018%20(2). pdf?fbclid=IwAR0Y6Wnr6e6qzv4IY_PRZPMfJ-OugwkIaF5XhVIN-HQydtA6BDj-aMa42aY, accessed 26 February 2019.

Brooks, M, Barclay, L & Hooker, C 2018, 'Trauma-informed care in general practice: Findings from a women's health centre evaluation', *Australian Journal of General Practice,* vol. 47, no. 6, pp. 370–5.

Glass et al. 2008, 'Non-fatal strangulation is an important risk factor for homicide of women', *The Journal of Emergency Medicine,* vol. 35, no. 3, pp. 329–35.

Forsdike, K, Tarzia, L, Hindmarsh, E & Hegarty, K 2014, 'Family violence across the life cycle', *Australian Family Physician,* vol. 43, no. 11, pp. 768–74.

The Royal Australian College of General Practitioners 2014, *Abuse and violence: Working with our patients in general practice,* 4th ed, RACGP, Melbourne, Vic.

Case 87
Marcus Petrovic

Instructions for the doctor

This is a short case.

Please take a history from Marcus and then request appropriate examination findings from the facilitator. Outline your diagnostic impressions and problem list to the facilitator. Negotiate your management plan with Marcus.

Scenario

Marcus Petrovic is 28-year-old man who moved to your practice six months ago. He has a 10-year history of schizophrenia with frequent hospital admissions. In the last year he has been relatively stable on fortnightly Zuclopenthixol (Clopixol) depot injections and nightly quetiapine (Seroquel).

He is obese, has borderline hypertension and is not very physically active. He has a family history of diabetes, heart disease and dyslipidaemia. He smokes but does not drink alcohol. He is unemployed and is on a disability support pension.

Your previous impression has been that he seems quite blunted in affect and you suspect he has at least some moderate intellectual and/or developmental delay, which gives him a child-like manner. Six months ago, he moved to your town to live with his parents but he has recently moved into a flat with friends. He is on the waiting list to see a local psychiatrist but has yet to engage with local mental health services.

He takes his medication, recognising that it has probably contributed to his good run in recent years. He presents today in between his scheduled fortnightly appointments.

The following information is on his summary sheet:

Past medical history
Chronic schizophrenia
Intellectual disability
Gastro-oesophageal reflux disease

Medication
Zuclopenthixol (Clopixol) depot injection IMI 300 mg/mL every two weeks
Quetiapine (Seroquel) XR 300 mg nocte
Gaviscon tabs po prn

Allergies
Nil known

Immunisations
Unknown

Social history
Smokes 15 cigarettes per day
Non-drinker
Lives with friends.

Instructions for the patient, Marcus Petrovic

The area of redness and soreness in your right elbow began a couple of days ago and is getting bigger each day. Early on in the discussion you say, 'I think I must've used a dirty needle'.

You readily volunteer information about your drug use and are not embarrassed about it. You've been using either ice or heroin ('Harry') for the past month, initially irregularly but now daily. You have never used drugs before but have been introduced to them by your new group of friends. You have never paid anything as your new friends (from the motorcycle gang) supply them for free along with the needles and injecting equipment. If specifically asked, your friends sometimes get you to 'do a Sydney run'—to ride your bike to Sydney and back with a package, or to carry packages around town. You have no idea what you are carrying on these trips.

You have limited understanding about safe injecting or bloodborne viruses. You are not concerned about the risks of IV drug use but don't like this infection because it is painful and you can't use that area for injecting. You like the way the drugs make you feel relaxed and happy. Other than this infection you haven't experienced any negative effects from your drug use and haven't contemplated quitting.

You talk animatedly about your 'new' bike (a 1974 Honda CB750) that your new friends helped you buy and look after. You are proud of your new-found independence—living in a flat with friends instead of living with your parents. You are positive about your new group of friends in the motorcycle gang and are not aware that they might be taking advantage of you.

You trust the doctor and have a good relationship but struggle to understand anything even slightly complex. You don't understand any medical jargon and get easily lost if the doctor uses long words or speaks too quickly.

The following information is on your summary sheet:

Past medical history

Chronic schizophrenia

Intellectual disability

Gastro-oesophageal reflux disease

Medication

Zuclopenthixol (Clopixol) depot injection IMI 300 mg/mL every two weeks

Quetiapine (Seroquel) XR 300 mg nocte

Gaviscon tabs po prn

Allergies

Nil known

Immunisations

Unknown

Social history

Smokes 15 cigarettes per day

Non-drinker

Lives with friends.

Suggested approach to the case

Establish rapport. Use an open and non-judgemental approach

Recognise and manage cellulitis as a result of intravenous drug use

Recognise the broader risks of unsafe injecting

Identify Marcus's vulnerability with respect to drug trafficking.

Specific questions

Explore the history of drug use—its context and Marcus' awareness of risks/safe injecting

Assess mood and thought content as well as any psychotic symptoms and, if present, their relationship to the drug use

Explore Marcus's awareness of his current vulnerability with his new friends and with the police.

Examination

General appearance
Vital signs
Examine right antecubital fossa for possible abscess; examine both antecubital fossae for track marks
Cardiovascular examination.

Management

Manage the presenting complaint (cellulitis) with appropriate antibiotics, e.g. flu/dicloxacillin to cover *Staphylococcus aureus,* which is the likely causative organism. Add in a topical skin wash such as chlorhexidine.

Outline the health risks of IV drug use to Marcus in words he understands. Explain the need for safe injecting as well as testing for bloodborne viruses and offer immunisation against hepatitis B.

Gently introduce the idea that his friends may be taking advantage of him. Ensure follow-up.

Physical examination

General appearance: obese man of stated age in no distress
Vital signs
    HR 78/min regular
    BP 135/82 mmHg sitting
    Temp 36.8°C
    Height 178 cm
    Weight 121 kg
    BMI 38 kg/m^2
    RR 14/min
Right antecubital fossa has a round area of redness, warmth and induration of the skin with no evidence of any underlying abscess
Both antecubital fossae have several small marks consistent with fresh puncture wounds
Cardiovascular examination: normal
Respiratory examination: normal
Abdominal examination: normal
Mental state examination: normal apart from a blunted affect and limited insight
Surgery tests: ECG—sinus rhythm 75/min; BSL (random)—6.2; Urinalysis —normal
Remainder of physical examination is normal and further investigations are not available.

Diagnostic impressions/problem list

Cellulitis—likely related to intravenous drug use with non-sterile equipment
Intravenous use of opiates (heroin) and methamphetamine ('ice')
Risk of contracting bloodborne viruses
Risk of drug use causing psychosis
Social vulnerability—currently being used for drug transportation
Existing problems of chronic schizophrenia, intellectual impairment and obesity
At risk of metabolic syndrome in the future.

 CASE COMMENTARY

Although research findings vary, it seems most adults with intellectual disability are less likely to use substances than adults without intellectual disability.[1] This may be related to the fact that a substantial number of people with intellectual disability live with families or other caregivers who provide some degree of supervision.[2] With the move to integrate patients with intellectual disability into the community comes potential exposure to substances such as alcohol and drugs and these vulnerable patients can lack the skills to cope with this. Patients with intellectual disability who do use alcohol and illicit drugs are more likely to develop an abuse problem.[2] Additionally, many of the intellectual disability population do not engage well with standard interventions for substance misuse which frequently fail to meet their needs.[3] As a result, intellectual disability substance abusers are less likely to receive substance abuse treatment or remain in treatment.[3, 4] When intellectual disability patients also suffer mental illness, the risk of serious problems with substance abuse increases further.[3-5] This group is at greater risk of complications because they tend to be prescribed medications for co-existent mental illness that can negatively interact with alcohol and drugs.[3, 5]

Patients such as Marcus risk the 'triple whammy' of chronic mental illness, intellectual disability and substance abuse, resulting in significant disability and real barriers to effective treatment. The skilled general practitioner can provide individualised longitudinal care through a trusted relationship and can support engagement in services and build resilience over time.[6]

 COMMON PITFALLS

If the doctor adopts a judgemental or punitive role, the likelihood of Marcus adhering to treatment and remaining engaged with the GP is reduced. Also, if the candidate fails to target the advice and information to an appropriate level then the patient education is ineffective. Under the pressure of time in a short case we can try to cover all the content quickly and forget to check for patient understanding.

The other pitfall here is to focus on the simple condition of localised cellulitis or to only expand as far as addressing the risk of bloodborne viruses and safe injecting but to avoid the broader psychosocial issues as being firmly in the 'too hard basket'. The opportunity to list the identified diagnoses (or more broadly, problems) represents the chance to demonstrate the candidate's thinking regarding Marcus's health even though they will not get to address all these issues with Marcus within the time frame of the case.

Marcus is vulnerable and in need of advocacy and a holistic approach to his care.

The insightful GP will recognise that without significant intervention the next likely outcome will involve the authorities and will probably result in Marcus's incarceration. This would have further significant negative impacts on his health.

References

1   Carroll-Chapman, SL & Wu L 2012, 'Substance abuse among individuals with intellectual disabilities', *Research in Developmental Disabilities,* vol. 33, pp. 1147–56.

2   Emerson, E & Brigham, P 2013, 'Health behaviours and mental health status of parents with intellectual disabilities: Cross sectional study', *Public Health,* vol. 127, pp. 1111–16.

3   Day, C, Lampraki, A, Ridings, D & Currell, K 2016, 'Intellectual disability and substance use/misuse: a narrative review', *Journal of Intellectual Disabilities and Offending Behaviour,* vol. 7, no. 1, pp. 25–34.

4   Lin, E, Balogh, R, McGarry, C et al. 2016, 'Substance-related and addictive disorders among adults with intellectual and developmental disabilities: an Ontario population cohort study', *British Medical Journal Open,* vol. 6, p. e011638.

5   Chaplin, E, Gilvarry, C & Tsakanikos, E 2011, 'Recreational substance use patterns and co-morbid psychopathology in adults with intellectual disability', *Research in Developmental Disabilities,* vol. 32, no. 6, pp. 2981–6.

6   Samuel, S 2016, 'GPs and vulnerable populations' (editorial), *Australian Family Physician,* vol. 45, no. 10, p. 697.